TUMOR PROGRESSION

DEVELOPMENTS IN CANCER RESEARCH

TUMOR PROGRESSION

Proceedings of a Chicago Symposium, Chicago, Illinois, U.S.A., October 3–5, 1979

Editor:

RAY G. CRISPEN
Director of ITR Biomedical Research
904 W. Adams, University of Illinois, Chicago, Illinois, U.S.A.

Sponsored by:

University of Illinois at the Medical Center and Illinois Cancer Council

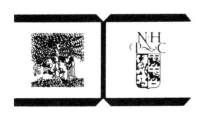

ELSEVIER/NORTH-HOLLAND
NEW YORK • AMSTERDAM • OXFORD

© 1980 by Elsevier North Holland, Inc.

Published by:

Elsevier North Holland, Inc.
52 Vanderbilt Avenue, New York, New York 10017

Sole distributors outside of the United States and Canada:

Elsevier/North Holland Biomedical Press
335 Jan van Galenstraat, P.O. Box 211
Amsterdam, The Netherlands

Library of Congress Cataloging in Publication Data

Main entry under title:

Tumor progression.
     (Developments in cancer research; v. 2 ISSN 0163-6146)

     Bibliography: p.
     Includes index.
     1. Cancer—Immunological aspects—Congresses. 2. Metastasis—
     Congresses. 3. Cancer—Chemotherapy—Congresses. 4. Immunotherapy—
     Congresses. I. Crispen, Ray G. II. University of Illinois at the Medical
     Center. III. Illinois Cancer Council. IV. Series. [DNLM: 1. Neoplasm metastasis
     —Congresses. W1 DE997VMv. 2 / QZ202 T924   1979]
RC268.3.T85   616.99'407   80-19458
ISBN 0-444-00432-7

Manufactured in the United States of America

Contents

Preface

The most important property of cancer cells is their ability to metastasize and spread to distant sites. Many more patients would be cured and cancer would not be such a "dreaded disease" if it were possible to control their growth. Until recently, little effort has been given to the difficult study of cancer cell dissemination. The processes involved in the release of tumor cells from a primary tumor and their development at distant sites are very complex. New developments in this area are presented in the chapters of this volume. Investigative research on the pathology of the metastatic process includes theories on host-stromal dependence, cell-cell interactions and cell surface properties associated with metastasis. Consideration is given to animal model systems and reports of experiments conducted to treat induced metastasis in mice and guinea pigs. Clinical trials have been initiated also to evaluate possible beneficial responses in patients receiving immunostimulation, in most cases as an additional component to chemotherapy and/or surgery. Clinical trials in the management of advanced lymphomas, acute leukemias, disseminated melanomas, advanced breast cancer, sarcomas and other cancers are discussed. Current theories regarding the use of immunological markers in detecting disease progression and evaluating tumor cell kill in relation to therapy are explored. It is our hope that the contributions in this text will encourage further research on the basic biology of tumor cell spread. Only when we learn more of the nature of metastasis will we be able to achieve a more effective therapeutic strategy. It is through the combined efforts of basic researchers and clinicians that the prognosis for the advanced cancer patient will be improved.

TUMOR PROGRESSION

Immunology and Immunotherapy of Experimental Metastasis

Host Response to Antigenic Tissues During Progression and Metastasis of Breast Neoplasia[a]

Glenn Slemmer

Department of Pathology, University of British Columbia, Vancouver, British Columbia

Summary

The cell biology and immunology of murine mammary neoplasia were studied using transplantation methods. Mammary glands comprising mosaics of cells of different genotypes permitted observation of interactions of separate cell types in normal and neoplastic tissues. Biologically-different types of neoplasia arose from different cell types. Neoplastic cells of some types retained dependence on normal cells of other types. Distant metastatic masses from such mosaic-dependent (M-D) carcinomas included large numbers of normal mammary cells. Neoplastic cells of M-D carcinomas retained dependence on normal cells through 15 metastatic generations. All types of mammary carcinomas invaded and metastasized in the form of large, organized structures comprising millions of cells.

The afferent limb of the cellular cytotoxic immune response was defective in normal and neoplastic mammary tissues. Antigenic cells persistent for periods of months induced tolerance to their antigens. M-D carcinomas grew normally in hosts histo-incompatible with their normal-cell components. The allogeneic normal cells participated in growth and metastasis and induced tolerance to their alloantigens. This indicated that failure of development of effective immunity is related more to the physiology of the neoplastic mass than to characteristics of the neoplastic

[a]Funded by Grant CA-18987 from the National Institutes of Health, DHEW, and by Grant MA 5856 from the Medical Research Council of Canada.

cells *per se*. Tolerance interfered with some immune responses but qualitatively different responses could break tolerance and cause rejection of established neoplasms.

Introduction

Knowledge of basic principles relevant to the cell biology and immunology of cancer remains inadequate for understanding the biology of development and the spread of primary neoplasms. In areas where basic principles are not understood, reductionist methods can result in misidentification of minor or even irrelevant principles as basic. I believe this has occurred in studies of metastasis and immunology of cancer.

Twenty-five years of study of the immunology of cancer have resulted in little prevention or cure. Classical excision-challenge experiments and extensive *in vitro* studies demonstrated immune phenomena that correlated poorly with the *in vivo* biology of progressive tumor growth. Obviously, basic processes operating *in vivo* were not understood.

The unicentric cellular theory of the origin and development of cancer holds that neoplasms develop and grow as the result of the acquisition of heritable alterations in clones of cells deriving from single ancestors. Neoplastic progression results from sequential accumulation of heritable alterations permitting increasing escape from normal growth regulation.

Experimental studies of metastasis have dealt primarily with high neoplastic tumor lines. These were usually of mesenchymal or neural crest origin—cell types likely to be capable of growing and spreading as solitary or small groups of cells. The view that neoplasms invade and metastasize by the process of movement of solitary or small groups of cells, essentially independent of the primary mass, is widely held by experimental investigators and clinicians. I believe the unicentric cellular theory of cancer to be essentially correct. It does not necessarily follow that all types of neoplastic cells can grow and spread independently of the cell associations characterizing the normal tissues of origin. Cells of epithelial tissues in particular depend on association with other cells of the epithelial structure and on the epithelial-stromal junctional complex. Studies of highly neoplastic cell lines may not be relevant to most primary carcinomas and thus to the majority of human cancers.

Research in the development and spread of cancer is shifting to relatively more holistic studies frequently involving series of premalignant and malignant tissues derived from the same original tissue or tissue types. These studies represent a logical approach to the elucidation of characteristics of primary neoplasms not masked by numerous secondary alterations present in highly neoplastic cell lines. The mammary gland transplantation system permits serial transplantation of normal tissues or tissues representing various stages of neoplastic development. Tissues are grown in their natural environment *in vivo,* where host factors relevant to biology and immunology are operational. Many investigators doing mammary tissue transplantation have used pure strain recipients and implanted experimental tissues at the time of removal of the host parenchymal rudiment which must be done at about 18–21 days of age. In the program established in this laboratory, F1 hybrids between several inbred strains are produced and their mammary fat pads cleared of host parenchyma. They are then placed in stock for later use as experimental tissue recipients. When a transplantation procedure is carried out, test recipients of several different genotypes are available simultaneously to receive identical tissues. This simple logistic difference in experimental procedure accounts for the fact that it has been possible to extend the system to new applications.

A research program to study the cell biology and immunology of normal and neoplastic mammary glands has been developed over a period of years. New methodology uses tissues comprising mosaics of cells or tissues of different genotypes. Tissues for serial transplantation are selected and handled with care to preserve original cellular relationships. This approach has resulted in observation of interactions and interdependence of different cell types in normal breast and in neoplastic tissues during progression and metastases. Phenomena significant for understanding the immunology of neoplasia and of tissue transplantations have been observed. I believe these methods provide results relevant to the biology of primary neoplasms. Previous publications[1,2] reported results of studies of the immunology and cell biology of early stages of breast neoplasia. This paper will deal with recent results particularly in reference to the immunology of the development and spread of cancer.

Materials and Methods

Experimental Animals

Pure strains BALB/c AnNIcr(C), C3H/HeNIcr(C3), C57B1/6JNIcr(B6) and DBA/2AnPrIcr(D2) were maintained by brother-sister mating. F1 hybrid females B6D2, B6C3, B6C, D2C3, C3B6, C3D2, C3C, CD2, and CC3 were produced and their inguinal mammary fat pads cleared of host parenchyma at 18–21 days of age. Cleared animals were then placed in stock and used as transplant recipients when they were about 8 to 12 weeks of age.

Experimental Tissues

Lungs of tumor hosts and slices of tumor masses were studied with transmitted light using a high resolution stereoscopic microscope. Slices about 1 mm in thickness perpendicular to the tumor surface were made in carefully selected areas. Patterns of growth and stereomicroscopic morphology could be correlated with cellular composition. Solid pieces of tumor preserving the structure and composition of the original tumors were transplanted. These techniques permitted maintenance of desired forms through many serial transplant generations. Metastatic growths present in pulmonary arterial branches were frequently not visible on the lung surface. When lung lobes were studied with transmitted light, affected arteries appeared transparent against the opaque background of the refractile air-filled alveoli. Carcinoma tissues extending through small arterial branches protruded from cut surfaces.

Genotypically Mosaic Tissues

These were produced by associating normal or neoplastic cells of one genotype with normal parenchyma of a second.[2] This procedure is accomplished at will quickly and simply by present methods. The symbol [//] is used to denote associated tissues. Thus [C3//C] indicates C3 cells associated with C cells. I believe the cell types in mammary parenchyma (MP)[a] to be myoepithelial (ME), alveolar epithelial (AE) and ductal epithelial (DE).[2] An asterisk(*) is used to denote neoplastically transformed cells. Thus the composition of a C3 tumor to which C normal cells had been added would be designated thus: [C3-AE*//C-ME+ DE+AE], if all components of normal gland were present.

Mosaic tissues were maintained by serial transplantation in F1 hybrid hosts histocompatible with both genotypic components. The genotype and cell type composition of tissues during neoplastic progression and metastasis was determined by transplantation to animals histocompatible with one but not both genotypes. MHC-histoincompatible components were rejected. Histocompatible populations gave rise to growth characteristic of the component cell types.

Grading Metastasis to Lungs

Since lung involvement resulted from embolization and extension through pulmonary arteries, counting numbers was practical only by recording involved lobes. The following scheme was used. One lobe involved grade +1, 2 lobes +2, all but one lobe +3, all lobes +4.

Statistical Analyses

The 2 × 2 chi-square test with correction for continuity or exact treatment of 2 × 2 contingency tables were used.

---

[a]Abbreviations used in this paper are: AE—alveolar epithelial mammary cells; DE—ductal epithelial mammary cells; ESJ—epithelial-stromal junction; FP—mammary fat pad; LM—metastasis to lungs; M-D—mosaic dependent; ME—myoepithelial cells; MHC—major histocompatibility gene complex, i.e., H2; MP—mammary parenchyma; MTV—mammary tumor virus.

Immunology

In previous studies of host response to developing neoplasia,[1] I reported that antigenic *in situ* premalignant mammary lesions failed to induce effective immunity. The hypothesis that the intact epithelial-stromal junction (ESJ) could block the afferent limb of the cellular cytotoxic immune response was suggested in these studies and by reports in the literature. Billingham and Medawar [3] in studies, subsequently shown to involve survival of transplanted allogeneic cells, [4] found that allogeneic melanocytes survived and grew indefinitely in the epidermis of guinea pigs. Woodruff and Woodruff [5] and Merwin and Hill [6] found that subcutaneous transplants of allegeneic thyroid gland sometimes failed to elicit immunity. These studies and my own had in common the fact that the antigenic cells were separated from the host by an intact epithelial-stromal junction. Ozzello [7] found that the ESJ separating epithelial cells from vascular stroma consisted of a complex structure which included lamina lucida, basal lamina, a layer of avascular connective tissue and a layer of delimiting fibroblast cytoplasm. In order to recognize antigenic antigenic epithelial cells, specific T lymphocytes would have to transverse these complex structures.

Allogeneic Transplantation

To test this hypothesis, I carried out experiments as illustrated in Figure 1. The gland-free mammary fat pad of one pure strain either D2 or C^b was transplanted to the hybrid between these strains. Pure-strain normal or neoplastic mammary parenchyma of the opposite type was then transplanted into these transplanted fat pads. Resulting outgrowths consisted of mammary parenchyma of one genotype growing in stroma of the second. Small portions of these outgrowths were dissected and transplanted as primary allografts to recipients histocompatible with the stroma. It was necessary to cut through the parenchymal units to accomplish this. Barker and Billingham[8] found that exposure to allogeneic tissue for periods of four to six days was required for initiation of immune responses. Cut parenchymal units could heal within this time period. Thus, if the intact ESJ could block the afferent limb of the cellular cytotoxic immune response some allograted tissues might survive. Results shown in Table 1 demonstrated that significant numbers of the primary allografts survived. The experimental genotype of growths was determined by transplantation to recipients syngeneic with the original parenchyma donor or allogeneic and preimmunized against the parenchyma. Growth in the former and rejection in the latter confirmed

[b]These strains share major histocompatibility genes ($H2_d$) but differ at several minor histocompatibility loci.

8

Figure 1. Method of allogeneic transplantation.

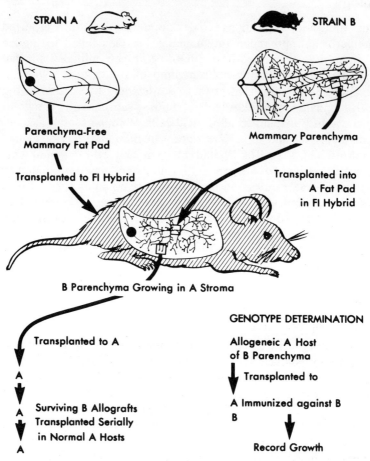

STRAIN A   STRAIN B

Parenchyma-Free
Mammary Fat Pad

Mammary Parenchyma

Transplanted to Fl Hybrid

Transplanted into
A Fat Pad
in Fl Hybrid

B Parenchyma Growing in A Stroma

GENOTYPE DETERMINATION

Transplanted to A

Allogeneic A Host
of B Parenchyma

A

Transplanted to

A

A Immunized against B

Surviving B Allografts
Transplanted Serially
in Normal A Hosts

B

A

Record Growth

A

the genotype. Serially transplanted allogeneic tissues (generations 2 and later) also survived with significant frequency. The fact that serial allografts survived significantly less frequently than transplants of these same tissues to syngeneic recipients (Table 2) demonstrates the mammary parenchymal tissues, in the apparent absence of donor-type stromal and lymphoid cells, can elicit allograft immunity.

Active Tolerance Induced by Persistent Antigenic Tissues

Hosts of allografts which had been present for periods of less than about four months retained the capacity to develop immunity to mammary tissues of the donor types. Fresh immunizing challenge grafts of allogeneic parenchyma in allogeneic stroma elicited immunity which destroyed them and the original allogeneic growth as well. Hosts of allogeneic

Table 1. Allogeneic Transplantation

Parenchyma Genotype	Tissue Type	Recipient Genotype	Surviving/Total Transplants (%) Generations		Syngeneic Recipients
			1	2 and later	
BALB/c	Normal	D2	1/20(5)	0/2(0)	85/88(97)
		C3D2F1	12/47(26)	2/4(50)	
		B6D2F1	2/14(14)	0/8(0)	
	Early Neoplasia	D2	0/15(0)		120/120(100)
		C3D2F1	10/48(21)	9/11(82)	
		B6D2F1	2/49(4)	8/46(17)	
DBA/2	Normal	C	0/29(0)		61/65(94)
		CC3F1	1/40(3)	0/2(0)	
		B6CF1	2/42(5)	9/16(56)	
	Early Neoplasia	C	0/26(0)		
		CC3F1	0/23(0)		
		B6CF1	0/33(0)		

growths that had been present for about four months or more behaved differently. Fresh grafts of allogeneic parenchyma in allogeneic stroma were accepted. With the passage of time what had initially been a failure of recognition evolved into an inability to respond effectively.

Transfer of Tolerance to Normal Adults

During the early stages of development of tolerance, host response to the immunizing grafts involved considerable lymphoid cell infiltration, inhibition of growth and damage to the allogeneic parenchyma as is illustrated in Figure 2. Transplants of 1 mm segments of parenchymal units from these growths to allogeneic recipients which were challenged simultaneously at a distant site with fresh allografts resulted in acceptance of both grafts. Apparently the lymphoid cells infiltrating these grafts transferred the tolerance. It was of interest to determine the distribution of this activity in lymphoid tissues of the body. Lymphoid tissues from tolerant donors were transferred along with fresh allografts to normal adult recipients (Figure 3.) Factors transferring tolerance were detected in lymphoid tissues throughout the body (Table 3).

Time-Dependent Evolution of Tolerance

In recipients of early tolerance responses, immunity capable of causing damage to the parenchyma gradually diminished with the passage of time (Figure 4). Lymphoid tissues of such hosts were sometimes capable of transferring this complete tolerance to normal adults (Figure 5). Recent results indicate that in long term (12 to 18 months) hosts with fully-

Table 2. Syngeneic Transfer of Tolerance

Parenchyma Inducing Tolerance	Tolerance Donor and Recipient Genotype	Lymphoid Tissue	#/Total[a]
BALB/c Normal	C3D2F1	Local LN2	15/30 (50%)
		Distant LN	1/3 (33%)
		Spleen	9/23 (39%)
		Infiltrating[b]	3/4 (75%)
		Thymus	3/7 (43%)
	B6D2F1	Local LN	2/5 (40%)
		Distant LN	2/3 (67%)
		Spleen	2/4 (50%)
		Thymus	2/3 (67%)
BALB/c Neoplastic	C3D2F	Local LN[c]	24/53 (45%)
		Distant LN	19/38 (50%)
		Spleen	34/80 (43%)
		Thymus	17/31 (55%)
	B6D2F1	Local LN	4/10 (40%)
		Distant LN	4/7 (57%)
		Spleen	7/33 (21%)
		Thymus	5/10 (50%)
DBA/2 Normal	CC3	Local LN[c]	0/4 (0%)
	B6C	Local LN	1/12 (8%)
		Infiltrating	0/9 (0%)
		Spleen	0/7 (0%)

[a] Number accepting fresh mammary allograft/total transfer attempts (%).

[b] Infiltrating: allogeneic growth with lymphoid infiltration.

[c] LN: lymph node.

developed tolerance, no factors capable of transferring these responses were associated with the experimental tissues. Transferring factors were also apparently less prominent in the lymphoid tissues of these animals. Thus, the response appeared to evolve into a form of mimicking normal self-tolerance.

Protection of Tissues Bearing Strong Antigens in Addition to the Tolerated Specificities

A fascinating, recent observation is that fully-developed tolerance induced by $C(H2^d)$ mammary parenchyma in $D2(H2^d)$ will prevent immunity to $B6CF1$ $(H2^{d + b})$ mammary parenchyma. In pilot experiments 0

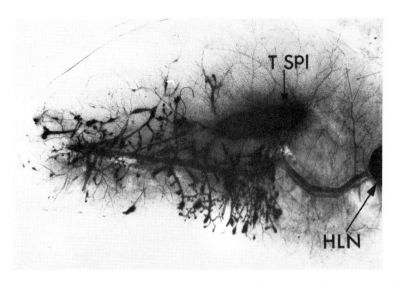

Figure 2. Hematoxylin-stained whole mount of mammary fat pad containing a transplant of spleen from a partially tolerant donor and mammary outgrowth from a fresh allograft. Note lymphoid infiltration and damage of experimental parenchyma 15 weeks after implantation. TSp1 = transplanted spleen; HLN = host lymph node.

of 12 B6CF1 implants survived in hosts tolerant for less than six months but six of nine survived (confirmed by genotyping transplants) in recipients tolerant for from six to 12 months. Thus, tolerance induced across a non-MHC barrier protected MHC-incompatible tissues. This is a potentially valuable observation as it could permit development of methods for easily preventing immunity to allografts. This phenomenon may also explain some aspects of the failure of immune control of neoplasms expressing neoantigens. Self-tolerance directed toward normal antigens might protect associated neoantigens.

Breaking Tolerance

The capacity of tolerance induced by mammary parenchyma to protect skin allografts was tested. Hosts tolerant of mammary allografts for periods of from six to 12 months rejected skin grafts of the tolerated parenchyma genotype. The resulting immune responses also caused the destruction of the long-established mammary allografts. Skin grafts and inoculations of spleen, lymph node or thymus of the tolerated parenchyma genotype caused rejection or inhibition of growth of previous tolerated tissues in many cases (Table 3). Established carcinomas as large as 2 cm were rejected. Skin and lymphoid tissues express determinants of the I region of the MHC. Tolerance induced by MP could protect tissues

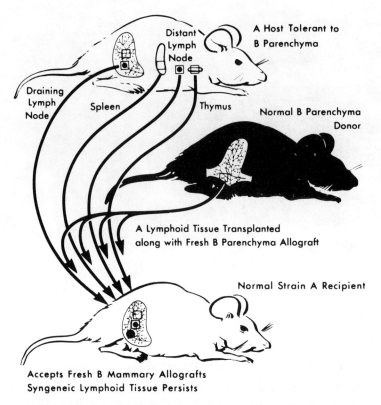

Figure 3. Transfer of tolerance to recipients syngeneic with the donor.

expressing non-I region MHC alloantigens. I region determinants may induce responses that can break this tolerance. Qualitatively-different antigen combinations may induce qualitatively-different immune responses.

Progression and Metastasis in the Allogeneic Host

Lines of early C neoplasia such as that illustrated in Figure 6 were maintained by serial transplantation in allogeneic hosts. These tissues survived for the duration of the life span of the host, induced tolerance to their alloantigens, progressed to malignancy, invaded veins and formed invasive metastatic growths in the lung (Figure 7). Although there was sometimes evidence of immunologic response characterized by lymphoid infiltration as in Figure 7, this did not prevent progression and metastasis.

Table 3. Immunotherapy of Established Growths in Tolerant Hosts

Experimental Tissue	Complete Rejection	Control of Growth[a]	Uninterrupted Progression	Total
Normal	2	2	7	11
Premalignant	3	11	1	15
Malignant	4	12	51	67

[a] Diminution of mass and/or growth rate by 50 percent or more.

Cell Biology

Neoplastic Development and Classification

Types of Cells in Mammary Glands

A number of investigators using histochemical techniques or electron microscopy have reported evidence they interpreted to indicate that the various types of cells in normal and neoplastic mammary tissues are interchangeable or derive from common stem cell precursors. My studies indicate that the different cell types have separate origins in adult tissues.

Figure 4. Recipient of tolerant lymph node and fresh allograft shows evidence of past immune damage with isolation of peripheral parenchymal units after destruction of intervening segments of ducts. The specimen illustrates fully-developed tolerance 11 months after tissue implantation. TLN = transplanted lymph node.

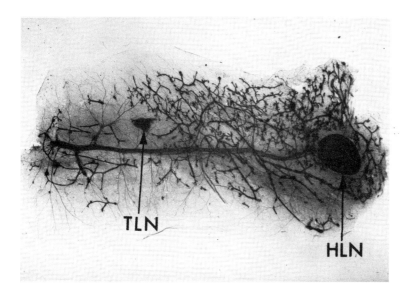

14

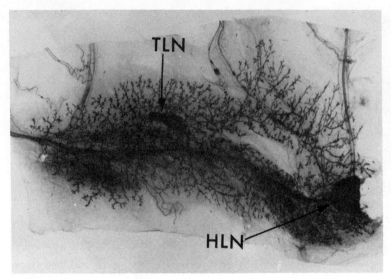

Figure 5. Recipient of tolerant lymph node and fresh allograft shows no evidence of immunity 9 months after implantation. A portion of the host lymph node was transplanted to maintain the line of tolerance.

Figure 6. Hyperplastic outgrowth of early neoplasia 12 weeks after implantation × 6.

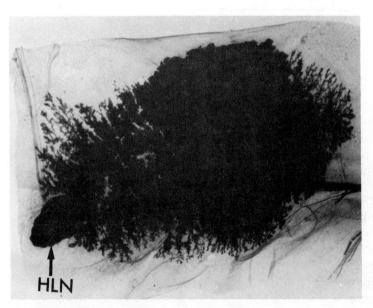

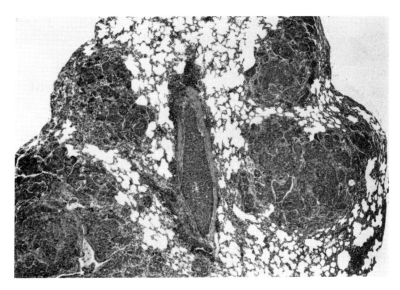

Figure 7. Lung of allogeneic C3D2F1 recipient of precursor C early neoplasia as in Figure 6, seven months after implantation. Metastatic malignant variant masses in pulmonary arterial branches and extending through lung parenchyma. Moderate lymphoid infiltration is apparent around large artery.

If this is correct, it could be significant for the understanding of breast neoplasia. It appears that in normal and neoplastic tissues—particularly during rapid growth—the separate cell types are not distinguishable morphologically. The transplantation methods developed here facilitate determination of cellular composition and may permit analysis of cellular functions and interactions which could not be determined by other methods.

Classification of Mammary Tumors

Dunn's established classification system for mammary tumors of mice[9] is generally accepted and considered reliable. My studies[2] indicate, however, that Dunn's system does not separate tumors which arise from different types of cells. Thus, neoplasms having different origins, etiology, epidemiology and general biology are grouped together because of a histologic resemblance. I have found that each of the three major classes of Dunn includes neoplasms arising from at least two and usually three separate cell types.

Mode of Origin of Neoplasia

Willis[10] rejected the view that neoplasms arise from small foci of cells and develop by multiplication of these and their descendents. A chapter in his book purports to show ". . . . that tumors arise from small or large fields of tissue and enlarge not only by cellular proliferation but also by progressive neoplastic conversion of tissues within those fields." He further claims that "Careful microscopic study of early tumors of many kinds affords clear evidence of such progressive change, with plain transitions from normal to neoplastic tissue." Ewing[11] and Foulds[12] observed, however, that collateral hyperplasia, the hypertrophy and hyperplasia that occur in biologically normal tissues adjacent to neoplasms, is sometimes indistinguishable histologically from neoplasia.

Interactions of Different Mammary Cell Types in Normal and Neoplastic Tissues

I previously reported[2] evidence indicating interactions and interdependence of cell types in various mammary tissues. Genotypically mosaic normal or neoplastic mammary tissues were maintained by serial transplantation in hosts histocompatible with both components. By observing the character of growths resulting from transplants to recipients compatible with one but not both components, it was possible to infer the cellular composition of the original. Results indicated that norma mammary glands are composed of at least three separate populations of cells representing different cell types: alveolar epithelial (AE), ductal epithelial (DE) and myoepithelial (ME) cells. During neoplastic progression the abnormal cells of some types retained association with normal cells of other types. With the passage of time and during the process of neoplastic progression, normal cell components aged and lost their growth potential. If sublines lacked normal cells of the genotype of the neoplastic cells then growth frequently did not occur in that strain. The neoplastic cells apparently retained dependence on normal cells. When all normal cell components had lost their growth potential, the tumor line became a benign, atrophic lesion difficult to maintain. Addition of young normal mammary cells to such a tumor resulted in rejuvenation of the growth.

Transplantation and Histopathology in Analysis of Tumor Composition

The neoplastic growths in Figures 8–11, for example, are composed of [AE*//ME+DE+AE] yet, there is little indication in most areas of these sections of anything other than malignant cells. In some areas, epithelial and myoepithelial cells were distinguishable (Figure 8). The biologically normal cell components took on morphologic characteristics of the neoplastic cells with which they were associated. They remained, however, biologically normal and, when separated from the neoplastic cells, produced normal growth (Figures 12, 13). I observed normal B6 AE cells in fields where cells are recruited into the developing neoplasm is wrong. serial tumor transplantation *in vivo* that never showed any sign of neoplastic transformation. Thus Willis's[10] concept of neoplasia arising

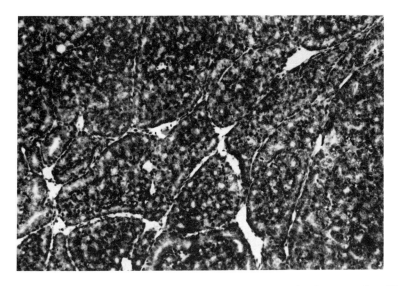

Figure 8. Section of M-D AE carcinoma five months after implantation. Bilayered units of epithelial and myoepithelial cells. H and E × 100.

in fields where cells are recruited into the developing neoplasm is wrong. What he saw may have been the collateral hyperplasia discussed by Ewing [11] and Foulds [12] which explains the observations made here.

Normal Cells Interacting with Neoplastic Cells During Metastasis 0f M-D AE Carcinomas

While studying the M-D carcinoma C3-5, I observed an interaction of the malignant cells with the lung structure. Extensive involvement resulted from extension through pulmonary arteries (Figure 11). When these lung masses were transplanted to mammary fat pads, resulting growths were identical to the original M-D forms. When these FP growths from LM or when LM themselves were transplanted to recipients compatible with the normal components, entirely normal growth resulted (Figure 13). Such growth indicates that literally millions of normal cells were involved in the transplant of the lungs, as smaller numbers would have limited growth potential.

Requirement of Neoplastic AE Cells for Association with Normal Cells

The data in Table 4 illustrate the fact that implants of malignant M-D AE carcinomas in recipients incompatible at MHC loci with the normal components frequently failed to produce any growths. These results indicate that many neoplastic AE cells require association with normal cells for survival.

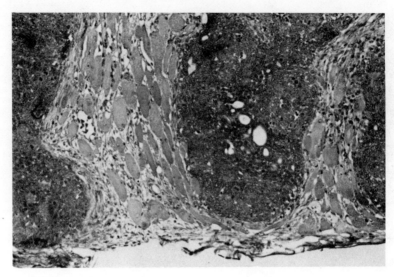

Figure 9. Section of large, organized masses of M-D AE carcinoma invading muscle.

Figure 10. Section of M-D AE carcinoma invading muscle. Apparently-isolated cells were attached to organized structures. H and E × 100.

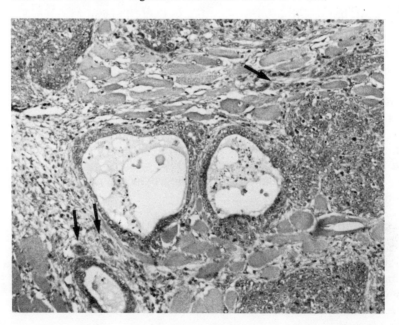

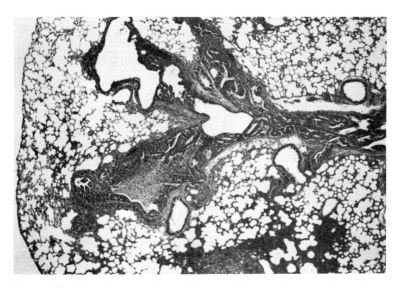

Figure 11. Histologic section of lung of host of mosaic-dependent alveolar epithelial (M-D AE) carcinomas eight weeks after implantation of the tumor in the mammary fat pad. Metastatic growth extending through pulmonary arterial branches. H and E × 50.

Figure 12. Whole mount of fat pad of B6CF1 recipient of [C3*//C] M-D AE carcinomas growing in C3D2F1 host. Normal lactating outgrowth in post partum host × 6.

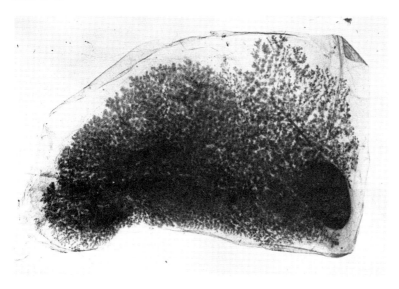

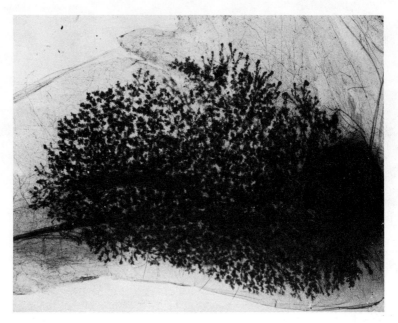

Figure 13. Fat pad of B6CF1 recipient of metastatic lung masses from [C3//C] M-D AE carcinoma growing in C3D2F1 host. Normal lactating outgrowth in post partum host × 8.

Requirement of Neoplastic AE Cells for Association with Normal Mammary Cells for Metastasis

The growths that did occur in recipients MHC-incompatible with the normal components developed very slowly and metastasized to lungs with significantly lower frequency than the parent M-D tumors. These results are shown in Table 4. Sublines of these tumors have retained dependence on associated normal components through as many as 15 serial metastatic generations. Recent results indicate that metastasizing populations may be select subpopulations of dependent cells. In one such subline, no growths have occurred in 74 recipients MHC-incompatible with normal components after an observation period of six months.

Control for Nonspecific Killing of Neoplastic AE Cells

Is it conceivable that nonspecific immune factors were responsible for killing AE cells in recipients incompatible with the normal components. To control for this, neoplastic AE cells were inoculated mixed with allogeneic normal cells to which the recipient had been preimmunized with or without admixed compatible normal cells. In 18/18 cases where compatible normal cells were present, rapid M-D growth occurred; this

Table 4. Growth of C3-5 in Recipients Histocompatible and Histoincompatible with Normal Components

Recipient	Incidence	Growth Rate[a]		LM
		Range	Mean	
Syngeneic	667/685 (97%)	2-21	5.1	331/568 (58%) 2.4[b]
Allogeneic MHC-compatible: [C3*//C] in C3D2F1	196/264 (74%)[c]	3-50	6.5	27/69 (39%) 2.2[d]
MHC incompatible	205/485 (42%)[e]	3-50	15.2	24/62 (39%) 2.15[f]
MHC incompatible from allogeneic C3D2F1 donor	25/70 (36%)	3-50	17.4	NR[g]

[a] Time in weeks rèquired to reach 2 cm.

[b] Lung metastasis: incidence, grade in the 45 percent of all syngeneic hosts studied for metastasis.

[c] 196/264 vs 667/685 P<0.001.

[d] 331/568 vs 27/69 P< 0.01.

[e] 205/485 vs 667/685 P<0.001.

[f] 331/568 vs 24/62 P<0.001.

[g] NR, not recorded.

compares with 0/24 cases where compatible cells were not included. These results indicate that nonspecific cytotoxicity plays little role in the results observed in these experiments.

Mechanisms of Metastasis

Metastasis of Mammary Carcinomas

I found that all types of mammary carcinomas invaded normal tissues and metastasized as large, organized structures (Figures 9,10,14). In veins draining carcinomas, I found large masses of organized cells as in Figure 14. Pieces of these structures broke off and embolized pulmonary arteries. Massive involvement of the lung resulted from growth by extension through the branches of the pulmonary arteries (Figure 11) and, in the case of some types of mammary neoplasia, extension through the lung parenchyma (Figure 7).

Literature Review—Metastasis

Willis[13] studied metastasis of carcinomas in humans. He observed that detachment of considerable fragments of malignant growth must be the rule and that of isolated cells the exception. He measured pulmonary

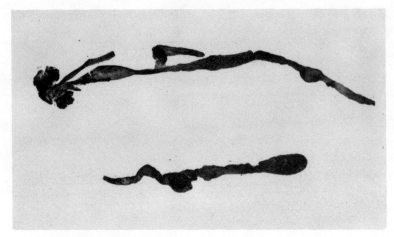

Figure 14. Hematoxylin-stained whole mount of intravenous extension from M-D AE carcinoma. From the site of vein penetration deep within the tumor where a portion of the original tumor is still attached at upper left, the mass extended into the vena cava.

arterioles occluded by emboli or growths of metastatic carcinomas. He found the average diameter was over 200 μ and the range 15 to 650 μ. He found that it was chiefly when growth gained entry to large veins that prolific metastasis resulted. He castigated investigators and clinicians who assumed that showers of solitary tumor cells are predominantly responsible for cancer metastasis. Similar observations were made in previous editions of his book.[14,15]

Weiss[16] cited Willis, then stated that cancer cells are shed into circulation by an "essentially exfoliative process." He noted that the histologic evidence for active movements of single cancer cells in invasion is "not impressive" and that active movements of single malignant cells in malignant infiltration are not of "great demonstrable importance." He then presented a detailed physical-chemical analysis of interactions of solitary cells and the supposed relationship of these to cancer metastasis.

Most experimental studies of metastasis have used highly neoplastic cell lines mostly of mesenchymal or neural crest origin. Fidler's studies [17,18] dealth primarily with the B16 melanoma. Hart and Fidler [19] studied sarcomas and melanomas. Kripke et al.[20] studied sarcomas. Baserga et al.[21] chose the Erhlich ascites cell lines for their studies of tumor growth in lungs following intravenous inoculation. Gullino[22] studied metastasis of a mammary cell line capable of growing in ascites form and found convective currents within these tumors played a major role in promoting the release of solitary neoplastic cells into the blood stream. Van de Velde et al.[23] used a mammary tumor line that had been passaged through 61 generations. They felt it was an excellent model for human disease because it was capable of metastasizing to lymph nodes in mice. Pollack[24] carried this reductionism to extremes in his paper on *in vitro* analysis of the metastatic process.

Mechanisms of Invasion

Erdlandson and Carstens[25] observed that the presence of intact basement membranes cannot be used as a criterion for noninvasive mammary carcinoma. Leighton[26] observed that cells of epithelial lines grew *in vitro* as integrated units in the propagation of similar groups of cells. Tickle et al.[27] found that cells of carcinomas, in contrast to neoplasms of mesenchymal and neural crest origin, did not move into the mesenchyme of developing chick wing but remained in contact with the epithelial cells.

In the studies here, organized structure of M-D carcinomas invaded normal tissues (Figures 9,10). Foci of apparent microinvasion by small clusters or solitary cells (Figure 10) were histologic artifacts. In adjacent sections these were found to be attached to organized structures. These protrusions from organized structures may be one characteristic pathologists have observed to be correlated with metastasis and mistakenly assumed to be microinvasion. The neoplastic cells of these tumors are dependent on association with normal mammary cells. It is unlikely that they would survive outside of the integrated structures. Hager et al.[28] found no correlation between invasion of tissues surrounding tumors and metastasis. This probably is because metastasis results from invasion of the larger veins within the tumor (Figure 14) rather than the smaller vessels in surrounding tissues.

The assumption of single cell invasion and spread is implicit in the discussion of metastasis by Prehn and Prehn.[29] McDivitt et al.[30] provide an unconvincing discussion under "Assessment of Noninfiltration and its Therapeutic Implications." They state that "Having examined multiple duct carcinomas that. . . . everywhere appeared noninfiltrative yet had metastasized to axillary lymph nodes, we do not feel that we can ever eliminate the possibility of microinfiltration of stroma." Clearly, they are assuming that invasion by solitary cells is required for metastasis. Elsewhere, however, they report finding tissues composed of epithelium associated with myoepithelium in lymph nodes draining neoplasms. Some tumors are described as being " . . . largely intraductal, but somewhere infiltration . . . will usually be found." I found that apparent "infiltration" and "microinvasion" can be seen when they are sought in neoplasms where the biology indicates they are very unlikely to exist.

Lymph node metastasis from tumors equivalent to human carcinomas would not be expected in mice because the diameter of the lymphatic vessels is too small to permit entry and passage of the organized structures. Van der Velde et al.[23] are therefore wrong in their assessment of their highly neoplastic tumor line as a "very attractive" model for human cancer. The fact that their tumor line can metastasize to mouse lymph nodes indicates that it differs from most human primary carcinomas in its modes of invasion and spread. In terms of resistance to invasion by carcinomas, murine veins resemble human lymphatic vessels. Thus, metastasis to lungs of mice could be an appropriate model for lymphatic metastasis in humans.

Synthesis of Cell Biology and Immunology

I reported evidence indicating, that while premalignant derivative malignant variant tissues expressed qualitatively and quantitatively similar neoantigenicity, implants of malignant tissue were relatively resistant to immune destruction.[1] The hypothesis was advanced that defects in immune responses resulted from physiologic factors within tumors. Spitalny and North[31] observed that immunity to bacteria was defective within tumors. Barker and Billingham[8] reported evidence which indicated that the development of allograft immunity in vivo required periods of at least four to six days. This suggested that a series of events requiring time might be necessary—proliferation and differentiation of specific T cells under the influence of appropriate regulator cells for example.

Based on observations of defects in the afferent response in epithelial and endocrine tissues, I hypothesized that similar defects might occur in nidi of neoplasia because of abnormal physiology.[32] To test this hypothesis, M-D AE carcinomas were implanted in recipients histoincompatible at non-MHC loci with the normal components of the tumors.

Allogeneic Normal Cells Survive in Tumors

Results of these experiments are shown in Table 4, in which it may be seen that tissues composed of [C3*//C] implanted in C3D2F1 hosts produced rapid growth in 196 of 264 cases (74%) compared with 97 percent of 685 implants of this tumor line in recipients syngeneic with both components. In constrast, slow growth occurred in only 42 percent of 485 recipients MHC-incompatible with the normal component. Transplants of the tumor tissues consisting of [C3//C] growing in C3D2F1 gave morphologic evidence of persistence of normal C cells by producing of normal mammary structures in 59 of 118 recipients compatible with C but not with C3. In 39 percent of these, sufficient normal cells were present to produce entirely normal extending, functional growths (Figures 13,14). The data in Table 5 also illustrate the fact that the allogeneic

Table 5. Normal Components of Mosaic-Dependent Carcinomas in MHC-Compatible Allogeneic Hosts Compared with Those in Syngeneic Hosts

		Generations After Adding Normal Component	
		2-5	6-8
Allogeneic Donors	Negative	24 (36%)	15 (47%)
	Epithelium in transplant site	11 (17%)	9 (28%)
	Normal outgrowth	31 (47%)	8 (25%)
	Total	66	32
Syngeneic Donors	Negative	71 (26%)	35 (47%)
	Epithelium in transplant site	70 (25%)	22 (29%)
	Normal outgrowth	136 (49%)	18 (24%)
	Total	277	75

normal components were similar in quantity to the normal components of these same tumors growing in histocompatible hosts. The mean growth rate of these tumors in non-MHC allogeneic hosts (6.5 weeks) compares with 5.1 in syngeneic and 17.4 when these same tissues were transplanted to MHC-incompatible recipients. Thus C normal components apparently survived and participated in growth in most of the 74 percent of the C3D2F1 hosts in which growth occurred.

Participation of Allogeneic Normal Cells During Metastasis

Transplants of metastatic masses directly from the lungs of allogeneic hosts to recipients compatible with the normal components produced entirely normal mammary growths (Figure 13). Thus, allogeneic normal components participated in metastasis. Metastasis was significantly inhibited in these animals, however, occurring in only 27 of 69 non-MHC allogeneic hosts as compared with 331 of 568 syngeneic hosts (P < 0.01). The mechanism of this inhibition of metastasis requires study.

Induction of Tolerance by Allogeneic Normal Components of M-D Carcinomas

Active tolerance to fresh allografts of C mammary parenchyma was transferred to normal adult C3D2F1 by lymphoid tissues of C3D2F1 hosts of [C3//C] carcinomas. One of the 15 recipients of lymphoid tissues from primary allograft donors accepted the C allograft versus seven of 32 recipients of tissues from second generation allografted tissues (P = 0.19). Experiments of the evolution of tolerance during serial transplantation in this model are continuing.

Discussion

Cunningham[33] reviewed evidence indicating that self-tolerance may be mediated by active suppressor mechanisms. Stumpf et al.[34] in studies of low-zone tolerance found that suppressor T cells were stimulated at lower antigen doses than helper T cells. These studies indicate that the initial responses to low levels of antigen such as occur in differentiation of tissue-specific antigens or in neoplastic development could be expected to be protective rather than immune. The studies reported here indicate that antigens persistent for long periods of time induce protective responses. It may be that the body naturally protects persistent antigens as self components. Phylogenetically, it is more important to protect against autoimmunity which can develop early in life, than it is to protect against neoplasia which usually arises after the reproductive period.

Thus neoantigens of gradually-evolving neoplasia may induce active tolerance as an initial response. This then could interfere with development of immunity. In the studies here allogeneic normal and early neoplastic tissues having known antigenicity, presumably as strong as the neoantigenicity of any neoplasm, induced protective responses which made that high antigenicity nearly undetectable in some serially-transplanted lines. Neoplastic progression and metastasis was not inhibited in spite of this high antigenicity. It is necessary in light of these observations to reassess tumor antigenicity and host response. Neoplasms with very high antigenicity could appear to be nonimmunogenic if active tolerance responses were an integral part of their composition. Various lymphoid cells, frequently comprising significant components in neoplasms, could have protective rather than immune functions.

Active tolerance responses induced by one combination of antigens may be broken by immune responses induced by different antigen combinations. It may be that qualitatively-different immune responses, possibly involving activation of differing lymphoid cellular subpopulations, may exist. Spontaneous, apparently immune-mediated, remission of cancer may result from such responses. Effective adjuvant immunotherapy may operate through similar mechanisms. Mammary tissues are advantageous for these studies in that they, like most organs and tissues, do not express I-region determinants. For this reason they are more suitable than skin for studies of organ and tissue transplantation immunology and the immunology of cancer.

The widely held concept that metastasis of cancer results from invasion and transport of solitary neoplastic cells may derive from misinterpretation of the implications of the unicentric cellular concept of the origin of cancer—the idea that cancers arise from single defective ancestral cells—and from experimental studies using neoplasms of types capable of growing as solitary cells.

If cancers develop as a result of accumulation of heritable alterations in cell clones, it does not follow that those neoplastic cells are necessarily capable of survival, growth or metastasis in the absence of association with other neoplastic cells or with mosaics of normal and neoplastic cells of the tissue of origin. Thousands of cells are usually required to transfer neoplasms of recent origin—particularly carcinomas—even if recipients are immunodepressed. The studies cited above[25–27] of the behavior of neoplastic epithelial tissues, the studies of Willis[13] and the work reported here indicated that carcinomas metastasize in the form of organized structures because of interactions and interdependence of their constituent cells.

Many experimental studies of cancer metastases have used highly neoplastic tumor lines—frequently of mesenchymal or neural crest origin (sarcomas, melanomas). Cells from these lines frequently are capable of growing and metastasizing as solitary cells. Such studies may be relevant to metastasis of the small percentage of human cancers arising from cells of these types. Those studies may not be relevant to metastasis of most human cancers which are carcinomas.

The neoplastic cell lines probably were chosen for technical reasons and not because they are particularly appropriate models for human disease. Ease of maintenance *in vitro* or ease of *in vivo* transfer were probably primary factors in their choice. Cell suspension methods of passaging mammary tumor lines would select against interdependent cell populations. Hager et al.[28] found that one mammary tumor could not be maintained in serial transplantation when drastic methods for cell suspension preparation were used. Tumor lines that can be easily passaged and maintained could be expected to differ in their biology from most primary tumors.

The results reported here demonstrate that some neoplastic epithelial cells are dependent not only on other similar cells but on normal cells of other types as well. The neoplastic cells of these tumors are not themselves cancer cells but components of cancer *tissues*. Cancer tissues may comprise various components in addition to neoplastic cells including many biologically-normal cells. Metastasis of cancer tissues requires passage of the intact integrated structure to the distant site. Medical intervention in the form of surgery or other manipulation might have little or no influence on metastasis of malignant tissues of these types.

Results demonstrating survival of normal components in allogeneic hosts and indicating their participation in metastasis are consistent with the hypothesis that immune responses are defective in nidi of neoplasia and indicate that the failure of the immune system to control the development and spread of cancer is related more to the physiology of the neoplastic mass than to characteristics of the neoplastic cells *per se*.

Hypothesis—Host Response to Developing Neoplasia

These studies indicate that there may be four factors that interfere with immune control of neoplastic development and spread exclusive of characteristics of the neoplastic cells themselves—if any exist:

1. There is an efferent block of epithelial and certain other tissues which prevents the entry of lymphoid cells capable of recognizing antigenicity.
2. The physiology of the neoplastic mass interferes with the afferent limb of the cytotoxic cellular immune response. This may involve an inability of the antigen recognition cells to proliferate and differentiate *in situ*.
3. There is an efferent blockade. Because of the characteristics of the neoplastic mass, effector cells cannot survive or function.
4. Persistent antigen induces active tolerance.

References

1. Slemmer, G: Host response to premalignant mammary tissues. *Nat. Cancer Inst. Monogr.* 35:57–71, 1972.
2. Slemmer, G: Interactions of separate types of cells during normal and neoplastic mammary gland growth. *J. Invest. Derm.* 63:27–47, 1974.
3. Billingham, RE, Medawar, PB: Pigment spread in mammalian skin: serial propagation and immunity reactions. *Heredity* 4:141–164, 1950.
4. Billingham, RE, Silvers, WK: Further studies on the phenomenon of pigment spread in guinea pigs' skin. *Ann. N.Y. Acad. Sci.* 100:348–360, 1963.
5. Woodruff, MFA, Woodruff, HG: The transplantation of normal tissues: with special reference to auto- and homotransplantation of thyroid and spleen in the anterior chamber of the eye, and subcutaneously in guinea pigs. *Phil. Trans. Roy. Soc. Lond.* B 234:559–582, 1950.
6. Merwin, R, Hill, EL: Fate of vascularized and nonvascularized subcutaneous homografts in mice. *J. Nat. Cancer Inst.* 14:819–839, 1954.
7. Ozzello, L: Epithelial-stromal junction of normal and dysplastic mammary glands. *Cancer* 25:586–600, 1970.
8. Barker, CF, Billingham, RE: The role of afferent lymphatics in the rejection of skin homografts. *J. Exp. Med.* 128:197–221, 1968.
9. Dunn, TB: Morphology of mammary tumors in mice. In: Homberger, F, ed. *The Physiopathology of Cancer.* Second Edition, pp. 238–292, Hoeber-Harper Inc., New York, 1959.
10. Willis, RA: *Pathology of Tumors.* Fourth Edition, p. 105–124, Butterworths, London, 1967.
11. Ewing: *Neoplastic Development.* Saunders, Philadelphia, 1928.
12. Foulds, L: The histological analysis of tumors: a critical review. *Am. J. Cancer* 39:1–24, 1940.
13. Willis, RA: *The Spread of Tumors in the Human Body.* Butterworths, London, 1973.

14. Willis, RA: *The Spread of Tumors in the Human Body.* Second Edition, Butterworths, London, 1952.

15. Willis, RA: *The Spread of Tumors in the Human Body. Baker Inst. Monogr. 2.,* J. & A., Churchill, London, 1934.

16. Weiss, L: Cell detachment and metastasis. *Gann Monogr. Cancer Res.* 20:25–35, 1977.

17. Fidler, IJ: Patterns of tumor cell arrest and development. In: Weiss, L. ed. *Fundamental Aspects of Metastasis,* p. 275–289, Amsterdam: North-Holland Pub. Co., 1976.

18. Fidler, IJ: Tumor heterogeneity and the biology of cancer invasion and metastasis. *Cancer Res.* 38:2651–2660, 1978.

19. Hart, R, Fidler, IJ: An *in vitro* quantitative assay for tumor cell invasion. *Cancer Res.* 38, 3218–3224, 1978.

20. Kripke, ML, Gruys, E, Fidler, IJ: Metastatic heterogeneity of cells from an ultraviolet light-induced murine fibrosarcoma of recent origin. *Cancer Res.* 38:2962–2967, 1978.

21. Baserga, R, Kisieleski, WE, Halvorsen, K: A study on the establishment and growth of tumor metastasis with tritiated thymadine. *Cancer Res.* 20, 910–917, 1960.

22. Gullino, PM: *In vivo* release of neoplastic cells by mammary tumors. *Gann Monogr. Cancer Res.* 20:49–55, 1977.

23. van de Velde, CJH, van Putten, LM, Zwaveling, A: A new metastasizing mammary carcinoma model in mice: model characteristics and applications. *Europ. J. Cancer* 13:555–565, 1977.

24. Pollack, R: A strategy for the *in vitro* analysis of the metastatic process. *Gann. Monogr. Cancer Res.* 20:37–46, 1977.

25. Erdlandson, RA, Carstens, PHB: Ultrastructure of tubular carcinoma of the breast. *Cancer* 29:987–995, 1972.

26. Leighton, J: Pathogenesis of tumor invasion II. Aggregate replication. *Cancer Res.* 20:575–586 and 6 plates, 1960.

27. Tickle, C, Crawly, A, Goodman, M: Mechanisms of invasiveness of epithelial tumors: ultrastructure of the interactions of carcinoma cells with embryonic mesenchyme and epithelium. *J. Cell Sci.* 33:133–156, 1978.

28. Hager, JC, Miller, FR, Heppner, GH: Influence of serial transplantation on the immunological-clinical correlates of BALB/Cf C3H mouse mammary tumors. *Cancer Res.* 38:2492–2500, 1978.

29. Prehn, RT, Prehn, L: Pathobiology of neoplasia. *Amer. J. Path.* 80:529–550, 1975.

30. McDivitt, RW, Stewart, FW, Berg, JW: Tumors of the breast. *AFIP Atlas of tumor pathology,* Series 2, Fascicle 2, Washington, D.C. 1968, (Armed Forces Institute of Pathology).

31. Spitlany, George, L, North RJ: Subversion of host defense mechanisms by malignant tumors: an established tumor as a privileged site for bacterial growth. *J. Exp. Med.* 145:1264–1277, 1977.

32. Slemmer, G: Qualitatively-different cellular immune responses to antigenic cells. *Proc. Amer. Assoc. Cancer Res.* 19:776, 1978.

33. Cunningham, AJ: Self-tolerance maintained by active suppressor mechanisms. *Transplant Rev.* 31:23–43, 1976.

34. Stumpf, R, Heuert, J, Kolsch, E: Suppressor T cells in low zone tolerance. 1. Mode of action of suppressor cells. *Europ. J. Immunol.* 7:74–80, 1977.

Blood-Borne Tumor Metastasis: Some Properties of Selected Tumor Cell Variants of Differing Malignancies[a]

Garth L. Nicolson, Christoper L. Reading, Kenneth W. Brunson

Departments of Developmental and Cell Biology and Physiology, College of Medicine, University of California, Irvine, California

Summary

In vivo and *in vitro* selection techniques have been used to obtain malignant variants of the RAW117 lymphosarcoma system in BALB/c mice. This mouse model is similar to human lymphosarcoma in pathogenesis and organ involvement. Ten sequential selections for implantation, invasion, survival and growth in liver were used to obtain a lymphosarcoma cell line (RAW117-H10) that formed approximately 200 times as many gross liver tumor nodules than did the parental line (RAW117-P). *In vitro* selections for cell surface alterations were performed on the RAW117 lines by sequentially selecting for nonadherence to polystyrene-immobilized lectins. Selection for nonadherence to immobilized lectins were performed with concanavalin A, *Ricinus communis* agglutinin *I*, peanut agglutinin and wheat germ agglutinin. Parental line RAW117-P was sequentially selected ten times on immobilized concanavalin A resulting in a variant line which was dramatically more malignant and formed 10 to 100 times as many liver tumor colonies compared to RAW117-P in biologic assays. An examination of cell surface properties indicated that the selected lines with enhanced malignancy and metastasis *in vivo* show a reduction in binding of [^{125}I]-labeled concanavalin A and a decrease in the major concanavalin A-staining band (approximately 70,000 molecular weight) after sodium dodecylsul-

[a]These studies were supported by USPHS NCI Grant RO1-CA-22950, American Cancer Society Grant BC-211B and NCI Contract NO1-CB-74153 from the Division of Cancer Biology and Diagnosis.

fate polyacrylamide slab gel electrophoresis. Thus, both *in vivo* and *in vitro* selection techniques can yield variant lines with altered malignancies *in vivo* and modifications in their cell surface properties.

Introduction

Metastasis, or the spread of tumors, is the most life-threatening characteristic of malignant cells.[1-4] Metastasis usually begins when a primary tumor mass extends into or invades surrounding local tissues[5,6] indicating loss of proper cell positioning and cell-cell interactions.[7,8] Metastatic colonies can be near the primary site or they can form at some distance from the primary site, particularly in cases in which tumor cells penetrate the lymphatics or circulatory system. Malignant cells which enter the blood stream can be transported to distant sites and to major organs where subsequent implantation, survival and growth can occur.[1-5] However, few tumor cells survive during blood-borne transit and the overwhelming majority of malignant cells which enter the blood die in the circulation and do not survive to form secondary tumors. [1,3,9,10]

The successful colonization of distant sites by metastatic cells depends upon their ability to circulate successfully in the blood, implant in the microcirculation, extravasate or invade the capillary endothelium and establish a microenvironment for subsequent vascularization and growth.[2-5] During blood-borne transport the distributions of viable malignant cells are not necessarily based upon circulatory pathways or pattern of initial microcirculatory arrest,[11-13] and the mere presence of free tumor cells or their multicell emboli in the blood does not necessarily infer that distant metastasis will occur.[11,14] In addition, blood-borne malignant cells can be temporarily arrested in a capillary bed at one site and escape to recirculate and arrest at another site.[11-13,15] At the time of arrest the malignant cells either die, or they survive and grow at the site of implantation, detach and recirculate or extravasate and grow to form secondary tumors. Since the recirculation of blood-borne tumor cells after their initial arrest is common in experimental systems,[11-13,15,16] it is not unexpected that distributions of gross metastases are nonrandom.[11-13] These findings suggest that other factors besides anatomical or mechanical are involved in specific malignant cell arrest, survival and growth to form metastases. However, nonspecific trapping of large tumor cell emboli can occur. Zeidman[17] has shown that the rates at which tumor cells and emboli pass through capillaries are related to their ability to be deformed while traversing the microcirculation and are not related to their relative diameter within certain limits.

Several experimental metastatic systems have been used to demonstrate that the sites of gross metastases can be nonrandom and not correlate with simple trapping in the first capillary bed. Using plasma-cytoma,[18] histiocytoma,[19] melanoma,[2,12,13,20,21] reticulum cell sarcoma,[22] lymphosarcoma[23,24] and others,[16,18] investigators have demonstrated that unique organs can be colonized after intravenous injection of malignant cells. We have proposed that the recognition of unique capillary vascular endothelial cell determinants by circulating malignant cells could be in part responsible for malignant cell arrest and extravasation at specific sites.[24] However, other factors are also involved.[2–5,8]

Malignant cells in the circulation undergo intercellular interactions with themselves as well as with circulating and noncirculating host cells as well as soluble blood components. The interactions of malignant cells with platelets,[26] lymphocytes,[27,28] other unidentified host blood cells and endothelial cells[25,29] can lead to enhanced tumor cell arrest in the microcirculation. Experimentally, it has been found that the larger the circulating tumor cell embolus the greater the rate of arrest and survival to form more secondary tumors,[30] since larger cell clumps or emboli are trapped more effectively in the capillaries than are single cells or small groups of cells. Self- or homotypic adhesion of malignant cells to form clumps may also be important during blood-borne transit,[30,31] and many malignant cells have high thromboplastic activities which allows them to be coated with fibrin and perhaps other deposits in the circulation which can alter their arrest properties.[32–34]

Extravasation or secondary invasion by malignant cells through the capillary endothelium and underlying basement membrane after arrest in the microcirculation is an important step in the metastatic process. Shortly after tumor cell or emboli arrest, malignant cells may become trapped in a fibrin matrix,[33,34] but this does not always happen.[34,35] The malignant cells must escape the fibrin matrix by dissolution of the thrombus and invasion of the endothelial cell layer.[34,37] Endothelial invasion appears to occur at sites where endothelial cells retract or have been retracted from the underlying basement membrane or extracellular matrix[33,35,36,39] or where the endothelial cells have been penetrated directly.[32] Cell surface or secreted degradative enzymes appear to be important in the destruction of the underlying basement membranes[38–40] and the escape of malignant cells from the circulation. Once they have escaped the circulation, tumor cells can proliferate in the extravascular environment; however, their growth is aided by the establishment of a new vascular system.[41,42] In fact, it is thought that vascularization of the secondary tumors allows them to grow into gross metastases at sites where adequate blood flow is limited.

During each step of the pathogenesis of tumor metastasis, malignant cells must escape nonimmune or immune host defenses.[1–5] In some cases, immunological surveillance against malignant cells accounts for inhibition of metastasis in secondary tumor growth.[43−45] But in many systems, host defenses are unable or inadequate to halt tumor progression in the formation of distant metastases.[46−48]

Experimental Models of Malignancy and Metastasis

Several experimental models for studying malignancy and metastasis now exist in a number of species. The successful development of these models depended upon the existence of mixed cell populations in the original tumors with heterogeneous metastatic properties of individual cells in the population. Therefore, variant cell lines could be selected or cloned from the original population that showed significantly different malignant properties when assayed *in vivo*.[1,49−51] Thus, tumor cell lines of low malignant or metastatic properties could be subjected to selection or cloning to obtain variant cell lines or clones which were highly metastatic when assayed. Several tumor systems have now been developed utilizing spontaneously-, virally- and chemically-transformed tumor cell lines of low metastatic potential to obtain variant cell lines and clones of high metastatic potential and enhanced organ preference or colonization. [2,3,51] Fidler [52] selected B16 melanoma lines for enhanced lung implantation, survival and growth after intravenous injection. With each selection the highly malignant tumor cells were enriched in the population, and after ten sequential selections for lung colonization, a line was obtained (B16-F10) which was significantly more metastatic when assayed for its ability to form gross lung tumor colonies after intravenous injection into syngeneic mice.[27,52] This B16-F melanoma system has proven particularly useful for studying tumor cell and host properties associated with metastasis.[2,3,51,53] That the preference of lung colonization of line B16-F10 was not due to simple mechanical trapping was demonstrated via introduction of [^{125}I]-labeled melanoma cells by tail vein by IV or left ventricle by i.c. injection. [12] By the latter route, extrapulmonary arrest, attachment and recirculation are necessary in order to reach the lung microcirculation. Organs and blood from groups of animals were analyzed for viable [^{125}I]-labeled B16 cells. Although the kinetic distributions of blood-borne melanoma cells were different in blood and all organs within two minutes after injection via these two routes, after one day the same number of viable B16-F10 cells were found in the lungs, independent of the route of melanoma cell entry into the circulation. When animals were sacrificed after two weeks and the gross numbers of melanoma nodules counted in the lungs and other sites, the same numbers of pulmonary metastases were found in mice who received the melanoma cells via the tail vein or left ventricle.[12] In B16-F10, extrapulmonary metastases were not found after two weeks which indicates that initial blood-borne tumor cell distribution and arrest may have little bearing on subsequent metastatic colonization. These experiments were confirmed using parabiosed pairs of syngeneic mice where the kinetic distributions of [^{125}I]-labeled melanoma cells in injected as well as uninjected parabiotic animals were followed at various times after IV introduction into one animal of each pair. [13] These results indicated that viable, blood-borne tumor cells temporarily arrest, recirculate and are capable of traversing the site of anastomosis from one to three hours post-injection and can form pulmonary tumors in either parabiotic pair of animals.

Utilizing an *in vivo* selection strategy, brain colonizing B16 melanoma variants have been obtained from the original B16 melanoma line by sequential *in vivo* selection for brain implantation, survival and growth.[20] In this case, B16-F1 cells were injected i.c. into the left ventricle of syngeneic mice and the resulting brain tumors were recovered and cultured to obtain cell line B16-B1. After 10 selections for experimental brain metastasis, lines B16-B10n (colonizing the rhinal and longitudinal fissures) and B16-B10b (less specific but colonizing the meninges in the cerebral cortex) were obtained.[20] Similarly, ovary-colonizing B16 melanoma variants have also been selected from B16-F1 by removing rare ovarian tumors formed after B16-F1 injection and culturing them for further selections for ovarian colonization. After 10 sequential selections for ovary tumor metastasis, line B16-O10 was obtained which forms more gross ovarian tumors compared to unselected lines.[21]

Another system now available utilizes a murine lymphosarcoma which is capable of forming some solid tumor nodules in livers, lungs and spleens of injected mice.[23] We have used the RAW117 lymphosarcoma line which forms solid lymphosarcoma tumors in BALB/c mice to select for RAW117 lines with enhanced liver colonization. After 10 sequential selections for liver colonization in the lymphosarcoma, cell line (RAW117-H10) was obtained which formed approximately 200–250 times more gross liver tumor nodules than the parental line in comparable biological assays and displayed enhanced malignancy when assayed by time of host death.[23] We have used the RAW117 system to study properties associated with malignancy and hepatic colonization. In addition, we have selected RAW117 cell variant lines *in vitro* on the basis of altered cell surface properties[24] in order to examine the role of the cell surface in metastasis.

Methods

Tumor Cells

Lymphosarcoma line RAW117 was induced *in vitro* from spleen cultures of BALB/c mice infected by Abelson leukemia virus[54] and was grown as previously described[23] in plastic Petri dishes using Dulbecco's modified Eagle's medium (DMEM) supplemented with 10 percent heat-inactivated (50°C, 30 min) fetal bovine serum without antibiotics. Cells were tested routinely for mycoplasma using a modification of the nucleoside-phosphorylase assay[55] and the uridine/uracil ratio assay[56] and were negative.

Biologic Assays

Lymphosarcoma cells were washed three times in serum-free DMEM and injected IV (5,000 cells) in 0.2 ml serum-free DMEM. After 14 days mice were anesthetized, the livers were perfused *in situ* with four percent formalin phosphate-buffered saline and excised. After fixation for 24 hr in buffered formalin, a small portion was removed for histology and the livers were stained in a hematoxylin solution as described[24] so that the lymphosarcoma surface tumor colonies appear as dark purple spots and could be easily counted with the aid of a dissecting microscope. Liver colony assays were confirmed by histology. Paraffin embedded sections (3–5 μm) were stained with hematoxylin and eosin before examination. Lungs were examined after tracheal inoculation of a formalin solution containing colloidal carbon.[23]

Lectins and Immobilized Lectins

Affinity purified peanut agglutinin (PNA),[57] *Ricinus communis* agglutinin *I* (RCA$_I$),[58] concanavalin A (Con A)[59] and wheat germ agglutinin (WGA)[60] were prepared according to published procedures. Lectins were radiolabeled with [^{125}I][61] and repurified by affinity chromatography. Quantitative lectin binding assays were performed by an assay[23] taken from Novodgrodsky et al.[62]

Lectins were covalently coupled via their free amino groups to the carboxylic acid groups exposed on polystyrene Petri dishes by a water soluble carbodiiomide[23] using previous procedures.[63] Once immobilized the lectin-coated plates could be stored for one year in the cold.

Selection in Vitro for Altered Binding to Immobilized Lectins

RAW117-P or RAW117-H10 lymphosarcoma cells (10^6) were washed in Dulbecco's phosphate-buffered saline by centrifugation, resuspended in the same buffer and incubated in 35 mm Petri dishes containing immobilized lectin for 30 min at 25°C with occasional rocking.[23] At this time a majority of the cells was bound to the surface of the lectin-coated Petri dishes, and the few cells that remained in suspension ($< 1\%$) were aspirated and washed by centrifugation as described previously.[23] The unbound cells were grown *in vitro* to a density of approximately 10^6/ml, harvested and the selection process was repeated on the same immobilized lectin to obtain lines RAW117-P Con A^{al}, RAW117-P WGA^{al}, RAW117-P PNA^{al} or RAW117-P RCA^{al} for cells selected once on immobilized-Con A, -WGA, -PNA or -RCA, respectively. The second round of selection on immobilized Con A yielded RAW117-P Con A^{a2} and so on. Similar sequential selections were performed on RAW117-H10.[23]

Analysis of Cell Surface Proteins and Glycoproteins

Cells were labeled by the lactoperoxidase-catalyzed [^{125}I]iodination technique as described.[23] The [^{125}I] surface-labeled cells were disrupted with 0.5% Nonidet P-40 (NP-40) and then centrifuged at 4°C to remove cell nuclei. The NP-40 supernatants were then completely solubilized by boiling in two percent sodium dodecyl sulfate containing two percent 2-mercaptoethanol. Aliquots were applied to 7.5 percent polyacrylamide slab gels and electrophoresed. Autoradiograms were prepared from the dried gels and these were scanned with a densitometer. [64]

Cell Agglutination with Lectins

Cells were washed twice with Dulbecco's phosphate-buffered saline and suspended with this buffer at a final concentration of 5×10^6 cells/ml in plastic wells at a final volume of 0.4 ml/well. Serial dilutions of lectins were added and suspensions were gently rotated for 10 min on a rotary shaker at 1.5 Hz, and the wells were scored for agglutination as described previously.[65]

Results

Selection for Liver Colonization

Sequential selection in vivo of lymphosarcoma cells for liver implantation, invasion, survival and growth resulted in tumor cell lines with markedly enhanced malignancy and organ colonization as demonstrated by decreased survival times in recipient mice and increased numbers of solid lymphosarcoma tumors formed in the liver per input tumor cell (Table 1). Difference in host survival rates were also noted between the unselected parental lymphosarcoma line and its selected variants. [23] The approximate times for 50 percent host death after IV injection of 5,000 viable lymphosarcoma cells were 40, 16 and eight days for lines RAW117-P, RAW117-H5 and RAW117-H10, respectively. [23] Although liver colonization potential increased with each succeeding in vivo selection, the numbers of lymphosarcoma nodules in the lungs were low in both parental and selected RAW117 lines (Table 1).

Some Cell Surface Properties of In Vivo Selected Lymphosarcoma Lines

Although there were few differences noted in lectin-mediated agglutination of parental compared to H10-selected lymphosarcoma lines (Table 2), there was a difference in quantitative lectin binding. The most

38

Table 1. Lymphosarcoma Tumors Formed After Intravenous Injection of RAW117 Variant Lines[a]

Line	No. of Liver Tumor Colonies per Animal	Median	(Range)	No. of Lung Tumors per Animal	Median	(Range)
RAW117-P	0,0,0,0,0,0,0,1,1 1,1,1,2,2,4	1	(0- 4)	0,0,0,0,0,0,0,0,0,0, 1,1,1,1,1,1	0	(0- 1)
RAW117-H10	0,1,1,2,2,2,4,5, 7,8	2	(0- 8)	0,0,0,0,0,0,1,1,1, 1	0	(0- 1)
RAW117-H5	9,10,15,18,23,23, 26,27,34,36	23	(9-36)	0,0,0,0,1,1,1,2,2, 2	1	(0- 2)
RAW117-H10	> 200, > 200, > 200, > 200, > 200, > 200, > 200, > 200, > 200, > 200[b], > 200[b], > 200[b]			1,1,1,1,1,1,1,2,2, 3,3,4,4,4	1	(1- 4)

[a] 5,000 viable RAW117 cells were injected i.v. in 0.2 ml medium, and mice were examined after ten days.

[b] Animal died before assay date.

dramatic difference was found in the binding of [^{125}I]-labeled Con A to parental and selected lines (Figure 1). Quantitative binding studies indicated that the H10-selected line bound less than half of the number of Con A molecules compared with the parental which suggests a modification in cell surface oligosaccharides. Surface proteins of lymphosarcoma cells were labeled by the lactoperoxidase-catalyzed [^{125}I]iodination techniques and were examined by sodium dodecylsulfate polyacrylamide gel electrophoresis autoradiography. Scanned autoradiograms prepared from the dried gels indicated that the most dramatic difference between the parental and selected lines was a decrease in protein migrating at approximate molecule weight of 70,000 (Figure 2).

In Vitro *Selection of Lymphosarcoma Variant Lines*

Since it was likely that the *in vivo*-selected lymphosarcoma lines possessed cell surface alterations, we selected cell surface variants of RAW117 lymphosarcoma *in vitro*.[24] Utilizing immobilized lectins, we sequentially selected for lectin attachment variants of RAW117 cells by nonadherence to polystyrene-immobilized lectins.[24] The parental lymphosarcoma line RAW117-P grows in suspension and is bound rapidly by immobilized lectins. After an attachment period where the majority of the cells bound to lectin-derivatized Petri dishes, the unattached cells (< 1%) could be removed by aspiration and subcultured. Selection by nonadherence to immobilized lectins was repeated seven to 10 times and the resulting cell lines were tested in BALB/c mice to determine their

Table 2. Lectin Agglutination of Lymphosacroma Cells[a]

Cell Lines	Lectin	μG/ML Lectin										
		1000	500	250	125	60	30	15	7	4	2	1
RAW117-P	PNA	+	+	+/−	−	−	−	−	−	−	N.D.	N.D.
	RCA$_I$	N.D.	N.D.	4+	4+	2+	+	+	+	+	+/−	−
	SBA	N.D.	N.D.	4+	2+	+	+	+	+/−	−	−	−
	WGA	N.D.	N.D.	2+	+	+	+	+	+/−	−	−	−
	WBA	N.D.	N.D.	4+	4+	4+	4+	2+	+/−	−	−	−
	Con A	N.D.	N.D.	+	+	+	+	+	+	+/−	−	−
RAW117-H10	PNA	+	+	+	+/−	−	−	−	−	−	N.D.	N.D.
	RCA$_I$	N.D.	N.D.	4+	4+	4+	2+	+	+	+/−	−	−
	SBA	N.D.	N.D.	4+	4+	+	+	+	+/−	−	−	−
	WGA	N.D.	N.D.	2+	2+	4+	4+	4+	+	+/−	−	−
	WBA	N.D.	N.D.	2+	2+	4+	4+	4+	+	+/−	−	−
	Con A	N.D.	N.D.	+	+	+	+	+	+/−	−	−	−

[a] Tumor cells were suspended at a concentration of 5×10^6 cells/ml in PBS and inoculated into Linbro FP-54 wells (final volume, 0.4 ml) containing serially diluted lectins. After 10 min at room temperature, agglutination was scored as follows: −, no agglutination ($<$ 2%); +/−, 10% agglutinated cells; +, 10–25% agglutinated cells; 2+, 25–50% agglutinated cells; 3+, 50–75% agglutinated cells; 4+, $>$ 75% agglutinated cells; N.D., not determined.

malignant potentials (Table 3). Sequential selection of parental cell lines RAW117-P five or six times on immobilized-WGA, -PNA, RCA$_I$ did not alter significantly the *in vivo* malignant properties of *in vitro*-selected cell lines compared with the parental RAW117-P line (Table 3). However, selection of lines RAW117-P by nonadherence to immobilized-Con A resulted in variants of increased malignancy, and after ten selections to obtain line RAW117-P Con A^{a10} the median numbers of liver tumor colonies compared with RAW117-P was increased approximately 100 times.

When several animals injected with lymphosarcoma variant lines were examined by histology, microscopic examination confirmed the gross observations in all cases.[24] Liver tumor colonies were rarely found in RAW117-P injected animals and the liver tissue appeared normal (Figure 3). Extensive lymphosarcoma tumors were apparent in most of the animals injected with the more malignant RAW117-H10 and RAW117-P Con A^{a9} (Figure 4) lines.

Discussion

The syngeneic lymphosarcoma model system based on the RAW117 tumor cell lines and their *in vivo*[23] and *in vitro*[24] selected variants is a useful system for studying cellular properties associated with enhanced

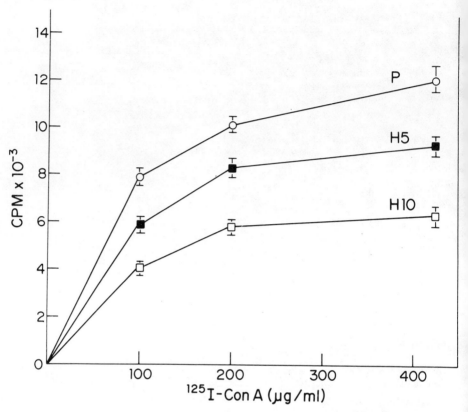

Figure 1. Quantitative binding of [^{125}I]-labeled Con A to *in vivo*-selected RAW117 lymphosarcoma cell lines. Parental RAW117 (o, RAW117-P) and cell lines sequentially selected five (■, RAW117-H5) and ten times (□, RAW117-H10) for liver colonization, respectively, were washed three times in PBS and suspended at a concentration of 5×10^6 cells/ml in PBS. [^{125}I]-labeled lectin was added at various concentrations to polypropylene tubes with or without 50 mM α-methyl-*D*-mannoside. After a 30 min incubation with gentle mixing, the cells were separated from unbound lectin on a dibutylphthalate: dioctylphthalate mixture.[24] Each point is the average of triplicate samples less controls which averaged 5%-10% of raw data.

malignancy and metastasis. Since the RAW117 lymphosarcoma was induced by an Abelson leukemia virus complex,[66] the resulting lympho-sarcoma lines probably represent nonthymus-derived tumors.[54,67] This system also appears to be relevant to clinical lymphosarcoma because the majority of human malignant lymphosarcomas are probably of the B-cell type[68] and the most commonly involved organs are the liver and spleen.[69]

In vivo selection of lymphosarcoma cells for liver implantation, inva-

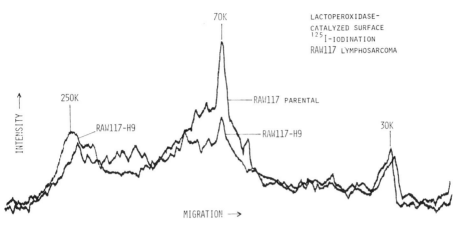

Figure 2. Densitometry scans of autoradiograms made from sodium dodecylsulfate polyacrylamide slab gel electrophoresis of cell lines surface labeled with lactoperoxidase-catalyzed [^{125}I]iodination techniques.[20] The major difference between parental RAW117-P and *in vivo*-selected RAW117-H9 cell lines is the loss of a major protein of approximate molecular weight 70,000.

sion, survival and growth results in tumor cell lines with markedly enhanced malignancy and specificity of liver colonization. The liver-selected line RAW117-H10 forms approximately 100 times the number of gross liver tumor colonies compared with the parental RAW117. Since several selections were required to yield lymphosarcoma variants with increased ability to colonize liver, enhanced malignancy in this system probably does not occur by temporal adaptation of the entire cell

Table 3. Liver Tumors From *In Vitro*-Selected Lymphosarcoma Cells Injected Intravenously (5,000 cells)[a]

Cell Line	Number of Tumor Colonies per Animal	Median (Range)
RAW117-P	0,0,0,0,0,0,0,0,0,0,0,0,0,0,0,0,0,0,0, 0,0,0,0,0,0,0,0,0,0,0,1,1,1,1,1,1,2, 4,10,20	0 (0- 20)
RAW117-P PNA[a5]	0,0,0,0,0,1	0 (0- 1)
RAW117-P RCA[a5]	0,0,0,0,5,5,20	0 (0- 20)
RAW117-P WGA[a6]	0,0,0,0,0,1	0 (0- 1)
RAW117-P Con A[a5]	1,15,20,25,215,243	15 (2- 243)
RAW117-P Con A[a7]	0,1,11,20,50	11 (0- 50)
RAW117-P Con A[a9]	0,0,3,10,10,10,57,99,208,213	10 (0- 213)
RAW117-P Con A[a10]	9,37,62,93,95,97,>200,>200,>200,>200	95 (9->200)

[a] Tumor cells (5,000 viable, single cells) were injected IV in 0.2 ml medium, and mice were examined after ten days.

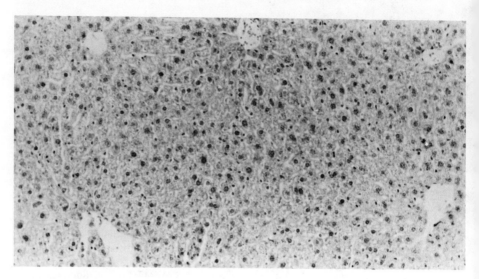

Figure 3. Histologic section at Day 10 of liver from a BALB/c mouse injected with 5,000 parental RAW117-P cells. Hematoxylin-eosin staining, × 130.

population to a different growth environment as suggested by the results of Sutkoff and Bosmann.[70] These authors[70] used combinations of *in vivo* growth in the peritoneal cavity and *in vitro* growth to obtain a cell line with differing malignancy with only one *in vivo* passage. In contrast to the RAW117 tumor model system when the L5187Y leukemia cells were grown *in vitro,* they gradually lost malignancy when subsequently assayed *in vivo.* By two months of *in vitro* growth L5187Y cells were nontumorigenic when injected i.v. In addition, the RAW117 lymphosarcoma shows long term stability during *in vitro* growth, and malignant variants can be obtained by a completely *in vitro* selection process. Using a selection procedure based upon the failure of RAW117 cells to rapidly attach to lectins derivatized onto Petri dishes, we have selected variants of RAW117.[24] The most interesting variant line was selected repeatedly for nonadherence on immobilized Con A to obtain the line RAW117-P Con A^{a10}. This immobilized Con A-selected line shows a reduction in Con A-binding components and enhanced malignancy and liver colonization when assayed *in vivo.* That the selection process was specific is suggested by our inability to select RAW117-P sublines with differing malignancy on immobilized lectins with specificities different from Con A and the fact that all of these cell lines are stable during growth in tissue culture. Recently we have been able to perform *in vitro* selections on immobilized WGA using the highly malignant RAW117-H10 lines and have obtained variant lines (RAW117-H10 WGA^{a8}) with

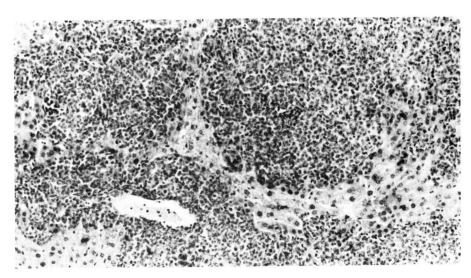

Figure 4. Histologic section at Day 10 from a BALB/c mouse injected with 5,000 *in vitro*-lectin adherence selected RAW117-P Con A^{a9} cells. Hematoxylin-eosin staining, × 130.

decreased malignancy *in vivo*.[24] Our results are somewhat similar to Tao and Burger[71] who utilized a B16 melanoma line and selected subpopulations resistant to cytotoxic concentrations of WGA. They found these to be less malignant compared with unselected parental cells.[71]

However, selection of other tumor systems can lead to quite different results. Killion and Kollmorgen[72] found that L1210 lymphoma cells which were not retained by a column of immobilized Con A were less malignant and more immunogenic than those retained on the columns and eluted with Con A-inhibitory sugars. In the RAW117 system the parental lymphosarcoma line of low malignancy was selected for nonadherence on immobilized Con A to obtain RAW117-P Con A^{a10} which shows a dramatic increase in malignancy and liver tumor colonization.[24]

The *in vivo* and *in vitro*-selected RAW117 cell lines show similarities in surface properties which correlate with their malignancy in BALB/c mice. These are the loss of Con A-reactive surface components measured by the binding of [^{125}I]-labeled Con A and a decrease in the major Con A labeling band on sodium dodecylsulfate polyacrylamide gels.[24] This component of approximate molecular weight 70,000 is also lost in the *in vivo*-selected, highly malignant RAW117-H10 line but reappears on the *in vitro*-selected RAW117-H10 WGA^{a8} line which has lost *in vivo* malignancy. Lactoperoxidase-catalyzed surface iodination and metabolic labeling with [^{14}C]glucosamine also detected loss of a component of approximately 70,000 molecular weight on the RAW117-H10 line.[73] Since cell surface labeling techniques, metabolic labeling and staining polyacrylamide gels with [^{125}I]-labeled Con A all demonstrate a dramatic reduction in the 70,000 mol. wt. Con A-reacted component, it is likely that this component is decreased in amount on the *in vivo-* and *in vitro-*selected lines of low malignancy.

The identity of the approximately 70,000 mol. wt. Con A-reacted component has been established using immunological techniques. These suggest that the 70,000 mol. wt. glycoprotein is a major RNA virus envelope glycoprotein gp70. Using a competition radioimmune assay with [^{125}I]-labeled Moloney gp70, we have detected a 10-fold decrease in gp70 between RAW117-P and the *in. vivo-*selected H10 line.[73] In addition, *in vitro-*selected lines of high malignancy such as RAW117-P Con A^{a10} show lowered amounts of gp70, while *in vitro-*selected lines of lowered malignancy such as RAW117-H10 WGA^{a8} show higher levels of gp70 when compared with RAW117-H10. These results are reminiscent of the results of Mora et al.[74] who found that tumor forming SV40-transformed Al/N fibrosarcomas in mice have lost SV40 surface antigens due to immunological selection. In the RAW117 model the host immune system may also eliminate the cells with strong viral antigens present on their surfaces thus allowing tumors to form with lowered amounts of gp70.[73]

One question remaining is the origin of RAW117 cells with decreases in specific cell surface components such as gp70. These could be the result of sequential mutation events occurring during growth of the cells after each selective cycle *in vivo* or to the selection of pre-existant variants in the tumor cell population. In other systems, cloning experiments have established that fibrosarcoma, sarcoma, adenosarcoma and melanoma tumor cell lines contain clones of widely different malignant and metastatic potentials.[1,49–51,75] Even in recently established fibrosarcoma lines,[50] clones can be obtained that show dramatic differences in malignancy and metastatic properties. Therefore, in the RAW117 system malignant variants may exist in the unclaimed parental population and these could be enriched in the *in vivo-* or *in vitro-*selected cell lines. That subpopulations exist in the RAW117 system has been shown recently by cell cloning experiments.[73] In these studies, clones were obtained from the parental RAW117 lymphosarcoma line as well as *in vivo-* and *in vitro-*selected variant populations. Each RAW117 clone was unique in its malignant properties. We are currently examining clones from RAW117 lines and are evaluating them as to the stability of their malignant properties in relationship to gp70 and other cell surface markers.

References

1. Fidler, IJ: Tumor heterogeneity and the biology of cancer and metastasis. *Cancer Res.* 38:2651–2660, 1978.

2. Nicolson, GL: Experimental tumor metastasis: characteristics and organ specificity. *BioScience* 28:441–447, 1978.

3. Fidler, IJ, Gersten, DM, Hart, IR: The biology of cancer invasion and metastasis. *Adv. Cancer Res.* 28:149–150, 1978.

4. Sugarbaker, EV: Cancer metastasis: a product of tumor-host interactions. *Curr. Prob. Cancer* 3:1–59, 1979.

5. Fidler, IJ: Mechanisms of cancer invasion and metastasis. In: Becker, FF, ed. *Biology of Tumors: Surfaces, Immunology, and Comparative Pathology,* Vol. 4 of *Cancer: A Comprehensive Treatise,* pp. 101–131, Plenum Publishing Corp., New York, 1975.

6. Nicolson, GL, Birdwell, CR, Brunson, KW, Robbins, JC: Cellular interactions in the metastatic process. In: Marchesi, VT, ed. *Membranes and Neoplasia: New Approaches and Strategies.* Alan R. Liss, Inc., New York, 1976.

7. Nicolson, GL, Poste, G: The cancer cell: dynamic aspects and modifications in cell-surface organization. *New Engl. J. Med.* 295:197–203 (Part 1); 253–258 (Part 2), 1976.

8. Weiss, L: A pathobiologic overview of metastasis. *Sem. Oncol.* 4:5–19, 1977.

9. Salsbury, AJ: The significance of the circulating cancer cell. *Cancer Treat. Rev.* 2:55–72, 1976.

10. Fidler, IJ: Patterns of tumor cell arrest and development. In: Weiss, L, ed. *Fundamental Aspects of Metastasis,* pp. 275–289, North-Holland Publishing Co., Amsterdam, 1976.

11. Sugarbaker, EV: The organ selectivity of experimentally induced metastasis in rats. *Cancer* 5:606–612, 1952.

12. Fidler, IJ, Nicolson, GL: Organ selectivity for implantation, survival and growth of B16 melanoma variant tumor lines. *J. Natl. Cancer Inst.* 57:1199–1202, 1976.

13. Fidler, IJ, Nicolson, GL: Fate of recirculating B16 melanoma metastatic variant cells in parabiotic syngeneic recipients. *J. Natl. Cancer Inst.* 58:1867–1872, 1977.

14. Malmgren, RA: Studies of circulating tumor cells in cancer patients. In: Denoix, P, ed. *Mechanisms of Invasion in Cancer,* pp. 108–117, Springer-Verlag, New York, 1967.

15. Fisher, B, Fisher, ER: The organ distribution of disseminated[51] Cr-labeled tumor cells. *Cancer Res.* 27:412–420, 1967.

16. Proctor, JW: Rat sarcoma model supports both "soil seed" and "mechanical" theories of metastatic spread. *Br. J. Cancer* 34:651–654, 1976.

17. Zeidman, I: The fate of circulating tumor cells. I. Passage of cells through capillaries. *Cancer Res.* 21:38–39, 1961.

18. Potter, M, Rahey, JL, Pilgrim, HI: Abnormal serum protein and bone destruction in transmissible mouse plasma cell neoplasm (multiple myeloma). *Proc. Soc. Exp. Biol. Med.* 94:327–333, 1957.

19. Dunn, TB: Normal and pathologic anatomy of the reticular tissue in laboratory mice, with a classification and discussion of neoplasms. *J. Natl. Cancer Inst.* 14:1281–1422 1954.

20. Brunson, KW, Beattie, G, Nicolson, GL: Selection and altered tumor cell properties of brain-colonizing metastatic melanoma. *Nature* 272:543–545, 1978.

21. Brunson, KW, Nicolson, GL: Selection of malignant melanoma variant cell lines for ovary colonization. *J. Supramol. Struct.* (in press) 1979.

22. Parks, RC: Organ-specific metastasis of a transplantable reticulum cell sarcoma. *J. Natl. Cancer Inst.* 52:971–973, 1974.

23. Brunson, KW, Nicolson, GL: Selection and biologic properties of malignant variants of a murine lymphosarcoma. *J. Natl. Cancer Inst.* 61:1499–1530, 1978.

24. Reading, CL, Belloni, PN, Nicolson, GL: Selection and *in vivo* properties of lectin-

attachment variants of malignant lymphosarcoma cell lines. *J. Natl. Cancer Inst.* (submitted) 1979.

25. Nicolson, GL, Winkelhake, JL: Organ specificity of blood-borne tumor metastasis determined by cell adhesion? *Nature* 255:230–232, 1975.

26. Gasic, GJ, Gasic, TB, Galanti, N et al.: Platelet-tumor cell interaction in mice. The role of platelets in the spread of malignant disease. *Int. J. Cancer* 11:704–718, 1973.

27. Fidler, IJ: Biological behavior of malignant melanoma cells correlated to their survival *in vivo. Cancer Res.* 35:218–224, 1975.

28. Fidler, IJ, Gersten, DM, Budmen, MB: Characterization *in vivo* and *in vitro* of tumor cells selected for resistance to syngeneic lymphocyte-mediated cytotoxicity. *Cancer Res.* 36:3160–3165, 1976.

29. Kramer, RH, Nicolson, GL: Interactions of animal and human tumor cells with vascular endothelial cells *in vitro:* a model for metastatic invasion. *Proc. Natl. Acad. Sci. U.S.A.* (in press) 1979.

30. Fidler, IJ: The relationship of embolic homogeneity, number, size and viability to the incidence of experimental metastasis. *Eur. J. Cancer* 9:223–227, 1973.

31. Winkelhake, JL, Nicolson, GL: Determination of adhesive properties of variant metastatic melanoma cells to BALB/3T3 cells and their virus-transformed derivatives by a monolayer attachment assay. *J. Natl. Cancer Inst.* 56:285–291, 1976.

32. Baserga, R, Saffiotti, U: Experimental studies on histogenesis of blood-borne metastases. *Arch. Pathol.* 59:26–34, 1955.

33. Chew, EC, Jospehson, RL, Wallace, AC: Morphologic aspects of the arrest of circulating cancer cells. In: Weiss, L, ed. *Fundamental Aspects of Metastasis,* pp. 121–150, North-Holland Publishing Co., Amsterdam, 1976.

34. Wood, S Jr: Experimental studies of the intravascular dissemination of ascitic V2 carcinoma cells in the rabbit, with special reference to fibrinogen and fibrinolytic agents. *Bull. Schweiz. Akad. Med. Wiss.* 20:92–121, 1964.

35. Dingemans, KP: Invasion of liver tissue by blood-borne mammary carcinoma cells. *J. Natl. Cancer Inst.* 53:1813–1819, 1974.

36. Warren, BA, Vales, O: The adhesion of thromboplastic tumor emboli adherent to vessel walls *in vivo. Br. J. Exp. Pathol.* 53:301–313, 1972.

37. Dingemans, KP, Roos, E, van den Bergh Weerman, MA, van de Pavert, IV: Invasion of liver tissue by tumor cells and leukocytes: comparative ultrastructure. *J. Natl. Cancer Inst.* 60:583–598, 1978.

38. Liotta, LA, Kleinerman, J, Catanzaro, P, Rynbrandt, D: Degradation of basement membrane by murine tumor cells. *J. Natl. Cancer Inst.* 58:1427–1431, 1977.

39. Dresden, MH, Heilman, SA, Schmidt, JD: Collagenolytic enzymes in human neoplasms. *Cancer Res.* 32:993–996, 1972.

40. Hashimoto, K, Yamanishi Y, Dabbous, Y: Electron microscopic observations of collagenolytic activity of basal cell epithelium of the skin *in vivo* and *in vitro. Cancer Res.* 32:2561–2567, 1972.

41. Folkman, J: Tumor angiogenesis. *Adv. Cancer Res.* 19:331–358, 1974.

42. Folkman J: Tumor angiogenesis. In: Becker, FF, ed. *Biology of Tumors: Cellular Biology and Growth,* Vol. 3 of *Cancer: A Comprehensive Treatise,* pp. 355–388, Plenum Publishing Corp., New York, 1975.

43. Kim, U: Metastasizing mammary carcinomas in rats: induction and study of their immunogenicity. *Science* 164:72–74, 1970.

44. Milas, L, Hunter, N, Mason, K, Withers, HR: Immunological resistance to pulmonary

metastases in C3Hf/Bu mice bearing syngeneic fibrosarcoma of different sizes. *Cancer Res.* 34:61–71, 1974.

45. Vaage, J, Chen, K, Merrick, S: Effect of immune status on the development of artificially induced metastases in different anatomical locations. *Cancer Res.* 31:496–500, 1971.

46. Duff, R, Doller, E, Rapp, F: Immunologic manipulation of metastasis due to Herpesvirus transformed cells. *Science* 180:79–81, 1973.

47. Fidler, IJ, Nicolson, GL: Tumor cell and host properties affecting the implantation and survival of blood-borne metastatic variants of B16 melanoma. *Israel J. Med. Sci* 14:38–50, 1978.

48. Prehn, RT: Immunostimulation of the lymphodependent phase of neoplastic growth. *J. Natl. Cancer Inst.* 59:1043–1049, 1977.

49. Fidler, IJ, Kripke, ML: Metastasis results from pre-existing variant cells within a malignant tumor. *Science* 197:893–895, 1977.

50. Kripke, ML, Gruys, E, Fidler, IJ: Metastatic heterogeneity of cells from an ultraviolet light-induced murine fibrosarcoma of recent origin. *Cancer Res.* 38:2962–2967, 1978.

51. Nicolson, GL, Brunson, KW, Fidler, IJ: Specificity of arrest, survival and growth of selected metastatic variant cell lines. *Cancer Res.* 38:4105–4111, 1978.

52. Fidler, IJ: Selection of successive tumor lines for metastasis. *Nature New Biol.* 242:148–149, 1973.

53. Fidler, IJ, Nicolson, GL: The immunobiology of experimental metastatic melanoma. *Cancer Biol. Rev.* (in press) 1979.

54. Raschke, WC, Ralph, P, Watson, J et al.: Oncogenic transformation of murine lymphoid cells by *in vitro* infection with Abelson leukemia virus. *J. Natl. Cancer Inst.* 54:1249–1252, 1975.

55. Levine, EM: A simplified method for the detection of mycoplasma. *Meth. Cell Biol.* 8:229–248, 1974.

56. Schneider, EL, Stanbridge, EJ: A simple biochemical technique for the detection of mycoplasma contamination of cultured cells. *Meth. Cell Biol.* 10:277–290, 1975.

57. Lotan, R, Skutelsky, E, Danon, D, Sharon, N: The purification, composition, and specificity of the anti-T lectin from peanut (*Arachis hypogaea*). *J. Biol. Chem.* 250:8518–8523, 1975.

58. Nicolson, GL, Blaustein, J, Etzler, ME: Characterization of two plant lectins from *Ricinus communis* and their quantitative interaction with a murine lymphoma. *Biochemistry* 13:196–204, 1974.

59. Agrawal, BBL, Goldstein, IJ: Protein-carbohydrate interaction. VI. Isolation of concanavalin A by specific adsorption on cross-linked dextran gels. *Biochim. Biophys. Acta* 147:262–271, 1967.

60. Bloch, R, Burger, MM: Purification of wheat germ agglutinin using affinity chromatography on chitin. *Biochem. Biophys. Res. Commun.* 58:13–19, 1974.

61. Cuatrecasas, P: Interaction of wheat germ agglutinin and concanavalin A with isolated fat cells. *Biochemistry* 12:1312–1323, 1973.

62. Novogrodsky, A, Lotan, R, Ravid, A, Sharon, N: Peanut agglutinin, a new mitogen that binds to galactosyl sites exposed after neuraminidase treatment. *J. Immunol.* 115:1243–1248, 1975.

63. Edelman, GM, Rutishauser, U, Millette, CF: Cell fractionation and arrangement on fibers, beads, and surfaces. *Proc. Natl. Acad. Sci. U.S.A.* 68:2153–2157, 1971.

64. Nicolson, GL: Lectin interactions with normal and tumor cells and the affinity

purification of tumor cell glycoproteins. In: Sell, S, ed., *Cancer Markers: Developmental and Diagnostic Significance*. Humana Press, Clifton, N.J. (in press) 1979.

65. Nicolson, GL: Topography of cell membrane concanavalin A-sites modified by proteolysis. *Nature New Biol.* 239:193–197, 1972.

66. Abelson, HT, Rabstein, LS: Lymphosarcoma: virus-induced thymic-independent disease in mice. *Cancer Res.* 30:2213–2222, 1970.

67. Ralph, P, Nakoinz, I, Raschke, WC: Lymphosarcoma growth is selectively inhibited by B-lymphocyte mitogens: LPS, dextran sulfate, and PPD. *Biochem. Biophys. Res. Commun.* 61:1268–1275, 1974.

68. Lukes, RJ, Collins, RD: Immunologic characterization of human malignant lymphomas. *Cancer* 34:1488–1503, 1974.

69. Molander, DW, Pack, GT: Treatment of lymphosarcoma. In: Pack, GT, Ariel, IM, eds. *Treatment of Cancer and Allied Diseases. Lymphomas and Related Diseases,* Vol. IX, 2nd ed., pp. 131–167, Harper and Row, New York, 1964.

70. Sutkoff, DR, Bosmann, HB: Characterization of L5178Y leukemic cells which rapidly develop and lose implantation ability. *Biochem. Biophys. Res. Commun.* 68:277–283, 1976.

71. Tao, TW, Burger, MM: Non-metastasizing variants selected from metastasizing melanoma cells. *Nature* 270:437–438, 1977.

72. Killion, JJ, Kollmorgen, GM: Isolation of immunogenic tumor cells by cell-affinity chromatography. *Nature* 259:674–676, 1976.

73. Reading, CL, Brunson, KW, Torrianni, M, Nicolson, GL: Malignancy in murine lymphosarcoma variants is correlated with decreased display of RNA cell surface tumor virus envelope glycoprotein gp70. *Proc. Natl. Acad. Sci. U.S.A.* (submitted) 1979.

74. Mora, PT, Chang, C, Couvillion, L et al.: Immunological selection of tumor cells which have lost SV40 antigen expression. *Nature* 269:36–40, 1977.

75. Suzuki, N, Withers, HR, Koehler, MW: Heterogeneity and variability of artificial lung colony-forming ability among clones from mouse fibrosarcoma. *Cancer Res.* 38:3349–3351, 1978.

Correlation of Metastatic Behavior with Tumor Cell Degradation of Basement Membrane Collagen[a]

L. A. Liotta, S. Garbisa, K. Tryggvason, M. Wicha

Laboratory of Pathophysiology, National Cancer Institute, National Institutes of Health, Bethesda, Maryland

Summary

Basement membranes (BM) are extracellular matrices which separate organ parenchymal cells from underlying stroma. The BM serves as a scaffold for organization of tissue structure. Normal cells remain attached to their respective sides of the BM. In contrast, tumor cells do not respect this orientation and readily invade the BM to traverse tissue boundaries. Tumor cells cross epithelial and endothelial basement membranes during the successive stages of the metastatic process. We have therefore compared normal and malignant cells for their attachment and degradative properties for type IV collagen. These data show: (a) normal breast epithelial cells require basement membrane collagen (type IV collagen) for attachment and growth *in vitro* whereas malignant mammary carcinoma cells do not; (b) tumor cell lines of high metastatic potential secrete a protease which preferentially degrades type IV collagen; (c) the relative amount of type IV collagen degradation correlates with the spontaneous metastatic behavior of the tumor cell lines studies and can possibly serve as an *in vitro* biochemical marker for metastatic potential.

Introduction

Basement membranes are continuous extracellular matrices which separate organ parenchymal cells from underlying connective tissue stro-

---

[a]Laboratory of Developmental Biology and Anamolies, National Institute of Dental Research, National Institutes of Health, Bethesda, Maryland

ma.[1] The basement membrane (BM) is composed of type IV collagen (40–60%),[2] glycoproteins,[3] and glycoaminoglycans[4] and serves a variety of functions[1,5,6,7] listed in Table 1. Vracko[1] has proposed that the BM forms a scaffolding for organization of organ cells. When the BM remains intact following tissue injury, organ parenchymal cells can reestablish the organ architecture by migrating along the preexisting BM. However, if the BM is damaged healing can only occur through scar formation.[1] Normally, organ cells and stroma cells remain attached to their respective sides of the BM. Special attachment proteins may be utilized by cells which are anchored to a BM.[8] Metastatic tumor cells, however, do not respect this barrier and readily penetrate the BM to traverse tissue boundaries. Tumor cells penetrate BMs during many stages of the metastatic process starting with the transition from *in situ* to invasive carcinoma where dissolution of the epithelial BM occurs and tumor cells in single cell form or in clusters enter the stroma to gain access to blood vessels and lymphatics (Table 2).[9–13] Tumor cells traverse the endothelial basement membrane during entry into and egress from the circulation. Careful electron microscopy studies of Babai and Vlaeminck et al.[14,15] have shown local dissolution of the BM at the point of contact with tumor cell pseudopodia and have suggested an enzymatic mechanism for degradation of BM. Wallace et al.[16] have observed local destruction of the endothelial BM in the lung by individual tumor cells injected intravenously. Leung and Babai have shown that tumor cell invasion is probably not solely a result of mechanical growth pressure.[17]

In view of the above findings, we have searched[18] for an enzymatic activity related to metastatic tumor cells which degrades basement membrane type IV collagen. Type IV collagen is a major structural protein of basement membranes and is chemically and genetically distinct from stroma collagen type I and III and cartilage collagen type II. Previously characterized animal collagenases which cleave collagen types I, II, and III fail to degrade type IV collagen.[19]

Table 1. Functions of Basement Membranes

---

1. *Tissue architecture*
   Organizes cells for reconstitution of tissue during healing (Vracko, *A.J. Path.*, 1974)

2. *Induction and restriction of cell multiplication*
   During parenchymal cell turnover (Vracko, *Path. Anat.*, 1972)

3. *Selective permeability*
   (Caulfield, *J. Cell Biol.*, 1974)

4. *Structural stability*
   Capillaries and tubules of kidney (Murphy, *Microvasc. Res.*, 1975)

Table 2. Examples of Basement Membrane Dissolution Seen During Transition from *in Situ* to Invasive Carcinoma

Tissue	Tumor	Investigator
Uterine cervix	Squamous carcinoma	Rubio and Biberfield (1975)
Mammary gland	Infiltrating ductal carcinoma	Ozzello (1959, 1971)
Colon	Adenocarcinoma	Frei (1978)
Oral cavity	Squamous carcinoma	McKinney et al. (1977)

We have recently purified[19,20,21] about 1,000-fold and characterized a neutral protease activity preferential for type IV collagen from metastatic tumor cells and shown it (a) to produce specific degradation products, (b) to have a molecular weight of 65,000, (c) not to be plasmin, cathepsin or an acid protease by pH and inhibitor studies, and (d) not to degrade significantly other collagens or fibronectin. This enzyme is secreted in latent form requiring trypsin or plasmin activation. This is similar to mammalian collagenases which also exist in latent form.[19] In this study we extend this finding by quantitating the ability of several murine tumor cell lines of known metastatic potential to degrade type IV collagen. We have also studied the growth of normal and metastatic mammary epithelium on type I (stromal) and type IV (basement membrane) collagen.

Materials and Methods

Tumor Cell Lines

The metastatic murine tumor cell lines used here were variants of the B16 melanoma and the T241 sarcoma. Cell lines F_1 and F_{10} selected from the B16 melanoma by Fidler exhibit a ten-fold difference in metastatic efficiency[22,23] (number of lung colonies per cell following tail vein injection). Line B16-BL6 is a variant with increased invasive capacity *in vitro* and *in vivo* selected from F_{10} by Ian Hart. Line PMT was selected from a pulmonary metastasis of the T241 sarcoma as described previously.[24]

Ducts and alveoli liberated from the mammary glands of perphenazine stimulated, virgin, Sprague-Dawley rats by partial collagenase digestion were separated from adipocytes, blood cells and fibroblasts by sedimentation through Ficoll gradients as previously described.[25] Studies of cell attachment and growth were performed utilizing medium 199 containing 5 percent fetal calf serum plus insulin (0.1 μg/ml), prolactin (300 ng/ml), hydrocortisone (0.5 μg/ml), estradiol 17-β (1 ng/ml) and progesterone (1 ng/ml) plus gentamicin (50 μg/ml) as described. A metastasizing DMBA induced mammary carcinoma transplantable in F344 rats was maintained in culture with RPMI 1640 media, no hormones and 10 percent FCS.

Labeled Substrate

[^{14}C]Proline-labeled type IV collagen was prepared in organ cultures of EHS sarcoma essentially as described elsewhere.[26] The benign basement membrane-producing tumors were grown in C57BL/6J mice as reported previously[26] and harvested after two weeks of growth. The excised tissue was minced, washed with PBS, and preincubated for 30 min in a proline-free Dulbecco-Vogt medium containing 20 percent dialyzed fetal calf serum, 75 μg/ml ascorbate (Sigma) and 50 μg/ml β-aminoproprion-tirile (Aldrich Chemical Co.) in a moist atmosphere containing 5 percent CO_2 and 95 percent air. After the preincubation period [^{14}C]proline (> 285 mCi/mmol), Amersham was added to a final concentration of 5 μCi/ml and the incubation continued for 5 hr. The tissue was homogenized (1 ml tissue/9 ml solution) in ice cold 0.5 M acetic acid containing 20 mM EDTA (Sigma) and 8 mM NEM (Sigma), and extracted overnight in the same solution. The mixture was then clarified and the supernatant precipitated with 10 percent NaCl, pH 3.0. The precipitate formed was redissolved in 0.5 M acetic acid, clarified and dialyzed against 0.05 M Tris-HCl, 0.5 M NaCl, pH 7.4 and the small amount of precipitated material was removed by centrifugation. The supernatant was then dialyzed against 0.05 M Tris-HCl, 1.71 M NaCl, pH 7.4, and the precipitate formed was redissolved in 0.5 M acetic acid and dialyzed against the enzyme reaction buffer (0.05 M Tris-HCl, pH 7.6, containing 0.2 M NaCl, 5 mM $CaCl_2$) and stored frozen until use. Each substrate preparation was studied for purity on polyacrylamide slab gels by autoradiography.

Assay for Type IV Collagen Degradation

A. Degradation by Living Cells

Costar tissue culture cluster wells were coated with [^{14}C]proline-labeled type IV collagen by applying 0.2 ml (2.5 $\times$ 10^3 cpm) of a solution of the collagen in 0.01 M acetic acid to each well followed by evaporation. Cells in log phase of growth were harvested by 0.1% EDTA with 80 percent viability and first washed with complete medium (RPMI 1640 + 10% FCS) and then with serum-free medium. Cell viability was judged by trypan blue exclusion. From 1 $\times$ 10^3 to 3 $\times$ 10^6 viable cells were inoculated into coated wells in a volume of 2 ml serum-free medium. After ten hours 1 ml of medium from each well was harvested, centrifuged at 2,000 rpm for 10 min at 4°C and soluble radioactive digestion products were counted in a scintillation counter.

Culture medium alone released 45 $\pm$ 20 [^{14}C] cpm/well or approximately

2.0 percent of applied counts. Purified bacterial collagenase (10 units) released 2,200 ± 50 cpm or 90 percent of applied counts.

B. Degradation by Enzyme Activity Derived from Media of Cultured Cells

Tumor cells and control cells were grown to log phase in T75 tissue culture flasks. The culture media were replaced with 20 ml of serum-free RPMI 1640 media and incubated for 72 hours. The media were collected and the enzyme activity was precipitated with 25–50 percent ammonium sulfate and the precipitate was dissolved in and dialyzed against the reaction buffer (0.15 M Tris-HCl, 0.2 mM NaCl, 10 mM $CaCl_2$, pH 7.6) in such a volume that it became 20 ml/10^6 viable cells to assess direct comparison between cell number in original cultures. The reaction was preceded by trypsin activation of the enzyme by 0.25 volumes of trypsin (10 μg/ml) at 37°C for four min followed by trypsin inhibition by 0.25 volume of soybean trypsin inhibitor (50 μg/ml). The enzyme reaction was carried out with various volumes of the activated enzyme at 37°C for four hours in a final volume of 1.6 ml containing 50 μl (2500 cpm) of [^{14}C]-proline-labeled type IV collagen in the reaction buffer. The undigested substrate was precipitated with 200 μl of a solution of 10 percent TCA, 0.5 percent tannic acid using 20 μl of bovine serum albumin (1 mg/ml) as a carrier. After precipitation at 4°C for 30 min the tubes were spun at 2500 rpm for 15 min and aliquots of the supernatants were counted in a liquid scintillation counter.

The relative activity of the cell lines was computed from the linear portion of the dilution curve. Trypsin (1.0 μg/ml) digested 14.0 percent of the substrate. If digestion in an individual assay was less than trypsin or plain media controls it is shown as "none detected."

Results

When normal rat mammary epithelium was plated on type IV collagen coated dishes it exhibited a three-fold growth stimulation compared with growth on plates coated with type I collagen. This was, in part, because

Table 3. Mammary Epithelium and Mammary Carcinoma Growth on Collagen-Coated (1 μg cm^2) Dishes at 5 Days (Cells/Dish) x 10^3

Collagen	Epithelium	Carcinoma
Type IV	450[a]	640[a]
Type I	160[a]	590[a]

[a]S.D. less than 10 percent of mean.

Table 4. Latent Type IV Collagenolytic Activity in Media

Epithelium	Carcinoma
None detected ($<$ 40 cpm/10^6 cells)	814 $\pm$48 cpm/2 x 10^5 cells

of the special adhesive characteristics of these cells and type-specific collagen-dependent growth.[25] Metastatic rat mammary carcinoma cells, however, showed no preference for growth on either type of collagen (Tables 3-4). When media taken from growing cultures of these two cell types were assayed for latent type IV collagenolytic activity, the metastatic cells exhibited latent enzyme activity while the normal cells did not (Tables 3-4).

When highly metastatic cells were plated on labeled type IV collagen,

Figure 1. Time course of degradation of (^{14}C) proline labeled type IV (basement membrane) collagen coated in plastic tissue culture wells inoculated with living cells (* = no. of cells). Bovine endothelial cells are control cells ($\triangle$ 0.25 10^5 cells inoculated) which normally rest on basement membrane *in vivo*. BL6 ($\bullet$) is a highly invasive variant of the F10 melanoma line of I. Fidler. Melanocytes normally rest on a basement membrane *in vivo*.

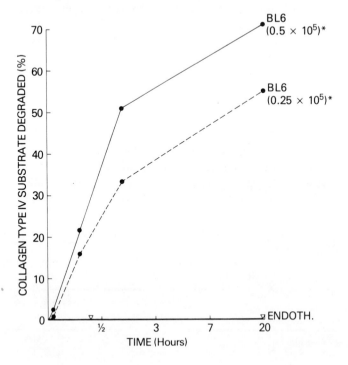

Table 5. Degradation of $[^{14}C]$ Proline-Labeled Basement Membrane Collagen (Activated Enzyme from Media)

Cell Type	Type IV Collagen Degradation[a] $(cpm/10^6$ cells)	Incidence of Spont. Metas. After i.m. Injection of 25,000 Cells and Amputation of Primary Tumor
Adult mouse fibroblasts	No detectable activity	None
Tumor Cells:		
F_1	398 ± 36	None
F_2	714 ± 62	30% (within 4 weeks)
BL6	2274 ± 136	80% (within 4 weeks)
PMT	8230 ± 214	100% (within 2 weeks)

[a] Digestion 37° C 4 hr, pH 7.6.

90 percent of the cells attached within one hour. Degradation of the substrate could be detected after one hour and increased with time and cell concentration. In contrast, normal endothelial cells attached to the substrate at the same rate but subsequent degradation was not observed (Figure 1). When a series of tumor cell lines of known spontaneous metastatic propensity was studied, the tumor cells with the highest incidence of metastasis exhibited the greatest enzyme activity (Tables 5-6). Tumor cells grown on labeled type IV collagen could elaborate latent (requiring activation) type IV collagenolytic activity into the media but could degrade the substrate to which they were attached without activation.

These data support the hypothesis that a specific enzymatic process plays a role in tumor cell penetration of basement membranes. Normal cells which *in vivo* rest on a basement membrane may possess a specific affinity for this matrix as suggested by the results shown in Tables 3 and

Table 6. Effect of Protease Inhibitors on Partially Purified Metastatic Tumor Enzyme[a]

Enzyme Treatment	Type IV Collagen Degradation[b]
Non-activated	720 cpm
Activated	2880 cpm
+ EDTA 30 mm	15 cpm
+ NEM 30 mm	2920 cpm
+ PMSF 30 mm	2850 cpm
+ Cystein 30 mm	780 cpm

[a] Digestion 37° C 4 hr, pH 7.6.
[b] Maximum substrate cpm = 3200.

4 and previous studies by Murray et al. and Wicha et al. The normal turnover of basement membranes is an extremely slow and poorly understood process. It is probable that the epithelial and endothelial cells resting on the basement membrane elaborate small amounts of proteolytic enzymes required for normal remodeling of these structures. Tumor cells retain the capacity, probably repressed in their normal cell counterparts, to express enzyme activity which degrades type IV collagen. *In vivo* this activity may be membrane bound and probably may be activated locally at the contact point of tumor cells with basement membranes. Assay for such activity might serve as a biologic marker *in vitro* for predicting the metastasizing capacity of tumor cells including human tumor samples. Even though the metastatic process is highly complex, with many sequential steps, interference of such enzyme activity may modify the process to inhibit metastases.

References

1. Vracko, R: Basal lamina scaffold-anatomy and significance for maintenance of orderly tissue structure. *Amer. J. Pathol.* 77:314–346, 1974.

2. Kefalides, NA, Denduchis, B: Structural components of epithelial and endothelial basement membranes. *Biochemistry* 8:4613–4621, 1969.

3. Kefalides, NA: Basement membranes: structural and biosynthetic considerations. *J. Invest. Dermatol.* 65:85–92, 1975.

4. Bernfield, MR, Cohn, RH, Banerjee, SD: Glycosaminoglycans and epithelial organ formation. *Amer. Zool.* 13:1067–1083, 1973.

5. Caulfield, JP, Farquhar, MG: The permeability of glomerular capillaries to graded dextrans. *J. Cell Biology* 63:883–903, 1974.

6. Murphy, ME, Johnson, PC: Possible contribution of basement membrane to the structural rigidity of blood capillaries. *Microvascular Research* 9:242–245, 1975.

7. Welling, LW, Grantham, JJ: Physical properties of isolated perfused renal tubules and tubular basement membranes. *J. Clinical Investigation* 51:1063–1075, 1972.

8. Murray, JC, Stingl, G, Kleinman, HK et al.: Epidermal cells preferentially adhere to type IV basement membrane collagen. *J. Cell Biology* 80:197–202, 1979.

9. Ozzello, L: The behavior of basement membranes in intraductal carcinoma of the breast. *Am. J. Pathol.* 35:887–899, 1959.

10. Ozzello, L, Sanpitak, P: Epithelial-stromal junction of intraductal carcinoma of the breast. *Cancer* 26:1186–1198, 1970.

11. Rubio, CA, Biberfeld, P: The basement membrane of the uterine cervix in displasia and squamous carcinoma: an immunofluorescent study with antibodies to basement membrane antigen. *Acta Pathol. Microbiol. Scand. A.* 83:744–748, 1975.

12. Frei, JV: Objective measurement of basement membrane abnormalities in human neoplasms of colorectum and of breast. *Histopathology* 2:107–115, 1978.

13. McKinney, R, Singh, B: Basement membrane changes under neoplastic oral mucous membrane. *Oral Surg.* 44:875–888, 1977.

14. Babai, F: Etude ultrastructural sur la pathogenie de l'invasion du muscle strie par des tumeurs transplantables. *J. Ultrastr. Res.* 56:287–303, 1976.

15. Vlaeminck, MN, Adenis L, Mouton Y, Demaille, A: Etude experimentale de la diffusion metastatique chez l'oeuf de poule embryonne. Repartition, microscopie et ultrastructure des foyers tumoraux. *Int. J. Cancer* 10:619–631, 1972.

16. Wallace, AC, Chew, E, Jones, DS: The arrest and extravasation of cancer cells in the lung. In: Weiss L, Gilbert, HA, eds., Chpt. 3, pp. 26–42. Pulmonary metastasis, G.K. Hall, Boston, 1978.

17. Leung, TK, Babai, F: Etude ultrastructurale de l'invasion des cultures primaires du foie par des cellules cancereuses. *Virchows Arch. B Cell Path.* 29:267–280, 1979.

18. Liotta, LA, Kleinerman, J, Catanzaro, P, Rynbrandt, D: Degradation of basement membrane by murine tumor cells. *J. Natl. Cancer Inst.* 58:5.1427–1431, 1977.

19. Liotta, LA, Abe, S, Gehron-Robey, P, Martin, GR: Preferential digestion of basement membrane collagen by an enzyme derived from a metastatic murine tumor. *Proc. Natl. Acad. Sci. USA* 76.5:2268–2272, 1979.

20. Liotta, LA, Garbisa, S, Tryggvason, K et al.: Purification and characterization of a tumor-derived collagenase which degrades basement membrane (type IV) collagen. *Am. Assoc. Cancer Res. Proc. 15th Annual Meeting,* p. 235, 1979.

21. Liotta, LA, Tryggvason, K, Garbisa, S et al.: Partial purification and characterization of a neutral protease which cleaves type IV collagen. Submitted to *Biochemistry.*

22. Fidler, IJ: Selection of successive tumor lines for metastases. *Nature (New Biol)* 242:148–149, 1973.

23. Fidler, IJ, Gersten, DM, Hart, IR: The biology of cancer invasion and metastasis. A-V. *Cancer Res.* 28:149–250, 1978.

24. Liotta, LA, Vembu, D, Saini, RK, Boone, C: *In vivo* monitoring of the death rate of artificial murine pulmonary micro-metastases. *Cancer Research* 38:1231–1236, 1978.

25. Wicha, MS, Liotta, LA, Garbisa, S, Kidwell, WR: Basement membrane collagen requirements for attachment and growth of mammary epithelium. *Exper. Cell Res.* (in press).

26. Timpl, R, Martin, GR, Bruckner, P, et al.: Nature of the collagenous protein in a tumor basement membrane. *Eur. J. Biochem.* 84:43–52, 1978.

Active Specific Immunotherapy of Residual Micrometastasis: Conditions of Vaccine Preparation and Regimen[a]

M.G. Hanna, Jr., L.C. Peters, J.S. Brandhorst

Cancer Metastastis and Treatment Laboratory, NCI Frederick Cancer Research Center, Frederick, Maryland

Summary

Although recognized as being biologically sound as well as having enormous potential applicability for treatment of resident disseminated micrometastatic disease, active specific immunotherapy is burdened by technical limitations. In this chapter we review the various conditions of vaccine preparation and administration which contribute to effective active specific immunotherapy in a weakly immunogenic hepatocarcinoma of the inbred guinea pig model. Significant and reproducible immunotherapy is achieved when BCG plus tumor cell vaccines are prepared under defined conditions. Although it is not possible to directly extrapolate the results regarding optimal operational dose and conditions of adjuvant and tumor cells from this guinea pig model to other tumor systems, these results are relevant to the major issues of active specific immunotherapy. Most human immunotherapy trials have been performed with what these results suggest are suboptimal vaccine preparations.

Introduction

The success of immunotherapy in both experimental animals and in man depends upon the stage of the tumor at the time of treatment. The major potential for immunotherapy is its use as an adjunct to chemotherapy or after surgery of the primary tumor when there is only minimal regional

[a]This research was sponsored by the National Cancer Institute under Contract No. NO1-CO-75380 with Litton Bionetics, Inc.

lymph node metastasis and micrometastatic disease in the visceral organs. Nonspecific immunomodulation directed toward enhancement of immune reactivity against disseminated minimal residual malignancy has been attempted clinically with agents such as *Mycobacterium bovis* strain BCG,[a] *Corynebacterium parvum*, several polynucleotides, levamisole and, more recently, interferon. The unsuccessful or equivocal results of these problematic, albeit feasible, clinical protocols may be partly attributable to the low degree of antigenicity of human cancer, whereas the successful animal models for nonspecific immunotherapy involved relatively antigenic transplantable murine tumors. Although immunopotentiators can enhance immune responses in general, the complicated host–tumor relationship indicates that in the immunocompetent host the immune response has a finite capacity to counteract any given antigen. Thus, it is unlikely that *generalized* or *nonspecific immunopotentiation* will result in a sufficiently elevated immunological capacity to alter significantly the growth of a weakly antigenic tumor or affect micrometastases.

There has also been a substantial effort to actively immunize autochthonous or syngeneic hosts with irradiated or chemically modified tumor cells in an attempt to achieve *active specific immunotherapy.* Inherent in this approach is the assumption that tumor cells express immunogenic tumor-specific transplantation antigens. Treatment of tumor cells with a variety of unrelated agents such as X-irradiation, mitomycin C, lipophilic agents, neuraminidase, viruses, or admixture of the cells with bacterial adjuvants has yielded nontumorigenic tumor cell preparations that are immunogenic upon injection into syngeneic hosts.[1–5] Basically, these results support the concept that antigens not found in normal adult tissues are frequently found in tumors and that the immunogenicity of these tumor cells can be expressed and even enhanced in normal and tumor-bearing hosts. These experimental results have validated the rationale of active specific immunotherapy of neoplasia.

Beginning with the pioneering studies of Mathé et al.,[6] who treated acute lymphocytic leukemia with BCG or killed leukemic blasts, or both, similar protocols for treatment of acute or chronic granulocytic leukemia,[7,8] malignant melanoma[9] and lung tumor[10] have produced encouraging results by prolonging disease-free intervals. However, as of now, none of the treatments has significantly increased patient survival. Not all immunotherapy trials have been successful, even with respect to maintenance of disease-free intervals, as shown by recent studies of

[a]Abbreviations used: HBSS, Hanks' balanced salt solution; BCG, bacillus Calmette Guérin; FBS, fetal bovine serum; DMSO, dimethyl sulfoxide; CMF, calcium magnesium free.

stage IIB malignant melanoma in which allogeneic or autochthonous tumor cells were used.[11] Although recognized as biologically sound, active specific immunotherapy is burdened by technical limitations that must be overcome before being practical in the laboratory or clinic.[12]

The weakly immunogenic L10 hepatocarcinoma of strain 2 guinea pigs has proven to be a useful experimental model for examining certain aspects of active specific immunotherapy and has provided a system to evaluate a potent immunostimulant, *Mycobacterium bovis* (BCG). Intra-tumoral injection of viable BCG produced regression of established tumors of limited size growing in the skin and the elimination of regional lymph node metastases;[13,14] it also conferred immunity to a second intradermal (i.d.) challenge with L10 tumor cells.[15,16] Also, more recent studies have shown that vaccines composed of viable BCG organisms admixed with metabolically active but nontumorigenic L10 cells were effective in eliminating established visceral micrometastases.[17-20] These observations imply that admixture of BCG with tumor cells, either through intratumoral injection or vaccine administration, provides an effective immune stimulus despite the weak antigenicity of the tumor cells. In this guinea pig model, the resultant tumor-specific immune response can eliminate established micrometastases. It is important to note that a feature common to both the elimination of localized tumor by intratumoral BCG alone and immunization by BCG-tumor cell vaccines is the regional development of a chronic inflammatory reaction culmi-nating in epithelioid granuloma formation[21,22] and development of sys-temic tumor-specific, cell-mediated immunity.[23] The relationship be-tween the chronic BCG-induced granulomatous inflammation[24,25] and the induction of systemic, tumor-specific immunity in this experimental guinea pig model is unclear.

Of the two therapeutic approaches, intratumoral BCG or BCG plus tumor cell immunization, the latter would appear to be more generally applicable in cancer treatment. In this chapter we will review the various conditions of vaccine preparation and administration that contribute to effective active specific immunotherapy.

Materials and Methods

Animals

Inbred male guinea pigs (Sewall-Wright strain-2) shown to be histocom-patible by skin grafting were obtained from Frederick Cancer Research Center's Animal Production Area, Frederick, MD. They were housed 7-10/cage, and were given kale daily and Wayne chow and water *ad libitum.*

Tumors

Both the induction of the primary hepatocarcinomas (L1 and L10) by diethylnitrosamine feeding and the antigenic and biological properties of the derived transplantable ascites tumors have been described previously.[26,27] The cell lines are maintained by serial passage in the peritoneum of weanling guinea pigs. To induce L10 disseminated micrometastases in various visceral organs of experimental animals, freshly harvested ascites cells were washed three times in HBSS, suspended at desired concentrations per 1 ml dose and injected into the dorsal penile vein of guinea pigs weighing 400 to 500 g. To induce L10 regional primary tumor growth and disseminated nodal metastases, we injected ascites cells, treated as above, at 0.1 ml per dose i.d. in the upper right dorsal quadrant.

BCG

Phipps TNC 1029 (1×10^9 per ml) fresh-frozen BCG was obtained from the Trudeau Institute (Saranac Lake, N.Y.) and stored in the gas phase of a LR-301A Linde Liquid Nitrogen Freezer. Tice IL105(s)19 (1×10^9 per vial) lyophilized BCG and Tice 381S (9.2×10^8 per ml) fresh-frozen BCG were obtained from Dr. R. Crispen, University of Illinois Medical Center, Chicago, IL., and stored at $-70°C$. Connaught ($5-6.85 \times 10^8$ per vial) lyophilized BCG was received from Dr. J. Paul Davignon, National Cancer Institute, Bethesda, MD, and stored at 4°C. All frozen BCG preparations were rapidly thawed in a 37°C water bath. Lyophilized preparations were diluted to 1×10^9 organisms/ml in buffered saline BCG diluent (Connaught 48.1-1).

Vaccine Preparations

For fresh tumor cell vaccines, L10 or L1 ascites cells, grown *in vivo*, were collected, washed three times in HBSS, resuspended at 20 to 40 ml and exposed to 20,000 Rad X-irradiation with a Phillips MD-301 X-irradiation unit. The cells were then counted, washed again, resuspended at the appropriate concentration and admixed at appropriate ratios with the various BCG's tested. L10 tissue culture cells, grown in spinner flasks, were harvested and processed in the same way. For cryopreserved vaccines, L10 ascites cells were collected, washed and separated into two batches. One batch of 10^8 cells/ml was mixed with an equal volume of chilled HBSS containing 10 percent FBS and 15 percent DMSO. The rationale for this method of freezing has been described in detail elsewhere.[28,29] In the second batch, the cells were pelleted and an equal volume of HBSS containing 30 percent glycerol was added. Cells frozen by this method have been shown to be relatively ineffective in vaccines in the guinea pig model.[30] Both batches were separated into 1-ml samples per freezer vial. All samples were frozen simultaneously in a Linde controlled rate biological freezer (BF-2) at −1°C per min to −80°C, then stored in liquid nitrogen. When needed, the cells were rapidly thawed in a 37°C water bath, transferred to a 50-ml centrifuge tube and diluted slowly to 50 ml. The cells were washed, resuspended at 20 ml per sample, and exposed to 20,000 Rad X-irradiation. The vaccines were then prepared in the same way as ascites vaccines. For vaccines containing disaggregated L10 cells, tumors were grown intramuscularly in the flank, surgically excised when 1 to 3 cm in diameter, and dissociated with 0.14% collagenase type I (190 units/mg) and 0.03% DNase (1790 Kunitz units/mg) in HBSS. Both the dissociation and the freezing procedure have been described in detail elsewhere.[31] All BCG-tumor cell vaccines consisted of 0.2 ml volumes and were given i.d., first in the upper right dorsal quadrant and a week later in the upper left. All immunizations were performed within two hr after the vaccines were mixed.

Results

Efficacy of BCG Plus Tumor-Cell Vaccines for Therapy of Disseminated Micrometastatic Malignant Disease

Guinea pigs were injected IV with L10 cells and treated as shown in Protocol A, Figure 1.

Efficacy of Various Sources of BCG

Fresh-frozen Phipps and Tice as well as lyophilized Connaught and Tice BCG were compared for efficacy in an immunization regimen consisting of 10^8 viable BCG admixed with 10^7 irradiated (attenuated) L10 ascites cells. Immunizations were administered i.d., one and seven days after IV tumor challenge. The results are shown in Table 1.

Five × 10^3 tumor cells administered IV was fatal to 70 percent of untreated guinea pigs. In this tumor challenge group 100 percent survival was achieved with all four BCG types used in the vaccines. Of those animals given an IV tumor challenge of 5 × 10^4, all untreated died, whereas those treated with vaccines utilizing fresh-frozen Phipps and lyophilized Tice achieved 100 percent survival. Treatment with vaccines utilizing fresh-frozen Tice and lyophilized Connaught achieved 90 percent survival. Five × 10^5 tumor challenge was also fatal in 100 percent of untreated guinea pigs. Ninety percent survival was achieved in animals vaccinated twice with L10 cells admixed with fresh-frozen Phipps, whereas 80 percent and 70 percent survival was achieved in animals vaccinated with lyophilized or fresh-frozen Tice, respectively. Of those animals treated with lyophilized Connaught, 60 percent survival was achieved. Differences in survival between the four treated groups and the untreated animals were highly significant at all tumor challenges.

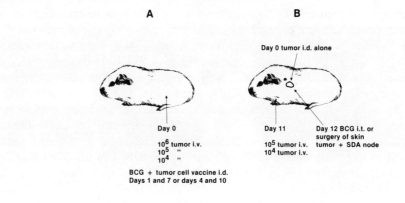

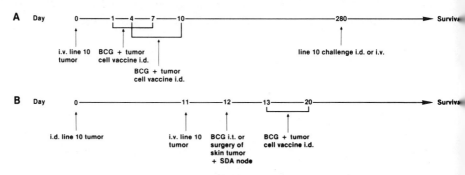

Figure 1. Protocols for experimental immunotherapy in guinea pigs with regional and/or disseminated tumor.

However, differences among vaccine treatment groups were not significant statistically. Thus, it is clear from this experiment that all four BCG preparations are effective in the specific immunotherapy protocol.

Comparison of Graded Doses of BCG and L10 Cells

BCG doses ranging from 10^5 to 10^8 viable organisms (Phipps 1029, fresh-frozen) were mixed with 10^7 irradiated L10 tumor cells and administered i.d. one and seven days after IV tumor injection. The tumor challenge consisted of either 10^4, 10^5 or 10^6 L10 cells. The results of the study are shown in Table 2.

In animals injected IV with 10^4 L10 cells, the difference between survival after treatment with vaccines containing 10^8, 5×10^7 or 1×10^7 BCG and survival of untreated controls is significant. At this tumor burden, there was no significant difference in survival among the three treated groups.

In animals injected IV with 10^5 L10 cells, a wider range of BCG doses

Table 1. Comparison of BCG Sources

IV L10 Tumor Challenge	Treatment[a] Days 1 and 7 After Tumor Challenge	Survivors/ Total[b]	Percentage Survival	Probability[c] (Compared with no Treatment)
5×10^3	Phipps BCG + L10	9/9	100	0.002
5×10^3	Tice IL105(S)19 BCG + L10	10/10	100	< 0.002
5×10^3	Tice 381S BCG + L10	10/10	100	< 0.002
5×10^3	Connaught BCG + L10	9/9	100	0.002
5×10^3	No treatment	3/10	30	
5×10^4	Phipps BCG + L10	10/10	100	< 0.001
5×10^4	Tice IL105(S)19 BCG + L10	10/10	100	< 0.001
5×10^4	Tice 381S BCG + L10	9/10	90	< 0.001
5×10^4	Connaught BCG + L10	9/10	90	< 0.001
5×10^4	No treatment	0/9	0	
5×10^5	Phipps BCG + L10	9/10	90	< 0.001
5×10^5	Tice IL105(S)19 BCG + L10	8/10	80	< 0.001
5×10^5	Tice 381S BCG +L10	7/10	70	0.001
5×10^5	Connaught BCG + L10	6/10	60	0.005
5×10^5	No treatment	0/10	0	

[a] All immunizations consisted of 10^8 BCG + 10^7 tumor cells.

[b] 180-200 day survival of guinea pigs with disseminated micrometastasis.

[c] Fisher's Exact Test, one-tailed.

Table 2. Comparison of Graded Doses of BCG

IV L10 Tumor Challenge	Treatment Days 1 and 7 After Tumor Challenge	Survivors/ Total[a]	Percentage Survival	Probability[b] (Compared with no Treatment)
10^4	10^8 BCG + 10^7 L10	15/15	100	< 0.001
10^4	5×10^7 BCG + 10^7 L10	15/15	100	< 0.001
10^4	10^7 BCG + 10^7 L10	14/15	93.2	< 0.001
10^4	No vaccination	2/9	22.2	
10^5	10^8 BCG + 10^7 L10	14/15	93.0	< 0.001
10^5	5×10^7 BCG + 10^7 L10	14/15	93	< 0.001
10^5	10^7 BCG + 10^7 L10	12/15	80	< 0.001
10^5	10^6 BCG + 10^7 L10	7/15	46.6	0.013
10^5	10^5 BCG +10^7 L10	1/15	6.6	
10^5	No vaccination	0/10	0	
10^6	10^8 BCG + 10^7 L10	9/20	45	0.017
10^6	5×10^7 BCG + 10^7 L10	7/15	46.6	0.019
10^6	10^7 BCG + 10^7 L10	4/15	26.6	
10^6	No vaccination	0/9	0	

[a] 180-200 day survival of guinea pigs with disseminated micrometastasis.

[b] By Fisher's Exact Test, one-tailed.

was used and a dose effect became very clear. Although treatments with 10^8 to 10^6 BCG doses resulted in significant increase in survival compared with untreated controls, no protection was achieved with 10^5 BCG. Application of the Cochran-Armitage chi-square test for trend indicates that as BCG dose increases there is a highly significant increase in survival ($P = < 0.001$).

Comparison of Graded 10:1 Ratios of BCG to Tumor Cells

Low ratios, ranging from 1:1 to 10:1 BCG to tumor cells, seem to be optimally effective vaccines. In these cases the dose of BCG was 10^7 or greater viable organisms. It has been suggested that the ratio *per se* of BCG to tumor cells may be as important as the actual dose of BCG.[32] To test this, guinea pigs challenged IV with tumor burdens of 5×10^3, 5×10^4 or 5×10^5 were treated with BCG/L10 vaccines of graded 10:1 ratios, in dosages of $10^8/10^7$, $10^7/10^6$, $10^6/10^5$ or $10^5/10^4$.

For all three IV tumor challenges, BCG dose-related rather than ratio-related effects on survival were measured (Table 3). Of animals receiving an IV tumor challenge of 5×10^3 L10, immunization with BCG doses of 10^6-10^8 achieved significant increases in survival compared with the untreated controls. For those animals receiving greater initial tumor

Table 3. Comparison of Graded 10:1 Ratios of BCG to L10

IV L10 Tumor Challenge	Treatment Days 1 and 7 After Tumor Challenge	Survivors/ Total[a]	Percentage Survival	Probability[b] (Compared with no Treatment)
5×10^3	10^8 BCG + 10^7 L10	9/9	100	0.002
5×10^3	10^7 BCG + 10^6 L10	10/10	100	< 0.002
5×10^3	10^6 BCG + 10^5 L10	9/10	90	0.01
5×10^3	10^5 BCG + 10^4 L10	5/10	50	
5×10^3	No vaccination	3/10	30	
5×10^4	10^8 BCG + 10^7 L10	10/10	100	< 0.001
5×10^4	10^7 BCG + 10^6 L10	9/9	100	< 0.001
5×10^4	10^6 BCG + 10^5 L10	2/10	20	
5×10^4	10^5 BCG + 10^4 L10	1/10	10	
5×10^4	No vaccination	0/9	0	
5×10^5	10^8 BCG + 10^7 L10	9/10	90	< 0.001
5×10^5	10^7 BCG + 10^6 L10	6/10	60	0.005
5×10^5	10^6 BCG + 10^5 L10	1/10	10	
5×10^5	10^5 BCG + 10^4 L10	0/8	0	
5×10^5	No vaccination	0/10	0	

[a] 180-200 day survival of guinea pigs with disseminated micrometastasis.

[b] By Fisher's Exact Test, one-tailed.

injections (5×10^4 or 5×10^5), the vaccines containing 10^6 or less BCG were ineffective. Thus, it is clear that the ratio of 10:1 is not a sufficient property of the vaccine and that the BCG dose is highly critical to vaccine efficacy. When these data are analyzed by the Cochran-Armitage chi-square test for trend, vaccination efficacy at all three tumor burdens had a high correlation with BCG dose. The effect was more pronounced with higher tumor burdens (5×10^3, P = 0.002; 5×10^4, P < 0.001; 5×10^5, P < 0.0001). At a 10^6 IV tumor burden 10^8 and 5×10^7 BCG are equivalent in efficacy (45 percent and 46.6 percent survival, respectively) and were significantly different from controls. Although 10^8 and 5×10^7 BCG were not significantly different from 1×10^7 BCG, the latter dose was not significantly different from no treatment.

Variables of Preparation of Tumor Cell Suspensions.
Comparison of Vaccine Preparations with a Different Syngeneic Hepatocarcinoma (L1), Tissue Culture L10, and L10 Irradiated with 12,000 or 20,000 Rads X-Irradiation

The L1 hepatocarcinoma is also syngeneic in strain-2 guinea pigs and grows progressively when transplanted at very high levels i.p. into weanling guinea pigs. However, in contrast to L10, when transplanted i.d. this tumor does not metastasize and regresses within two to four weeks. L10 and L1 share common embryonic antigens and show slight cross-reactivity. Yet, as shown in Table 4, these antigens were not of sufficient quantity and/or quality to promote any therapeutic effect when used as a vaccine against L10.

Tissue culture L10 was equally effective when compared with the ascites form of L10 and there is no appreciable difference in the efficacy of the BCG + L10 vaccine if the tumor cells are X-irradiated with 12,000 or 20,000 Rads.

Comparison of Cryopreservation Procedures: High- or Low-Viability Tumor Cell Vaccines

The DMSO-cryopreservation procedure, which yielded a high-viability tumor cell suspension (90%), was compared with the glycerol-cryopreservation procedure which yielded a low-viability tumor-cell suspension (30%). The vaccines were tested in guinea pigs inoculated IV with 10^5 or 10^6 L10 cells. Both doses were fatal in normal guinea pigs. The vaccines were administered on days one and seven post tumor challenge and contained 10^8 viable BCG organisms plus 10^7 frozen-thawed and X-irradiated L10 cells. Survival results are shown in Figure 2.

Compared with the 10^5 tumor challenge control animals with 100 percent mortality and a median survival of approximately 80 days, significant protection, 47 percent survival (P = 0.013) and a prolonged

Table 4. Survival of Guinea Pigs Injected i.v. with 10^5 Syngeneic Line 10 Hepatocarcinoma Cells: Comparison of Various Hepatocarcinoma Preparation and Radiation Doses

| | | Survival | |
| | | Vaccination Times (Days after i.v. Injection) | |
Treatment[a]	Tumor Cell Irradiation Dose	1-7	4-10
None	–	0/10	–
$(10^8$ BCG + 10^7 L1) $(10^8$ BCG + 10^7 L1)	20,000 rad	0/10	–
$(10^8$ BCG + 10^7 TC L10) $(10^8$ BCG + 10^7 TC L10)	10,000 rad	10/10	–
$(10^8$ BCG + 10^7 L10) $(10^8$ BCG + 10^7 L10)	12,000 rad	10/10	10/10
$(10^8$ BCG + 10^7 L10) $(10^8$ BCG + 10^7 L10)	20,000 rad	10/10	8/10

[a] FL10, frozen line 10; L1, Line 1 hepatocarcinoma, a regressor, syngeneic hepatocarcinoma with weak antigenic cross-reactivity with the line 10 progressor hepatocarcinoma; TC, tissue-culture-maintained cells that are tumorigenic in strain two guinea pigs.

median survival time (193 days), is achieved with the low-viability vaccine. However, the low-viability vaccine is significantly less effective (P = 0.005) than the high-viability vaccine (47 percent survival as compared to 100 percent survival).

The difference in protection afforded by low- and high-viability vaccines is further exemplified in the experiments in which animals were challenged with 10^6 tumor cells. With this tumor burden only one of 15 animals survived after treatment with the low-viability vaccine, whereas 53 percent of the animals survived in the high-viability vaccine group (P = 0.007).

Comparison of Enzymatic Procedures for Disaggregation of L10 Solid Tumors

Although the efficacy of the vaccine prepared from ascites cells is extremely encouraging, most human tumors are available in solid form. The purpose of the study presented here and in detail elsewhere[30] was to develop methods of dissociating solid tumor that would yield the largest number of viable cells per g tumor without destroying the immunogenic potential of the cells.

Utilizing the solid L10 tumor grown intramuscularly, we tested various modes and conditions of solid tumor disaggregation. The resulting cell suspensions were monitored for: sterility of preparation, cell yield per g tissue dissociated, percentage of viability by vital stain, cryobiological

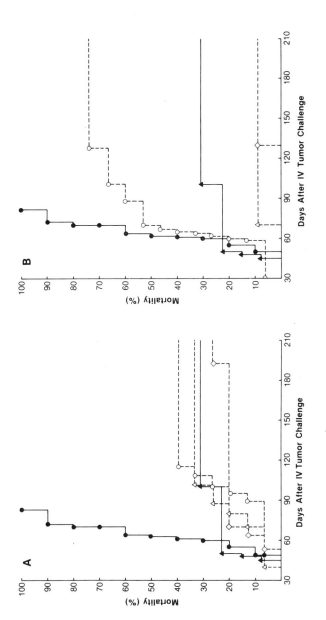

Figure 2. Cumulative mortality of animals inoculated IV with 10^5 or 10^6 tumor cells and immunized with 10^8 BCG plus 10^7 freeze-thawed irradiated high- or low-viability tumor cell vaccines. The response of unimmunized guinea pigs to tumor challenge is also shown.

preservation and recovery, metabolic activity and viability of tumor cells after 20,000 Rads X-irradiation, cell surface antigen utilizing tumor-specific antibody and immunofluorescence, and immunotherapeutic potential *in vivo* as a nontumorigenic vaccine used to immunize animals with established disseminated micrometastasis.

The combined data of several experiments comparing mechanical dissociation and enzymatic procedures for disaggregation of L10 solid tumors are presented in Table 5. The dissociation potential of trypsin, collagenase type I, collagenase type III, and collagenase type I plus hyaluronidase was evaluated on the basis of cell yield per g tumor and percentage of cell viability. Various collagenase type I concentrations were tested, and media were modified for calcium and magnesium, protease contaminants and temperature. Mechanical dissociation yielded 44×10^6 cells/g tumor with a viability of 10 percent, whereas tumor fragments dissociated in CMF-HBSS containing DNase and EDTA incubated at 37°C, with trypsin, collagenase type I, or collagenase type III yielded 52×10^6—96% viability, 39×10^6—94% viability, and 18×10^6—67% viability, respectively. Although trypsin gave the highest yield per g tumor, clumping of dissociated cells was a frequent occurrence, and there was a greater reduction of cell surface antigens[30] than found with the collagenases.

Dissociations at 37°C and room temperature were compared for both collagenase type I and type III. This approximately 10°C reduction in temperature reduced cell yield per g tumor more than 50 percent for both enzymes with a corresponding decrease in percentage of cell viability.

Collagenase type I contains some protease and peptidase activity, whereas collagenase type III is substantially free of these contaminants. Dissociations with both collagenase type I and type III were performed with 10 percent FBS (a protease inhibitor) in the medium. As a result, cell yield and viability were reduced for both collagenases. Thus, dissociation of L10 solid tumor with the more purified collagenase type III was not pursued further.

Although CMF media and EDTA are commonly used in enzyme dissociations, collagenase activity requires calcium. When HBSS was substituted for CMF-HBSS containing EDTA, cell yield reduction by the addition of FBS was abrogated and the time required for dissociation was cut by half.

Collagenase concentrations of 0.25 percent have been shown to cause widespread blebbing of the plasma membrane of liver cells. This blebbing is decreased significantly at 0.15 percent and below.[33] Our data showed effective dissociation can be achieved with collagenase type I concentrations of 0.10 percent or 0.14 percent.

Collagenase in combination with hyaluronidase has been shown to

Table 5. Comparison of Mechanical and Enzymatic Procedures for Disaggregation of L10 Solid Tumor

Method of Dissociation	Medium					Conditions		Results	
	HBSS	CMF HBSS	DNase 0.03%	EDTA 0.02%	Fetal Calf 10%	37°C	Room Temperature	Total Cells/g Tumor (x 10^6)	Viability (%)
Mechanical	+						+	44	10
0.14% trypsin		+	+	+		+		52	96
0.14% collagenase type I		+	+	+		+		39	94
0.14% collagenase type III		+	+	+		+		18	67
0.14% collagenase type I		+	+	+			+	16	84
0.14% collagenase type III		+	+	+			+	7	56
0.14% collagenase type I		+	+	+	+	+		18	87
0.14% collagenase type III		+	+	+	+	+		11	49
0.14% collagenase type I	+		+			+		36	91
0.14% collagenase type I	+		+		+	+		39	91
0.10% collagenase type I	+		+			+		35	90
0.05% collagenase type I	+		+			+		18	84
0.01% collagenase type I	+		+			+		12	75
0.01% collagenase type I + 3000 units hyaluronidase	+		+			+		14	68

have a synergistic effect at low concentrations in isolating parenchymal cells from rat liver[33] and in the preparation of isolated Ehrlich ascites carcinoma cells. It has been suggested that one enzyme aids the permeation of the other by unmasking reactive groups. The addition of hyaluronidase to collagenase did not alter cell yield with the L10 tumor, suggesting effective permeation with collagenase alone with this particular tumor.

Efficacy of BCG Plus Ascites L10 Cell Vaccines and BCG Plus Dissociated Solid Tumor L10 Cell Vaccine for Therapy of Micrometastasis

Guinea pigs were given IV injections of 10^4, 10^5, or 10^6 L10 cells and treated at one and seven days by i.d. immunizations with BCG plus L10 tumor cell vaccines. Fifteen animals from each tumor burden group were immunized with either 10^8 BCG admixed with 10^7 irradiated ascites L10 cells or 10^8 BCG admixed with 10^7 irradiated L10 cells dissociated from solid tumor. The L10 ascites cells used for vaccine were a combination of both frozen and freshly harvested cells, with a trypan blue exclusion index after irradiation of 97 percent and 95 percent. The L10 solid tumor-dissociated cells used for vaccines were a combination of five lots of frozen cells with a trypan blue exclusion index after irradiation of 82 percent and 84 percent. There were a few small clumps of aggregated cells and some cellular debris in these inocula. Survival results for these treated and untreated guinea pigs are shown in Figure 3.

In animals given IV injections of 10^4 L10 cells, 80 percent of the untreated controls died by 156 days after injection. In contrast all animals immunized at one and seven days with either 10^8 BCG plus 10^7 irradiated L10 ascites cells or 10^8 BCG plus 10^7 irradiated L10 solid tumor dissociated cells survived.

In animals given IV injections of 10^5 L10 cells, all untreated controls were dead within 96 days, with a 50 percent lethal dose of 68 days. Of the treated animals, one death occurred at 181 days among animals immunized with 10^8 BCG plus 10^7 irradiated L10 ascites cells and five deaths occurred among animals immunized with 10^8 BCG plus 10^7 irradiated L10 cells dissociated from solid tumor. Both treatments conferred insignificant protection as compared to the untreated controls (p = 0.0001 and < 0.0001, respectively). Although there were fewer survivors (10 of 15) in the group given solid tumor vaccine than those given ascites vaccine (14 of 15), this difference was not significant.

In animals given IV injections of 10^6 L10 cells, all untreated animals died by Day 63 after injection. The 50 percent lethal dose was less than 50 days. The number of deaths was the same (12 of 15) for each of the immunized groups. A nonstatistically significant shift in survival curves can be noted in this graph.

Overall survival achieved with immunizations of either BCG plus L10

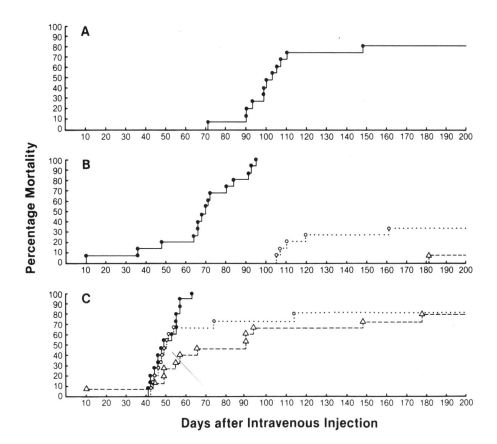

Figure 3. Adult guinea pigs were given i.v. injections of 10^4 (**A**), 10^5 (**B**), or 10^6 (**C**) L10 tumor cells. The next day the treatment groups were given i.d. injections of 10^8 BCG admixed with either 10^7 irradiated L10 ascites cells ($\triangle$) or 10^7 irradiated L10 cells dissociated from a solid tumor ($\circ$). Six days later, the vaccinations were repeated. Control groups ($\bullet$) were untreated. There were 15 animals per group.

ascites cells or BCG plus dissociated L10 solid tumor cells was statistically significant compared to untreated controls (p = 0.00001 for both treatment groups), and no significant difference overall could be determined between the two treatment groups.

Immunotherapy with BCG Plus Tumor Cell Vaccine After Surgery

The most critical evaluation of therapy with BCG plus L10 vaccine would be in guinea pigs with both regional and disseminated tumor (Protocol, Figure 1B). Guinea pigs were injected with 10^6 L10 cells i.d. on Day 0 followed by 10^5 L10 cells IV on Day 11. Treatment was started on Day 12. One group of animals was injected intratumorally with BCG; the skin tumor and SDA node were excised surgically in a second group; and the remaining animals were treated with BCG plus L10 vaccine one and seven days after the skin tumor and SDA node were excised. All animals treated by intratumoral BCG or surgery alone died (Figure 4A). However, an increased median survival time was achieved in the surgery treatment group relative to the intratumoral BCG treatment group. Approximately 30 percent of the animals treated by a combination of surgery and BCG plus L10 vaccine survived. In a second experiment using this same protocol, except 10^4 cells were injected IV 55 percent (5/9) of the animals survived after surgery and vaccine treatment, whereas no animals survived in the surgery alone treatment group (Figure 4B). This difference in survival is significant ($p = < 0.05$).

Discussion

Nonspecific immunotherapy of malignant diseases with BCG has been used extensively in human subjects over the past several years.[b] Several routes, schedules, doses and sources of BCG have been employed in these various clinical trials. The routes of administration include oral,[34] IV,[35,36] intralymphatic,[37] intratumoral,[9,38–40] i.d.,[38] Heafgun technique,[7] the tine plate method,[38] scarification,[41–44] and intrapleural.[45,46] Several strains of BCG and a variety of doses have been utilized; both of these parameters are considered important with regard to efficacy of therapy.[47–49] The use of BCG in immunotherapy has not been without untoward side effects.[50] There have been significant clinical problems and some fatalities.[51–55] These complications stem from the dissemination of BCG from the injection site,[54,56] resulting in systemic symptoms and signs similar to disseminated tuberculosis. In general, the severity of the complications is associated with the dose of BCG and the resistance of the host. Although the natural history and management of these complications are well documented, nonetheless such complications can interfere with active immunotherapy by direct immunodepression or antigenic competition. Current protocols of immunotherapy should evaluate the variables of BCG source and dose to develop the optimum operational dose of bacilli necessary to survive the immune reaction and stimulate general or specific tumor immunity.

Utilizing the syngeneic L10 hepatocarcinoma in inbred strain-2 guinea pigs, we have demonstrated that a BCG plus irradiated (attenuated) tumor cell vaccine can induce a degree of systemic immunity capable of eliminating disseminated visceral micrometastases.[17,18,23] Significant and

[b]International Registry of Tumor Immunotherapy: Compendium of Tumor Immunotherapy Protocols #4 NIH, NCI, Bethesda, MD.

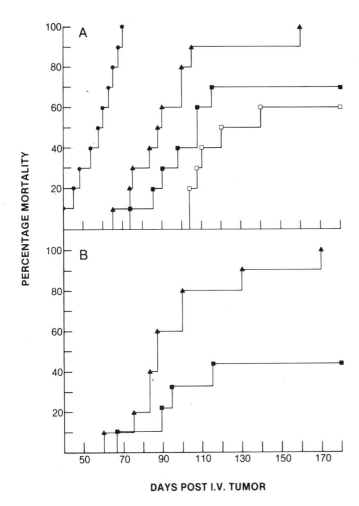

Figure 4. Percentage cumulative mortality in guinea pigs with regional and disseminated micrometastases, treated by intratumoral BCG or surgical excision of the primary skin tumor and SDA lymph node followed by vaccination with BCG plus L10 cells. There were 9–10 animals per group. (**A**) Experimental animals were injected i.d. with 10^6 L10 cells and 11 days later received 10^5 L10 i.v. One day later (Day 12) animals were either given intratumoral BCG (●—●); had surgical excision of the skin tumor and the SDA lymph node (△—△); had surgical excision of the skin tumor and the SDA lymph node and were treated with BCG plus fresh L10 cell vaccine at 13 and 20 days (■—■) or were given BCG plus frozen-thawed L10 cell vaccine at 13 and 20 days (□—□). (**B**) Experimental animals were injected i.d. with 10^6 L10 cells and 11 days later received 10^4 L10 cells i.v. One day later (Day 12) animals had surgical excision of the skin tumor and SDA lymph node (▲—▲) or had surgical excision of the skin tumor and SDA lymph node and were treated with BCG plus fresh L10 cell vaccine at 13 and 20 days (■—■).

reproducible immunotherapy is achieved when the BCG plus tumor cell vaccines are prepared under defined conditions. We examined the variables of the adjuvant, BCG, with respect to source, dose and ratio to tumor cells. Of the two lyophilized sources and two fresh-frozen sources of BCG, no significant difference could be detected with respect to adjuvant potential when they were mixed with attenuated tumor cells in a vaccine. This finding is of practical importance since only Connaught BCG and the lyophilized form of Tice IL105(S)19 are approved for human use. The BCG dose study clearly demonstrated that there is a BCG dose dependency with relation to induction of effective cell-mediated immunity or survival from disseminated micrometastatis disease. However, the lowest effective dose was a function of the tumor burden. Thus, at several levels of tumor growth the optimum operational BCG dose was 5×10^7 viable organisms.

It is not possible to use the results from this guinea pig model to recommend the optimal operational dose of BCG in other tumor systems. However, dosage of BCG is such an important consideration in clinical studies that more information is critical. Problems have evolved when empirical extrapolations of BCG doses from guinea pig studies to treatment in humans have been attempted.[54] Based on comparative studies of the relation of delayed sensitivity in man and the guinea pig, the quantities of cells required for transfer in the guinea pig are very large, whereas in the human relatively small amounts are needed.[57] This might indicate that in man lower doses of BCG could be used to achieve effects comparable with those in a guinea pig therapy model.

Various other prerequisites for preparation profoundly influence the efficacy of the vaccine in the inbred guinea pig immunotherapy model. The two most important variables are dose of BCG and the viability of injected tumor cells. It was shown that significant protection can be achieved with two vaccinations separated by one week and that the initial immunization requires 10^7 or greater viable BCG organisms admixed with 10^7 tumor cells. High tumor cell viability in the final vaccine preparation is also a requirement. Thus, any manipulations of the immunogenic preparation for cryobiological preservation or X-irradiation in order to develop nontumorigenic vaccines would have to incorporate these two major prerequisites. Using ascites L10 cells in the guinea pig experiment model, we have demonstrated that critical cryobiological preservation and 20,000 Rads X-irradiation of L10 cells can be accomplished and still maintain approximately 90 percent tumor cell viability at the time of immunization.

The method of cryopreservation of the tumor cells used in preparation of the vaccine is critical. In the guinea pig model, tumor cells that were frozen by an established procedure used for preservation of bone marrow in transplantation studies and assessed as an optimal procedure in several low-temperature biology studies were as effective in the vaccine as fresh ascites tumor cells. This is in contrast to results in the same model by Bartlett et al.[30] who, using a less critical cryopreservation procedure and achieving lower cell viability as a consequence of freezing and thawing, induced minimal cell-mediated tumor immunity in vaccine protection studies.

A clinical study that we feel emphasizes the need for critically performed cryopreservation and vaccine preparation was reported by McIllmurray et al.[58] In a controlled trial of active specific immunotherapy for Stage IIB malignant melanoma, eight of 15 patients were treated with one vaccination (over multiple sites). The preparation included Glaxo BCG and autologous irradiated tumor cells. Over a 24-month observation period, six of the eight vaccinated patients developed recurrent melanoma and five died; five of seven controls had recurrences and three died. At the 12-month time point, there was a suggestion of tumor enhancement in the vaccinated patients. The overall results indicate that active specific immunotherapy as performed in these patients was ineffective. The procedure for preparing the autologous tumor cell vaccine differed from the one described here in that the irradiated tumor cells, admixed with BCG in phosphate-buffered saline (0.05 M NaH_2PO_4-Na_2HPO_4 and 0.12 M NaCI, pH 7.4), were frozen at $-1°C$/min in liquid nitrogen. The vaccine was rapidly thawed at 37°C, and equal doses were injected i.d. in each limb and just below the umbilicus, each of the five sites receiving 10^7 tumor cells and 6×10^6 BCG organisms.[c] This irradiation and freezing procedure in our hands, using the L10 cells and freezing only in phosphate-buffered saline, results in greater than 90 percent cell death after the vaccine is thawed. These determinations on L10 cells were made by both fluorescein diacetate and trypan blue dye exclusion. On the basis of the results in the guinea pig model, we would have to assume that the single immunization, although at multiple sites, and the possible lack of viability as a result of inadequate cryopreservation abrogated the immunogenic potential of the BCG plus melanoma vaccine.

In another clinical study, Hedley et al,[11] treated patients with Stage IIB melanomas monthly with irradiated allogeneic melanoma cells and BCG, while the control patients receiving only BCG. Sixteen patients in the treatment group had a median relapse-free interval of five months compared with eight months in the 12 controls given chemotherapy and BCG. The authors concluded that immunotherapy composed of irradiated allogeneic melanoma cells as used in this study did not prolong survival in surgically treated patients with Stage IIB melanoma and may even have promoted early, local relapse. The guinea pig model is in agreement

[c]M.J. Embleton and R. W. Baldwin (personal communication).

with this study since syngeneic tumor (L1) used in a vaccine with BCG was ineffective in protecting animals with established disseminated L10 metastasis. We have an indication then that the immunity induced by the vaccine in the guinea pig model is tumor-specific. The L1 hepatocarcinoma, although syngeneic in strain-2 guinea pigs, is a regressor tumor upon i.d. challenge of 10^6 cells in contrast to the progressive growth of L10. Since in this tumor model the growth pattern and host response to the L1 tumor may be analogous in some respects to that seen with allogeneic tumors, some of the clinical procedures using allogeneic tumor cells should be questioned.

Our results are relevant to the major issues of active specific immunotherapy. Most human immunotherapy trials have been performed with what these results suggest are suboptimal vaccine preparations. The implication of the present study is that any negative clinical or animal experiments with suboptimal vaccine preparations should not be considered definitive and should be repeated with optimal vaccine preparations before any conclusions can be reached. The present experiments provide important information for the development of an optimal vaccine preparation to be used in active specific immunotherapy utilizing solid tumors surgically excised according to standard treatment. This experimental model in guinea pigs now lends itself to studies of combinations of modalities such as chemotherapy, surgery and active specific immunotherapy.

References

1. Barlett, GL, Zbar, B: Tumor-specific vaccine containing *Mycobacterium bovis* and tumor cells: safety and efficacy. *J. Natl. Cancer Inst.* 48:1709–1726, 1977.

2. Bekesi, JG, St. Arneault, G, Holland, JF: Increase of leukemia L1210 immunogenicity by *Vibrio cholerae* neuraminidase treatment. *Cancer Res.* 31:2130–2132, 1971.

3. Martin, WJ, Wunderlich, JR, Fletcher, F, Inman, JK: Enhanced immunogenicity of chemically-coated syngeneic tumor cells, *Proc. Natl. Acad. Sci. USA* 68:469–472, 1971.

4. Prager, MD, Baechtel, FS: Methods for modification of cancer cells to enhance their antigenicity. In: Busch, H, ed. *Methods in Cancer Research*, Vol. 9, pp. 339–400, Academic Press, New York, 1973.

5. Ray, PK, Thakur, VS, Sundaram, K: Antitumor immunity. I. Differential response of neuraminidase-treated and X-irradiated tumor vaccine. *Eur. J. Cancer* 11:1–8, 1975.

6. Mathé, G, Weiner R., Pouillart, P et al: BCG in cancer immunotherapy. Experimental and clinical trials of its use in treatment of leukemia minimal and/or residual disease. *Natl. Cancer Inst. Monogr.* 39:165–175, 1973.

7. Powles, RL, Crowther, D, Bateman, CJT et al.: Immunotherapy for acute myelogenous leukemia. *Br. J. Cancer* 28:365–376, 1973.

8. Sokal, JE, Aungst, CW, Grace JT Jr: Immunotherapy of chronic myelocytic leukemia. *Natl. Cancer Inst. Monogr.* 39:195–198, 1973.

9. Morton DL, Eilber, FR, Holmes, EC et al.: Present status of BCG immunotherapy of malignant melanoma, *Cancer Immunol. Immunother.* 1:93–98, 1976.

10. Hollinshead, AC: Active-specific immunotherapy. In: *Immunotherapy of Human Cancer*, 22nd Clinical Conference on Cancer, M.D. Anderson Hospital and Tumor Institute, pp. 213–233, Raven Press, New York, 1978.

11. Hedley, DW, McElwain, TJ, Currie, GA: Specific active immunotherapy does not prolong survival in surgically treated patients with stage IIB malignant melanoma and may promote early recurrence. *Br. J. Cancer* 37:491–496, 1978.

12. Prager, MD: Specific cancer immunotherapy. *Cancer Immunol. Immunother.* 3:157–161, 1978.

13. Zbar, B, Tanaka, T: Immunotherapy of cancer: regression of tumors after intralesional injection of living *Mycobacterium bovis*. *Science* 172:271–273, 1971.

14. Hanna, MG Jr, Zbar, B, Rapp, HJ: Histopathology of tumor regression and intralesional injection of *Mycobacterium bovis*. I. Tumor growth and metastasis. *J. Natl. Cancer Inst.* 48:1441–1455, 1972.

15. Zbar, B, Bernstein, ID, Bartlett, GL et al.: Immunotherapy of cancer: regression of intradermal tumors and prevention of growth of lymph node metastases after intralesional injection of living *Mycobacterium bovis (Bacillus Calmette-Guérin)*. *J. Natl. Cancer Inst.* 49:119–130, 1972.

16. Hanna, MG Jr, Snodgrass, MJ, Zbar, B, Rapp, HJ: Histopathology of tumor regression after intralesional injection of *Mycobacterium bovis*. IV. Development of immunity to tumor cells and BCG. *J. Natl. Cancer Inst.* 51:1897–1908, 1973.

17. Hanna, MG Jr, Peters, LC.: Immunotherapy of established micrometastases with *Bacillus Calmette-Guérin* tumor cell vaccine. *Cancer Res.* 38:204–209, 1978.

18. Hanna, MG Jr, Peters, LC: BCG immunotherapy: efficacy of BCG induced tumor immunity in guinea pigs with regional tumors and/or visceral micrometastases. In: *Immunotherapy of Human Cancer*. 22nd Clinical Conference on Cancer, M.D. Anderson Hospital and Tumor Institute, 111–129, Raven Press, New York, 1978.

19. Hanna, MG Jr, Peters, LC: Specific immunotherapy of established visceral micrometastases by BCG-tumor cell vaccine alone or as an adjunct to surgery. *Cancer* 42:2613–2625, 1979.

20. Hanna, MG Jr, Brandhorst, JS, Peters, LC: Active specific immunotherapy of residual micrometastasis: an evaluation of sources, doses and ratios of BCG with tumor cells. *Cancer Immunol. Immunother.* 7:165–173, 1979.

21. Snodgrass, MJ, Hanna, MG Jr: Histopathology of tumor regression after intralesional injection of *Mycobacterium bovis*. Ultrastructural studies of histiocyte-tumor cell interactions. *Cancer Res.* 33:701–716, 1973.

22. Hanna, MG Jr, Bucana, C: Active specific immunotherapy of residual micrometastasis: the acute and chronic inflammatory response in induction of tumor immunity by BCG-tumor cell immunization. *J. Reticuloendothel. Soc.* 26:439–452, 1979.

23. Hanna, MG Jr: Active specific immunotherapy of residual micrometastasis: a comparison of postoperative treatment with BCG-tumor cell vaccine to preoperative intratumoral BCG injection. In: Terry, W, Yamamura, Y, eds, *Immunobiology and Immunotherapy*. Elsevier North-Holland Publications, New York, pp. 331–350, 1979.

24. Adams, DO: The granulomatous inflammatory response: a review. *Am. J. Pathol.* 84:164–191, 1976.

25. Boros, DL: Granulomatous inflammations. *Progr. Allergy* 24:183–267, 1978.

26. Rapp, HJ, Churchill, WH Jr, Kronman, BS et al.: Antigenicity of a new diethylnitrosamine-induced transplantable guinea pig hepatoma: pathology and formation of ascites variant. *J. Natl. Cancer Inst.* 41:1–11, 1978.

27. Zbar, B, Wepsic, HT, Rapp, HJ et al.: Antigenic specificity of hepatomas induced in strain-2 guinea pigs by diethylnitrosamine. *J. Natl. Cancer Inst.* 43:833–841, 1979.

28. Mazur, P, Leibo, SP, Farrant, J et al.: Interactions of cooling rate, warming rate, and protective additive on the survival of frozen mammalian cells. In: Wolstenholme, GEW O'Connor, M, eds. *The Frozen Cell* p. 69–88, Churchill Livingston, London, 1970.

29. Leibo, SP: Comment on the loss of immunogenicity of tumor cells caused by freezing. *Cancer Immunol. Immunother.* 3:211–213, 1978.

30. Bartlett, GL, Katsilas, DC, Kreider, JW, Purnell, DM: Immunogenicity of "viable" tumor cells after storage in liquid nitrogen. *Cancer Immunol. Immunother.* 2:127–133, 1977.

31. Peters, LC, Brandhorst, JS, Hanna, MG Jr: Preparation of immunotherapeutic autologous tumor cell vaccines from solid tumors. *Cancer Res.* 39:1353–1360, 1979.

32. Bartlett, GL, Purnell, DM, Kreider, JW: BCG inhibition of murine leukemia: local suppression and systemic tumor immunity require different doses. *Science* 191:299–301, 1976.

33. Howard, RB, Christensen, AK, Gibbs, FA, Pesch LA: The enzymatic preparation of isolated intact parenchymal cells from rat liver. *J. of Cell Biol.* 35:675–685, 1967.

34. Falk, RE, Mann, P, Langer, B: Cell-mediated immunity to human tumor. Abrogation by serum factors and nonspecific effects of oral BCG therapy. *Arch. Surg.* 107:261–265, 1973.

35. Jurczyk-Procyk, S, Martin, M, Dubouch, P et al.: Toxicity studies of intravenously administered BCG in baboons. *Cancer Immunol. Immunother.* 1:55–61, 1976.

36. Khalil, A, Bourut, C, Halle-Pannenko, O et al.: Histologic reactions of the thymus, spleen, liver and lymph nodes to intravenous and subcutaneous BCG injections. *Biomedicine* 22:112–121, 1975.

37. Mangan, C, Jeglum, KA, Sedlackl: TV et al.: Intralymphatic BCG and the treatment of gynecologic malignancies. A Phase I study. *Cancer* 40:2933–2940, 1977.

38. Morton, DL, Eilber, FR, Holmes, EC et al.: BCG immunotherapy of malignant melanoma: summary of a seven-year experience. *Ann. Surg.* 180:635–643, 1974.

39. Nathanson, L: Regression of intradermal malignant melanoma after intralesional injection of *Mycobacterium bovis* strain BCG. *Cancer Chemother. Rep.* 56:659–665, 1972.

40. Pinsky, C, Hirshaut: Y: Oettgen, H: Treatment of malignant melanoma by intratumoral injection of BCG. *Proc. Am. Assoc. Cancer Res.* 13:21, 1972.

41. Bluming, AZ, Vogel, CL, Ziegler, JL et al.: Immunological effects of BCG in malignant melanoma: two modes of administration compared. *Ann. Int. Med.* 76:405–411, 1972.

42. Gutterman, JU, Mavligit, GM, McBride, CM et al.: Active immunotherapy with BCG for recurrent malignant melanoma. *Lancet* 1:1208–1212, 1973.

43. Gutterman, JU, Mavligit, GM, Kennedy, A et al.: Immunotherapy for malignant melanoma. In: *Neoplasms of the Skin and Malignant Melanoma.* p. 497–531, M.D. Anderson Hospital, Yearbook Medical Publishers, Chicago, IL.

44. Gutterman, JU, Rodriguez, V, McCredie, KB et al.: Chemoimmunotherapy of acute myeloblastic leukemia: 4-year follow up with BCG. In: Terry, WD, Windhorst, D, eds. *Immunotherapy of Cancer: Present Status of Trials in Man*, pp. 375–381, Raven Press, New York, 1978.

45. McKneally, MF, Maver, C, Kausel, HW: Regional immunotherapy of lung cancer with intrapleural BCG. *Lancet* 1:377–379, 1976.

46. McKneally, MF, Maver, C, Kausel, HW: Intrapleural BCG immunostimulation in lung cancer. *Lancet* 1:593, 1977.

47. Mackaness, GB, Auclair, DJ, Lagrange, PH: Immunopotentiation with BCG. I. Immune response to different strains and preparations. *J. Natl. Cancer Inst.* 51:1655–1667, 1973.

48. Hanna, MG Jr, Peters, LC, Gutterman, JU, Hersh, EM: Evaluation of BCG administered by scarification for immunotherapy of metastatic hepatocarcinoma in the guinea pig. *J. Natl. Cancer Inst.* 56:1013–1017, 1976.

49. Mathé, G, Halle-Pannenko, O, Bourut, C: BCG in cancer immunotherapy. II. Results obtained with various BCG preparations in a screening study for systemic adjuvants applicable to cancer immunoprophylaxis and immunotherapy. *Natl. Cancer Inst. Monogr.* 39:107–112, 1973.

50. Sparks, FC: Hazards and complications of BCG immunotherapy. *Med. Clin. N. Am.* 60:499–509, 1976.

51. Hortobagyi, GN, Richman, SP, Dandridge, K et al., Immunotherapy with BCG administered by scarification. Standardization of reactions and management of side effects. *Cancer* 42:2293–2303, 1978.

52. Stein, JA, Siletzki-Ciechanover, M, Gefel, A et al.: Untoward fatal hemorrhagic diathesis in a BCG-treated melanoma patient. *Cancer Immunol. Immunother.* 4:269–270, 1978.

53. Schwarzenberg, L, Simmler, MC, Pico, JL: Human toxicology of BCG applied in cancer immunotherapy. *Cancer Immunol. Immunother.* 1:69–76, 1976.

54. Rosenberg, SA, Seipp, C, Sears, HF: Clinical and immunologic studies of disseminated BCG infection. *Cancer* 41:1771–1780, 1978.

55. Sparks, FC, Silverstein, MJ, Hunt, JS et al.: Complications of BCG immunotherapy in patients with cancer. *N. Engl. J. Med.* 289:827–830, 1973.

56. Ritch, PS, McCredie, KB, Hersh, EM, Gutterman, JU: Disseminated BCG disease associated with immunotherapy by scarification in acute leukemia. *Cancer* 42:167–170, 1978.

57. Kabat, EA, Mayer, MM: *Experimental Immunochemistry, Delayed Hypersensitivity*, pp. 300–306, C.C. Thomas, Springfield, IL, 1961.

58. McIllmurray, MB, Reeves, WG, Langman, MJS et al.: Active immunotherapy in malignant melanoma. *Br. Med. J.* 2:579, 1978.

Time and Model Dependence of Cyclophosphamide Enhancement-Inhibition of Experimental Metastasis

Mao H. Tseng, Mong H. Tan, Constantine P. Karakousis

Department of Surgical Oncology, Roswell Park Memorial Institute, Buffalo, New York

Summary

The following experiments were conducted to delineate the mechanism of enhancement of metastases by cyclophosphamide (CPM). Experimental metastasis was induced by the injection of tumor cells intravenously into syngeneic C57BL/6J mice. CPM was administered 30 minutes (M30) before, or 24 hours (H24), seven days (D7) or 14 days (D14) after intravenous cell injection. CPM enhanced the intravenous metastases by 49 percent and 40 percent in the B16 melanoma and T241 sarcoma respectively, when given at M30. In contrast, it inhibited metastases when given at H24, D7, or D14. The number of lung metastases developing corresponded well with the initial cell-arrest curve in the lung, determined by the injection of 125 IUDR labeled tumor cells (Figures 1 and 2).

In the intradermally induced metastases model, the primary tumor was excised at three weeks. In the treated groups, CPM was given either one hour before or 24 hours after surgery. The effectiveness of CPM was evaluated four weeks later. Surgery alone mice, all contained lung metastases, whereas the CPM treated groups showed significant therapeutic response. CPM only enhances metastases when given prior to intravenous tumor cell injection.

Introduction

Cyclophosphamide (CPM) is a potent anti-tumor agent and is used broadly in the clinic. However, it has been shown to enhance metastasis formation in some laboratory models. This phenomenon has stimulated

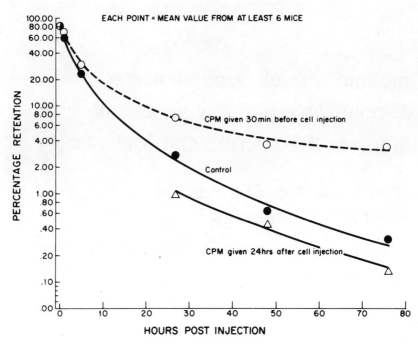

Figure 1. B16 melanoma: Cyclophosphamide (CPM) enhancement-inhibition of tumor cell retention in the lung.

a wide range of experimental studies and speculation,[1-4] and has raised the possibility that CPM therapy might produce certain unfavorable effects on the progression of human malignant disease particularly in the adjuvant setting. To provide further information on the enhancement versus inhibition of metastases, an artificial metastases model following intravenous tumor cells injection and a spontaneous metastases model using intradermally inoculation of tumor cells as a primary were developed. The former model demonstrated two opposite effects of CPM on the lung colonies formation, whereas the latter model which was designed to simulate clinical situation, only displayed inhibition of metastases.

Materials and Methods

Animals

Inbred C57BL/6J male mice, eight weeks old, were obtained from the Rosewell Park Memorial Institute Biology Laboratory.

Tumor Cell Lines and 125 IUdR Labeling Technique

B15 melanoma or T241 sarcoma cells, syngeneic to C57BL/6J mice, were grown in the falcon tissue culture flasks with RPMI 1640 media, supplemented with 10 percent heat inactivated fetal calf serum. 125 IUdR (125

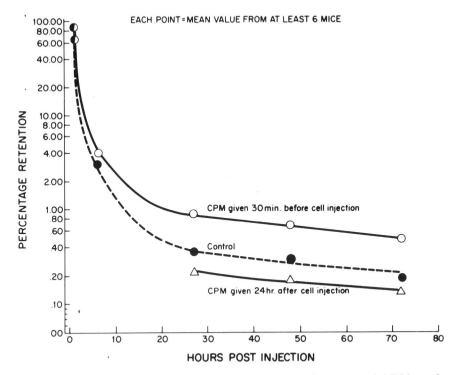

Figure 2. T241 sarcoma: Cyclophosphamide (CPM) enhancement-inhibition of tumor cell retention in the lungs.

I-5-iodo-z±-deoxyuridine) at a concentration of 0.5 μ Ci/ml of media was added into the culture media and incubated for 48 hours. At harvest, tumor cells were rinsed three times with 0.9% NaCl and then resuspended in growth media with a final single cell suspension at a concentration of $2 \times 10^4/0.1$ ml cells in B16 melanoma or $2 \times 10^5/0.1$ ml cells in T241 sarcoma, respectively for injection. Cell viability usually exceeded 95 percent by trypan blue exclusion test.

Measurement of the Cells Arresting in the Lung and Assessment of the Metastases

Three mice per group were killed at minutes 1-2, hours 1, 6, 27, 48, and 72 following tumor cells injection. The lungs were extracted in 70 percent ethanol, daily $\times$ 3. Radioactivity was assessed in a well type gamma-counter and expressed as:

$$\frac{CPM\ per\ organ\ -\ Background \times 100\%}{cpm\ per\ inoculum}.$$

In a concomitant study, unlabeled tumor cells were used and injected intravenously as mentioned above. All mice were killed at four weeks and the effectiveness of CPM was evaluated according to the number and size of lung colony formation.

Models of Metastases and the Administration of CPM

Intravenous metastases were studied by the injection of $2 \times 10^4/0.1$ ml of B16 or $2 \times 10^5/0.1$ ml T241 tumor cells into the tail vein. CPM 125 mg/ kg ip $\times$ 1, was given at either 30 minutes (M30) before or 24 hours (24H) or seven days (D7) or 14 days (D14) after cell injection. In the spontaneous metastasis model, the same concentration of B16 cells was injected intradermally to the abdominal wall of the mice. Three weeks later, tumors measuring 1.0–1.5 cm in diameter were excised. In treated groups, CPM was given either one hour before tumor excision or 24 hours after excision.

Results

As shown in Figures 1 and 2, tumor cells cleared exponentially after tail vein injection. At hour 24, 2-3 percent of B16 melanoma or 0.35 percent

Figure 3. B16 melanoma: Cyclophosphamide (CPM) enhancement-inhibition of lung colonies at 4 weeks post cell injection. Control: Not treated mice; −M30 CPM: CPM given 30 min before cell injection; H24 CPM: CPM given 24.hr after cell injection; D7 CPM: CPM given 7 days after cell injection; D14CPM: CPM given 14 days after cell injection.

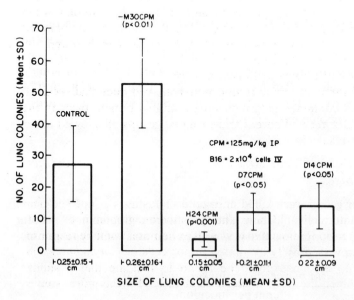

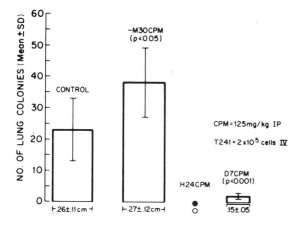

Figure 4. T241 sarcoma: Cyclophosphamide (CPM) enhancement-inhibition of lung colonies at 4 weeks post cell injection. Control: Not treated group; −M30 CPM: CPM given 30 min before cell injection; H24CPM: CPM given 24 hr after cell injection; D7 CPM: CPM given at 7 days after cell injection.

of T241 sarcoma were retained in the nontreated lung whereas 7 percent or 1% of B16 and 0.9% or 0.2% of T241 sarcoma were found retained, respectively, in the M30 and H24 CPM treated group.

The number of arrested cells corresponded well with lung metastases formation (Figures 3 and 4). CPM enhanced metastases by 49 percent and 40 percent, respectively, in B16 melanoma and T241 sarcoma when given 30 minutes prior to cell injection. On the contrary, it inhibited metastases by 87 percent or 54 percent or 46 percent in B16 and 100 percent or 91 percent in T241 tumor, respectively, when given at hour 24 or day seven or day 14 post cell injection.

Results using the intradermal tumor model showed mice that received surgery alone all contained lung metastases, and with metastases to the other organs in 3/9 mice. Whereas CPM treated groups all showed fewer mice with metastases (Table 1).

Discussion

The mechanism(s) by which CPM enhanced metastases is not yet clear from previous studies.[1–4] Using anti-lymphocyte globumin or whole body irradiation to suppress cellular as well as humoral immune response, or immunization with heavily irradiated tumor cells or *Corynebacterium parvum* (CP), no evidence could be found to indicate that a similar mechanism involved the CPM induced metastases. Furthermore, studies

Table 1. Intradermal Induced Metastases: Surgery Alone vs Adjuvant CPM Therapy at Four Weeks After Tumor Excision

Treatment	(Surgery Alone) Control	$-H_1$ CPM[a]	H_{24} H_{48} CPM[b]
Lung Metastases	9/9 (100%)	5/8 (62.5%)	3/8 (37.5%)
Other Metastases	3/9 (33.3%) Kidney, Chest Cavity	1/8 (12.5%) Chest Cavity	1/8 (12.5%) Peritoneum
Cure Rate	0/9 (0%)	3/8 (37.5%)	4/8 (50%)

[a] CPM 125 mg/kg i.p. x 1 given one hr before tumor excision.

[b] CPM 125 mg/kg i.p. x 2 given at 24 hr and 48 hr after tumor excision.

from Ruiter et al.,[2] showed that CPM promoted retention of living or dead cells, either osteosarcoma or embryonic cells, whereas *Corynebacterium parvum* can only reduce living sarcoma cells under these circumstances which means that the two drugs act in a different manner.

Our studies showed that initial rapid tumor cell clearance usually became slower and steadier after 24 hours and on, and the degree of radioactivity in the lung at this time usually reflects the eventual development of lung metastases. Therefore, any anti-tumor agent which can decrease the retention of cells at this period should achieve a therapeutic effect. The difference in the retention of tumor cells as shown in Figures 1 and 2, clearly indicated initially two to three times more B16 or T241 tumor cells retained in the CPM pretreated mice (M30), or the two to three times less of tumor cells retained in the CPM post-treated mice (H24) were responsible for the enhancement or inhibition of lung colonies observed four weeks later (Figures 3 and 4). Delay in giving CPM post

Table 2. Time Dependence of Cyclophosphamide (CPM) Enhancement-Inhibition of Tumor Metastasis[a]

Time[b] CPM Given	30 Min Before	24 Hr After	7 Days After	14 Days After
B16 Melanoma	46% Enhancement	87% Inhibition	54% Inhibition	46% Inhibition
T241 Sarcoma	40% Enhancement	100% Inhibition	91% Inhibition	Not Tested

[a] The enhancement or inhibition is calculated by comparison to concomitant control which did not receive CPM.

[b] Cyclophosphamide 125 mg/kg given i.p., at interval indicated before and after tumor cell injection.

tumor cell injection at D7 and D14 showed less therapeutic response possibly because of the tumor cells which lodged originally in the lung having increased in number (Table 2).

Studies of the effectiveness of adjuvant chemotherapy in the subcutaneous model for metastases[5] have demonstrated that the optimal therapeutic response of CPM was during the perioperative period. The present result, from using the intradermal metastatic model, again showed that the administration of CPM whether before or after primary tumor excision, in single dose or double dose, achieved therapeutic effect. There was no enhancement of metastases similar to that seen in the intravenous metastases model. This indicates that progression of tumor during the treatment of malignant disease is unlikely to occur if the CPM is effective to that particular tumor.

The general agreement that immune mechanisms, whether specific or nonspecific, are not involved in the enhancement of lung metastases induced by CPM. Our observations suggested that the possible explanation for that was caused by organ damage at the level of the endothelial lining of the vessels which render a higher chance of cells being trapped upon encounter as the main cause of enhancement of metastases.

References

1. Carmel, RJ, Brown, JM: The effect of cyclophosphamide and other drugs on the incidence of pulmonary metastases in mice. *Cancer Research* 37:145–151, 1977.

2. DeRuiter, J, Smink, T, Vanputten, LM: Studies on the enhancement by cyclophosphamide (NSC-26271) of artificial lung metastasis after labeled cell inoculation. *Cancer Treat. Rep.* 60:465–470, 1976.

3. Vanputten, LM, Kram, LKJ, Van Dierendonck, HHC et al.: Enhancement of drugs of metastatic lung nodule formation after intravenous tumor cell injection. *Int. J. Cancer* 15:588–595, 1975.

4. Peters, LJ, Mason, K: Enhancement of artificial lung metastases by cyclophosphamide: pharmacological and mechanistic considerations. In: Day, SB et al., ed. *Cancer Invasion and Metastasis: Biologic Mechanisms and Therapy.* Raven Press, New York, 1977.

5. Tseng, MH, Tan, MH, Holyoke, ED, Karakousis, CP: The effectiveness of immediate preoperative chemotherapy. Sumitted to *J.N.C.I.*

Selective Effect of Cytotoxic Chemotherapy on Immunoregulatory Suppressor Cells in Solid Tumor Cancer Patients[a]

D. P. Braun, M. A. Cobleigh, J. E. Harris

Department of Internal Medicine, Section of Medical Oncology, Rush-Presbyterian-St. Luke's Medical Center, Chicago, Illinois; Department of Internal Medicine, University of Indiana at the Medical Center, Indianapolis, Indiana

Summary

The level of immunoregulatory suppressor cell activity was measured in the peripheral blood leukocytes (PBL) of ten solid tumor patients prior to and following cytotoxic chemotherapy. Heightened pretreatment levels of suppressor cell activity were exhibited by PBL from 9/10 patients by demonstrating greater than normal levels of PHA-induced blastogenesis augmentation in 24-hour precultured and/or glass adherent cell depleted cells. Post-treatment "rebound-overshoot" recovery of lymphoblastogenesis occurred in eight patients and was associated with a diminution of suppressor cell activity. Moreover, recovery of suppressor cell activity resulted again in decreasing levels of lymphoblastogenesis. In the two patients who did not demonstrate "rebound-overshoot," one had increased suppressor cell activity at all assessment points while one never demonstrated suppressor cell activity. We conclude that "rebound-overshoot" recovery of immune function following chemotherapy results from selective drug-induced inhibition of suppressor cells at a time when lymphocytic responses are recovering.

Introduction

The final elimination of tumor cells during or following chemotherapeutic intervention for cancer might require a host immune response. In general, however, most anticancer drugs are cytotoxic to immunocytes.[1] This

[a]Partially supported by a grant from the Wadsworth Memorial Foundation.

may, in fact prove advantageous since under certain conditions, cytotoxic chemotherapy has been found to augment immune responses.[2-8] Thus, immunological monitoring of cancer patients receiving cytotoxic drugs has demonstrated that there may occur in the post-treatment interval following drug-induced immunosuppression, a "rebound-overshoot" recovery of immune reactivity to greater than pretreatment levels of function and that this phenomenon, when it occurs clinically, is associated with a more favorable prognosis.[9]

The explanation for this "rebound-overshoot" effect has not, as yet, been completely elucidated. One possibility that has been suggested is that the "rebound-overshoot" phenomenon results from a selective suppression of suppressor cell number and function and/or a differential rate of recovery between suppressor cells and effector cells.[9] We have tested this possibility by monitoring the effects of cytotoxic chemotherapy on glass adherent and 24-hour preculture-sensitive immunoregulatory suppressor cells in the peripheral blood leukocytes of solid tumor patients.

Materials and Methods

Patient Population and Chemotherapy

Immunoregulatory suppressor activity was quantitated in the peripheral blood mononuclear leukocytes (PBL) of ten solid tumor patients prior to and following the administration of cytotoxic chemotherapy by the method described below. No patient had received radiation or chemotherapy within six months or undergone a surgical procedure within three to six weeks of being entered on study (Table 1). Chemotherapy was as follows:

1. Four breast cancer patients, all of whom had undergone modified radical mastectomy and had been found to have axillary lymph node involvement received as adjuvant chemotherapy: phenylalanine mustard—4 mgm/M² orally for 5 days every 6 weeks and 5-fluorouracil—300 mgm/M² intravenously for 5 days every 6 weeks.
2. One breast cancer patient with disseminated disease who, on a 28 day cycle received: cyclophosphamide—100 mgm/M² orally Days 1–14; and adriamycin—30 mgm/M² intravenously Days 1 and 8; and 5-fluorouracil—500 mgm/M² intravenously Days 1 and 8.
3. Two head and neck cancer patients and one lung cancer patient received high dose methotrexate in one of the following ways:
   (i) methotrexate—1500 mgm/M² intravenously by 24-hour infusion weekly followed by leucovorin 25 mg orally every 6 hours × 2, to begin 30 hours after start of methotrexate infusion and 10 mgm orally

Table 1. Assessment of 24-hour Preculture Sensitive and Glass Adherent Cell Suppressor Activity in Peripheral Blood Mononuclear Leukocytes from Cancer Patients Prior to Chemotherapy

Patient	Age	Tumor	PHA-Induced Lymphoblastogenesis (CPM)[a]				
			Nonmanipulated Cells	24-hour Precultured Cells	(AI)[b]	Glass Nonadherent Cells	(AI)[b]
1	58	Breast II	45,751	60,201	1.31	89,986	1.97
2	61	Breast II	9,845	19,373	1.97	17,380	1.77
3	58	Breast II	23,434	13,970	0.60	42,958	1.83
4	58	Breast II	16,949	38,837	2.29	40,027	2.36
5	63	Breast IV	9,758	21,416	2.19	17,609	1.80
6	69	Head and Neck IV	9,835	4,772	0.49	47,157	4.79
7	46	Head and Neck III	13,194	10,134	0.77	52,104	3.95
8	59	Lung II	19,161	18,146	0.95	13,681	0.71
9	50	Lung IV	6,170	6,950	1.13	44,465	7.21
10	36	Colon D	7,893	18,465	2.34	23,019	2.92

[a] CPM is the mean counts per min/2 x 10^5 cells exhibited by triplicate samples.
[b] AI = Augmentation Index.

every 6 hours × 8 to start 6 hours after last 25 mgm dose (chemotherapy for disseminated laryngeal carcinoma, patient 6).

(ii) methotrexate—300 mgm intravenous "push" followed by 700 mgm infusion over 6 hours and leucovorin 12 mgm every 6 hours intramuscularly for 10 injections (adjuvant therapy for surgically resected Stage II lung cancer, patient 8).

(iii) methotrexate—60 mgm/M² intramuscularly every 6 hours × 4 followed in exactly 6 hours after last dose with leucovorin 24 mgm orally and then after 6 hours 9 mgm leucovorin orally every 6 hours × 7 (adjuvant presurgical chemotherapy for carcinoma of the tongue, patient 7).

4. One colon carcinoma (Dukes D) patient received: mitomycin C—10 mg/M² intravenously every 2 weeks and 5-fluorouracil—450 mg/M² intravenously Days 1 and 5 every 4 weeks.

5. One lung cancer patient (Stage IV) received as part of 21 day treatment cycle: hexamethylmelamine—50 mg three times daily by mouth for 14 days and mitomycin C—10 mg intravenously every 21 days.

Isolation of Peripheral Blood Mononuclear Cells (PBL)

Venous blood was aseptically drawn into sterile tubes containing preservative-free heparin, diluted with an equal volume of Hanks Balanced Salt Solution (HBSS) and layered over Lymphocyte Separation Medium (LSM, Bionetics, Kensington, MD.). After centrifugation, the mononuclear cell layer was recovered and washed twice in HBSS before further manipulation.

Lymphoproliferation Assay

PBL were resuspended in RPMI-1640 medium supplemented with 20% heat inactivated fetal calf serum (FCS), 100 U/ml penicillin and 100 μg/ml streptomycin to a concentration of 2×10^6/ml and 100 μl of cells were dispensed into triplicate wells of a sterile, 96 well Linbro microtiter plate. To individual wells, 100 μl of a 1:500 dilution of a 1 percent stock solution of PHA (Difco, lot #649848) were added and subsequently, cultures were incubated for 72 hours at 37°C in a humidified atmosphere of 5 percent CO_2 in air. During the last six hours of culture, cells were labeled by adding 1 μCi of ³H-thymidine to each well, following which, cells were harvested with the aid of a multiple automated sample harvester (MASH II, Beckman) and incorporated radioactivity was measured by liquid scintillation counting. Lymphoblastogenesis is expressed as mean counts per minute (cpm) for triplicate wells of individual cultures (standard deviation of the mean never exceeded 15 percent of CPM). Patients were considered to exhibit the ''rebound-overshoot'' phenomenon if, following cytotoxic chemotherapy, the level of PHA induced lymphoblastogenesis exhibited by their PBL was at least 50% greater than their pretreatment level.[9]

Assessment of 24-hour Preculture Sensitive Suppressor Activity in Patient PBL

For assessment of 24-hour preculture-sensitive suppressor activity, patient PBL were precultured for 24 hours prior to the addition of PHA stimulant. Briefly, cells were resuspended in RPMI-1640 medium supplemented with 10 percent FCS, 50 U/ml penicillin and 50 μg/ml streptomycin and 100 μl of cells were dispensed into culture plates as before. The next day, 100 μl of PHA suspended in RPMI-1640 medium containing 10 percent FCS, 50 U/ml penicillin and 50 μg/ml streptomycin were added to wells containing responder cells and the cultures were incubated an additional 72 hours prior to labeling and harvesting.

Assessment of Glass Adherent Suppressor Cell Activity in Patient PBL

For assessment of glass adherent suppressor cell activity, patient PBL were depleted of glass adherent cells prior to the addition of PHA stimulant. Briefly, PBL were resuspended in RPMI-1640 medium supplemented with 10 percent inactivated human AB serum, 50 U/ml penicillin and 50 μ/ml streptomycin to a final concentration of 2×10^6/ml and 5 ml of cells were dispensed into sterile glass tissue culture flasks. Flasks were incubated overnight at 37°C in a humidified atmosphere of 5% CO_2 in air following which nonadherent cells were recovered by gentle pipette aspiration and the percentage of monocytes remaining was determined by staining for alpha naphthyl acetate esterase (ANAE, Sigma). This procedure has been shown to adhere mononuclear phagocytes only, while permitting the release of polymorphonuclear phagocytes and adherent lymphocytes[10] and we have determined that this method reduces the percentage of ANAE positive cells in peripheral blood mononuclear cells from 10–20% to about 1–2%. Washed glass adherent cell depleted lymphocytes were then suspended to a concentration of 2×10^6/ml in RPMI-1640 medium supplemented with 20 percent fetal calf serum, 100 U/ml penicillin and 100 μg/ml streptomycin and 100 μl of cells were dispensed into triplicate wells of a 96-well microtiter plate. PHA stimulant was added and lymphocyte blastogenesis was assessed 72 hours later by methods described above.

Results

Assessment of 24-Hour Preculture Sensitive and Glass Adherent Cell Suppressor Activity in the Peripheral Blood Leukocytes of Cancer Patients Prior to Chemotherapy

PBL from cancer patients were subjected to an immediate stimulation with PHA and to a 24-hour precultivation or to depletion of glass adherent cells prior to stimulation with PHA. The level of lymphoblastogenesis obtained in nonmanipulated, 24-hour precultured and glass adherent cell-depleted cell cultures was determined 72 hours after the addition of stimulant (Table 1). The level of blastogenesis exhibited by nonmanipulated cell cultures from individual patients was compared to the mean level of blastogenesis obtained in a study of from six-ten normal individuals in the same decade of life as the patient. For purposes of this study, patients were considered to have an impaired PHA response if the level of blastogenesis exhibited by their PBL fell greater than 2 standard deviations below the mean level exhibited by their age-matched control group. The mean CPM/culture (± standard deviation) levels of blastogenesis exhibited by normal subjects was 60,640 ± 8575 for the fourth decade of life, 52,614 ± 9452 for the fifth decade of life, 49,680 ± 10,563 for the sixth decade of life and 42,997 ± 8817 for the seventh decade of life. Next, an augmentation index was calculated for each set of cultures by dividing the cpm per culture exhibited by 24-hour precultivated or glass adherent cell-depleted cells in the presence of PHA by the cpm per culture exhibited by nonmanipulated cells in the presence of PHA. These values were then compared to the augmentation indices exhibited by cells cultured under identical conditions from a group of 15 healthy subjects matched for age with the patient population. The mean augmentation indices (± standard deviation) exhibited by PBL from these normal individuals were 0.97 ± .33 and 1.10 ± .23 for 24-hour precultured and glass adherent cell-depleted cell cultures respectively. Augmentation indices greater than 2 standard deviations above or below the mean of these control group indices were considered to represent statistically significant differences in immunoregulatory suppressor activity in patient PBL. By these criteria, significantly depressed pretreatment PHA-induced lymphoproliferative responsiveness was seen in all patients except patient 1, significantly increased pretreatment 24-hour preculture-sensitive suppressor activity was detected in PBL from patients 2, 4, 5, and 10 while significantly increased glass adherent suppressor cell activity was detected in PBL from all patients except patient 8.

Assessment of the Effects of Chemotherapy on 24-Hour Preculture Sensitive and Glass Adherent Cell Suppressor Activity in PBL from Cancer Patients

At designated post-treatment assessment points (see Table 2), PBL from cancer patients were collected and assessed for their level of 24-hour preculture sensitive and glass adherent cell suppressor activity by the

Table 2. Effects of Cytotoxic Chemotherapy on 24-hour Preculture Sensitive and Glass Adherent Cell Suppressor Activity in Peripheral Blood Leukocytes from Cancer Patients

Patient	Days of Treatment	Blastogenesis (CPM)				
		Nonmanipulated	24-Hour Preculture	AI	Glass Nonad	AI
1	0	45751	60201	1.31	89986	(1.97)
	7	69632	54996	0.79	18346	(0.26)
	21	34893	50437	1.45	54144	(1.55)
2	0	9845	19373	1.97	17380	(1.77)
	14	37264	52433	1.40	33956	(0.91)
	28	12336	31272	2.54	47968	(3.89)
3	0	23434	13970	0.60	42958	(1.83)
	14	25819	33067	1.28	54577	(2.11)
	21	87910	53602	0.61	81379	(0.92)
4	0	16949	38837	2.29	40027	(2.36)
	7	50946	45751	0.90	36336	(0.71)
5	0	9758	21416	2.19	17609	(1.80)
	7	22529	14048	0.62	9499	(0.42)
6	0	9835	4772	0.49	47157	(4.79)
	3	4207	4220	1.00	23242	(5.50)
	7	7925	9410	1.19	49258	(6.22)
7	0	13194	10134	0.77	52104	(3.95)
	3	7954	8295	1.04	41459	(5.21)
	7	69683	61941	0.89	62510	(0.90)
8	0	19161	18146	0.95	13681	(0.71)
	3	8259	10937	1.32	6154	(0.74)
	7	21053	28022	1.33	17063	(0.81)
9	0	6170	6950	1.13	44465	(7.21)
	7	13064	35969	2.75	24929	(1.91)
	21	21193	28211	1.33	25115	(1.19)
10	0	7893	18465	2.34	23019	(2.92)
	7	12291	7615	0.62	13961	(1.14)
	21	8652	19391	2.24	5593	(2.96)

methods detailed above. Four of the breast cancer patients studied (patients 1-4) received a combination adjuvant chemotherapy regimen consisting of phenylalanine mustard and 5-fluorouracil and all exhibited post-treatment "rebound-overshoot" recovery of immune responsiveness in their nonmanipulated cell cultures (as evidenced by post-treatment values ranging from 1.5-3.8 fold greater than corresponding pretreatment values). The fifth breast cancer patient had disseminated disease and received therapy with adriamycin, 5-fluorouracil and cytoxan and also showed "rebound-overshoot" recovery of immune reactivity (post-treatment value was 2.3-fold greater than pretreatment value). In three of these patients (1, 4, and 5), "rebound-overshoot" occurred by Day seven post-treatment while in the other two patients (2 and 3) "rebound-overshoot" occurred on Days 14 and 21 respectively. The occurrence of "rebound-overshoot" was associated in each instance with a diminution of the augmentation indices exhibited by PBL subjected to 24-hour precultivation or glass adherent cell depletion from a pretreatment level that was significantly greater than normal (i.e., augmentation indices ranging from 1.97 to 2.36) to a post-treatment level that was well within, or even significantly below, normal limits (i.e., augmentation indices ranging from 0.26-1.40 at the time of "rebound-overshoot"). In addition, it was noted in two of these patients (1 and 2) that the reappearance of heightened augmentation indices was accompanied by a lowering of PHA-induced blastogenesis in the nonmanipulated cell cultures.

Of the three patients who received single agent chemotherapy with methotrexate (patients 6, 7, and 8) only one showed the "rebound-overshoot" phenomenon in their nonmanipulated cell cultures following treatment (this being patient 7 whose PHA-induced blastogenesis changed from 13,194 cpm prior to therapy to 69,683 cpm by Day seven post-treatment representing an increase of 5.3-fold of the pretreatment value). In that particular individual, "rebound-overshoot" was correlated with a substantial decrease in augmentation index in the glass adherent cell depletion test (e.g., 3.95 prior to therapy and 0.90 at the time of "rebound-overshoot"). In regard to the other two patients, patient 6 exhibited substantially increased augmentation indices in the glass adherent cell depletion test at each assessment point (4.79-6.22) while patient 8 exhibited normal augmentation indices at each assessment point. In each of these cases, therefore, the level of immunoregulatory suppressor activity appeared to be uneffected by chemotherapy and "rebound-overshoot" did not occur.

Each of the remaining two patients studied showed the "rebound-overshoot" phenomenon in association with a diminution of a previously heightened augmentation index to a normal augmentation index. Thus, for patient 9 lymphoblastogenesis changed from 6,170 cpm to 21,193 cpm (representing a rebound value 3.4-fold greater than pretreatment value) in association with a diminution in augmentation index for glass adherent cell depleted cultures of from 7.21 prior to therapy to 1.19 following therapy. For patient 10, lymphoblastogenesis rebounded from 7,893 cpm prior to therapy to 12,291 cpm by Day seven post-treatment (representing a rebound value 1.6-fold greater than pretreatment value) in association with a decline in augmentation indices from 2.34 and 2.92 to indices of 0.62 and 1.14 in the 24-hour preculture and glass adherent cell depletion tests respectively.

Discussion

This study demonstrates that drug-induced "rebound-overshoot" recovery of PHA-induced lymphoproliferative responsiveness in cancer patients is temporally associated with a diminution of 24-hour preculture sensitive and glass adherent cell suppressor activity. Of ten patients serially studied, eight exhibited the "rebound-overshoot" effect at a time following drug treatment when a previously heightened level of suppressor activity had diminished to a normal level. In the remaining two patients studied, "rebound-overshoot" was not observed nor was suppressor activity altered.

All of the patients entered on this study, with the exception of patient 8, exhibited a heightened level of either or both 24-hour preculture sensitive or glass adherent cell suppressor activity prior to therapy. Of these, 8/9 exhibited deficient PHA-induced lymphoblastogenesis. It would appear, therefore, that heightened levels of suppressor activity in this group of patients was responsible for the observed pretreatment immunodeficiency. However, pretreatment impaired immune responsiveness did not appear to be a prerequisite for the "rebound-overshoot" effect since for patient 1, "rebound-overshoot" occurred in the face of a normal pretreatment level of PHA-induced lymphoblastogenesis. Rather, it would appear from this study that a heightened pretreatment level of suppressor activity was a prerequisite for achieving "rebound-overshoot" following drug therapy. Thus, each of the eight patients who rebounded exhibited heightened pretreatment levels of suppressor activity while the one patient who did not (patient 8) never rebounded. Still, heightened pretreatment levels of suppressor activity alone did not guarantee that drug treatment would lead to "rebound-overshoot" since the other patient who did not rebound (patient 6) clearly exhibited heightened glass adherent cell suppressor activity but failed to rebound after receiving high dose methotrexate therapy. Further studies are needed to clarify these points.

The immunoregulatory mechanisms which were serially monitored in this study probably represent distinct but possibly overlapping phenomena.[11,12] Thus, glass adherent suppressor cells reportedly regulate human lymphoproliferative responses partly through synthesis of prostaglandins while the 24-hour preculture sensitive suppressor activity appear to be some form of regulation confined to the responding cells themselves, since fresh cells or exogenous prostaglandin cannot quantitatively overcome the augmented responsiveness of precultured cells.[11] In the present study, both kinds of suppressor activity appeared susceptible to cytotoxic chemotherapy (although differentially so) since the augmentation indices measured for each phenomenon substantially decreased following drug treatment in association with "rebound-overshoot".

The observation that immunosuppressive agents exert their effects on the immune system in a time-dependent manner has stimulated attempts to modulate immunity through the selective elimination of one or more lymphoid cell subpopulations. Thus, cytotoxic chemotherapy has been found, with appropriate manipulation of drug and antigen administration, to augment a variety of immunological reactions including antibody synthesis,[2] the development of delayed-type hypersensitivity,[3] the development of cell-mediated cytotoxicity,[4] mitogen responsiveness,[5] resistence to mycobacterial infections,[6] resistence to allogeneic or syngeneic tumor cells,[7,8] and resistence to adjuvant-induced disease.[5] In certain instances, it has been possible to ascribe the augmenting activity of drug treatment to a differential effect of the drug on immunoregulatory suppressor and effector cell functions. For example, cyclophosphamide reportedly can potentiate T cell-mediated immunity by eliminating blocking antibody[13] or suppressor T cells,[14] or by augmenting monocyte recruitment. [15] In contrast, oxisuram or 6-mercaptopurine may augment humoral immunity through the selective suppression of cell-mediated responses.[16,17] Methotrexate may restore depressed responsiveness to the T cell mitogens PHA and Con-A through a selective diminution of glass-adherent or plastic adherent suppressor cells in rat spleens[5] or by elimination of suppressor T cells in mice.[18] Furthermore, BCNU may augment cytotoxic cell development *in vitro*[4] by eliminating suppressor T cells which are selectively Con-A responsive and PHA nonresponsive.[19] The present study extends to the human situation the notion that immunoregulatory suppressor and effector functions may be differentially effected by cytotoxic drugs.

There are now a number of studies which suggest that effective chemotherapeutic treatment of cancer requires host immune responses. For example, cyclophosphamide therapy of chemically-induced murine sarcomas is more successful in immunostimulated hosts than in normal or immunodepressed hosts.[20] Similarly, the survival of leukemic mice treated with procarbazine is enhanced by immunostimulation if initiated within 48 hours following the cessation of drug treatment, but not if immunostimulation is delayed until longer periods of time.[21] In man, it has been observed that "rebound-overshoot" recovery of immune responsiveness to greater than pretreatment levels following cytotoxic chemotherapy is associated with a more favorable prognosis.[9] Since the present study indicates that post-therapy "rebound-overshoot" is due to drug-induced ablation of immunoregulatory suppressor activity, a knowledge of the effects of various single and combined agent regimens on suppressor and effector cell function should aid in the future drug scheduling design of chemotherapy trials.

The demonstration of suppressor cell mechanisms in patients following presumed definitive surgical resections for tumor (as with the four adjuvant chemotherapy breast cancer patients) may identify patients with true minimal residual disease. This might permit the selection of patients who could most benefit from adjuvant chemotherapy. For that chemotherapy to be effective it may be necessary that it not only exert cytotoxic effects on residual tumor, but also selectively inhibit abnormal immunoregulatory suppressor cell mechanisms that residual tumor may have activated. Treatment programs seeking to combine chemotherapy and immunotherapy will require careful assessment of cytotoxic drug effect on immunoregulatory suppressor cell mechanisms so as to most appropriately choose the time for optimum immunotherapeutic intervention.

The small number of patients studied in this preliminary investigation and the fact that more than half of those studied were receiving adjuvant chemotherapy does not permit any conclusion in this paper about the prognostic value of the "rebound-overshoot" phenomenon.

References

1. Hersh, EM: Immunosuppressive agents. In: Sartorelli, AC, Johns, DG, ed. *Antineoplastic and Immunosuppressive Agents I*, p. 577, Springer-Verlag, Berlin, Germany, 1974.

2. Duclos, H, Galanaud, P, Devinsky, O et al.: Enhancing effect of low dose cyclophosphamide treatment on the *in vitro* antibody response. *Eur. J. Immunol.* 7:679, 1977.

3. Polak, L, Rinck, C: Effect of the elimination of suppressor cells on the development of DNCB contact sensitivity in guinea pigs. *Immunology* 33:305, 1977.

4. Fass, L, Fefer, A: The application of an *in vitro* cytotoxicity test to studies of the effects of drugs on the cellular immune response in mice. I. Primary response. *J. Immunol.* 109:749, 1972.

5. Kourounakis, L, Kapusta, MA: Restoration of diminished T cell function in adjuvant induced disease by methotrexate: evidence for two populations of splenic T cell suppressors. *J. Rheum.* 3:346, 1977.

6. Alexander, J: Effect of cyclophosphamide treatment on the course of *Mycobacterium lepraemurium* infection and development of delayed-type hypersensitivity reactions in C57B1 and BALB/c mice. *Clin. Exp. Immunol.* 34:52, 1978.

7. Gerber, M, Andress, D, Pioch, Y et al.: Effect of cyclophosphamide and methylpred-

nisolone on *in vitro* cellular immune response to allogeneic tumor cells. *Transplant.* 26:142, 1978.

8. Falk, RE, Nossal, NA, Falk, JA: Effective antitumor immunity following elimination of suppressor T cell function. *Surg.* 84:483, 1978.

9. Harris, JE, Sengar, D, Stewart, T, Hyslop, D: The effect of immunosuppressive chemotherapy on immune function in patients with malignant disease. *Cancer* 37:1058, 1976.

10. Edelson, PJ, Cohn, ZA: Purification and cultivation of monocytes and macrophages. In: Bloom, BR, David, JR, eds. *In Vitro Methods in Cell-Mediated and Tumor Immunity,* 333, Academic Press, New York. 1976.

11. Rice, L, Laughter, AH, Twomey, JJ: Three suppressor systems in human blood that modulate lymphoproliferation. *J. Immunol.* 122:991, 1979.

12. Sohnle, PG, Collins-Lech, C: Differentiation of the effects of preincubation and indomethacin on lymphocyte transformation. *Clin. Immunol. and Immunopath.* 13:47, 1979.

13. Lagrange, PH, Mackaness, GB, Miller, TE: Potentiation of T cell-mediated immunity by selective suppression of antibody formation with cyclophosphamide. *J. Exp. Med.* 139:1529, 1974.

14. Mitsuoka, A, Morikawa, S, Baba, M, Harada, T: Cyclophosphamide eliminates suppressor T cells in age-associated central regulation of delayed hypersensitivity in mice. *J. Exp. Med.* 149:1018, 1979.

15. Milon, G, Marchal, G: Increased infiltration by monocytes in delayed type hypersensitivity site following cyclophosphamide treatment. *Immunol.* 35:989, 1978.

16. Freedman, HH: Selective immunosuppression of delayed hypersensitivity by oxisuram. In: Rosenthale, MF, Grossman, HC, eds., *Immunopharmacology.* Spectrum, New York, 1975.

17. Chanmougan, D, Schwartz, RS: Enhancement of antibody synthesis by 6-mercaptopurine. *J. Exp. Med.* 124:363, 1966.

18. Orbach-Arbouys, S, Castes, M: Augmentation of immune responses after methotrexate administration. *Immunol.* 36:265, 1979.

19. Stylos, WA, Chirigos, MA, Lengel, CR, Lyng, PJ: T and B lymphocyte populations of tumor-bearing mice treated with 1, 3 Bis(chloroethyl)–1–mitrosourea (BCNU) or Pryan. *Cancer Immunol. Immunother.* 5:165, 1978.

20. Moore, M, Williams, DE: Contribution of host immunity to cyclophosphamide therapy of a chemically-induced murine sarcoma. *Int. J. Cancer.* 11:358, 1973.

21. Amiel, JL, Berardet, M: Factor time for active immunotherapy after cytoreductive chemotherapy. *Europ. J. Cancer* 10:89, 1974.

Panel Discussion

MICHAEL HANNA: I have a question for Glenn Slemmer regarding the selective process of his model. When we do injection studies, do you think the metastatic clones of the lung have a lung stroma dependence? If so, is there a possibility that you are working with a selected clone which is a parenchymal cell that has a stromal dependence and that you are not working with a heterogeneous tumor anymore?

GLENN SLEMMER: Our studies of lung metastasis were done primarily with alveolar epithelial carcinoma mosaic-dependent cell types that required normal cells. They metastasize primarily to lungs, because they are confined to the arteries in the lungs, and are not likely to invade pulmonary veins to form systemic metastasis.

HANNA: In Josh Fidler's cloning system, he can show that within a tumor there are those cells that are highly metastatic and those that are less metastatic. In addition, he has some evidence indicating that there are also cells that have a certain propensity to certain organs. I don't know how solid this is but there is an indication that there may be both high or low metastatic cells which have a propensity for a certain site. In the model that you are studying, the cell that has the dependency on the mammary glands stroma, is it a selected clone and can you generalize from it?

SLEMMER: Metastatic populations have an increased probability of metastasizing in subsequent generations. This suggests, to some extent, that they are select sub-populations. The metastatic cells I showed are apparently a select sub-population in that they are totally dependent on normal cells. In the original tumor there are some cells that are not dependent on normal cells. The cells that are not dependent on normal cells do not metastasize. This suggests that the metastasizing sub-populations are select sub-populations which have characteristics that make them dependent on normal cells.

HANNA: What do you think this means to treatment? How would you view treatment then in disseminated disease?

SLEMMER: The neoplastic cells, that are part of the cancerous tissues, are totally dependent on this association with normal mammary cells. The evidence indicates this requires physical contact, but there could be some message that the myoepithelial cells, if that's what they are, are giving to the neoplastic epithelial cells and conceivably a drug could be developed that could block that interaction. If this were possible, then that form of metastatic breast carcinoma would be curable.

UNKNOWN: We have utilized another system which was chemically induced in the rat, the 13726 adenocarcinoma, and have used cloning techniques to derive cells from the parental tumor population. We took clones and implanted them in the mammary fat pad and they metastasized at a very high frequency. We could also directly inject these clones into the circulation and they colonized lungs with very high colonization potential. I think, within this system, the most malignant cells we could find within the population did not appear to require host-stromal cell or ductal cell component. I wonder whether you really have a tumor with a wide variety of different cell types, some of which require host cells for their livelihood and growth and others which are relatively autonomous. I think, in terms of tumor progression, we might be really selecting out the more autonomous cells within the population; those cells may have less of a tendency with time to require normal host cells. I believe that's consistent with your findings when you passage them.

SLEMMER: What I have observed is that mammary carcinomas represent different classes that have an entirely different biology. The alveolar epithelial carcinomas are dependent upon association with normal cells, apparently myoepithelial cells; while myoepithelial carcinomas represent an entirely different class of neoplasia. Biologically, breast cancer is at least three separate diseases. The different forms of cells are transformed by different etiologic factors, have different epidemiology, different biology, different cell biology, etc. Myoepithelial neoplasms are composed of pure populations of neoplastic cells, or at least the non-mosaic tumors I have studied, and tumors arising from these types of cells would be expected to behave like melanomas and sarcomas in terms of their biology and metastasis, particularly after they have been selected through many serial transplant generations. I believe then that the mammary carcinoma cell lines that have been studied for metastasis are probably all myoepithelial cell lines. The method used for transferring mammary tumors, i.e., cell suspensions method, selects against the mosaic-dependent carcinomas so you would lose those tumors. In fact, there are reports of tumors which could not be passaged serially by means of cell suspensions.

UNKNOWN: Based on our own experience, I think we have seen both types of populations morphologically existing in the same primary tumor. We have been able to clone out cells which look like myoepithelial cells when reinjected into animals and those cells are more metastatic if assayed in one of these metastasis assays. However, we do have cells which look like ductal epithelial cells *in vivo* and look like epithelial cells *in vitro,* and they also metastasize and do not seem to require host-stromal cells for that process. So, I think you could have both in those populations. I tend to agree with you, at least from our own experience in the one or two myoepithelial lines that we have, that they are more metastatic and that they grow at a slower rate than the cells that we think are epithelial cells.

UNKNOWN: I am a clinician and I do a little research. I always have some question in my mind whether what I am doing in the research world can be applied back to the clinic. Do you think there is clinical significance in the concept of heterogeneity?

HANNA: I think the clinical significance of heterogeneity was seen before the concept of heterogeneity was described. It was seen with chemotherapy of leukemias. When do they selectively clone naturally for chemotherapeutic resistant lines? I once heard Peter Nowell give a lecture on chemotherapy of leukemias and he pointed out that had they known the concept of heterogeneity they would have been able to strategize a little better and be a little less dumbfounded by some of the findings.

UNKNOWN: I think we are looking at sub-populations when we study these metastatic cells. The question in my own mind is, do we try and understand the biology of metastasis or simply treat it as a black box? I'm all for trying to understand some of the biologic mechanisms that occur during metastasis and studying cells which are highly successful. Sugarbaker once said, these are the marathon cells. They are capable of metastasizing and, therefore, I think very important to study. If we look at animal tumor models, where we selectively pulled out sub-populations and studied their various properties, it may well be they may not relate directly to the clinical situation. It's probably true, where you are dealing with a primary population that has both the highly malignant sub-populations and a lot of other cells too. I think it is a very minor sub-population that is highly malignant and highly metastatic that presents the most threat to patients and, therefore, these cell types are interesting.

HANNA: I think what we do in some cases with these models is to categorize the various phenotypes of the tumors. I have had this argument with Josh Fidler, we argue all the time. He tells me how important all of this is; I tell him how important could it be? I could take the line 10 tumor, I could stick it in the muscle, I could extract it to segregate it, mix it with BCG, stick it in the skin and cure those metastatic cells that are in the lung, which obviously had gone through and past the marathon and now have survived in the lung. How important can it be? Then he gets very confused and he swears at me in Yiddish and walks off. The point being though, it is important for certain types of treatment. For other types of treatment it may be less important. There are many phenotypes; a particular therapy that I am supporting now recognizes a commonality among the phenotypes. If you had to do a battery of treatments you would want to know their properties, you would want to know their differences, and you would want to know their points of similarity or commonalities. It is important that you have a data base regarding the malignancy before you attempt any type of therapy.

UNKNOWN: Dr. Hanna, what is the significance of heterogeneity for immunotherapy? Are we utilizing the wrong populations when we immunize against the primary tumor cells? If, as some investigators claim, metastatic tumor cells have different immunogenic properties, then preparing a vaccine from the primary tumor cells is wrong.

HANNA: I think that's the point I just made. We did prepare a vaccine.

UNKNOWN: What if you use the metastases?

HANNA: If I take the lung nodules out, in some cases I get 100% cure. The cures being that the animals are still alive after two years. Why would I go back and remove the lung nodules? Why would I want to do that? The point I was trying to make, and I think it is an important point, is that there are various phenotypes in a tumor and, based on certain approaches to controlling the malignancy, they could be used as a positive avenue to do something. There are also commonalities that all of the phenotypes are going to have and that is some weak tumor antigen. I have not seen any strong convincing evidence that cells that are metastatic are less antigenic, that cells that are less metastatic are more antigenic, or any combination you want to make. In fact, it would not be important if there were quantitative differences. You would have to have qualitative differences. You would have to have qualitative differences before it would make a difference in immunotherapy. I have seen no evidence that there are qualitative differences in terms of tumor antigens of the cells.

UNKNOWN: I think it is going to be hard to find qualitative differences between tumor cells. It is one thing that we ruled out many years ago. There are no explicit types of properties that occur on these cells; either compared to normal cells or compared to other tumor cells within a heterogeneous population. There are some experiments which have demonstrated different classes of antigens on metastatic cells; and perhaps these are not important in your guinea pig system but they may be important in other systems.

HANNA: I should qualify that to transplantation antigens.

UNKNOWN: Right, in that system it seems to be very important to immunize with metastases and not with the primary. You will prevent metastasis if you try to immunize with cells from the primary tumor but you can prevent it if you immunize with metastatic cells.

HANNA: One of the things that is happening in the clinics where this procedure is used is they are using primary cells and immunizing against distant lymph node metastases. Using this for the vaccine, I think, is a plus.

UNKNOWN: I think that's a step in the right direction. The main concern, at least in my own mind, is to the therapy that failed, not to the therapy that succeeds. If you have a therapy that succeeds, you can find a theory that will make it work. It's really the therapy that fails to cure metastases, and there are a lot of examples in tumor immunology, that is important.

UNKNOWN: I have a question regarding the timing of chemoimmuno-therapy. Do you feel that it is best to give immunotherapy at a depressed state or at the time of rebound?

HANNA: I'll let Joe Sokal answer that question.

JOSEPH SOKAL: It's an interesting question. The tendency has been among clinical immunotherapists to go for the rebound of immuno-logic reactivity and to give the immunotherapy seven to 14 days after the chemotherapy to take advantage of the immunologic reactivity. I don't know any one who could give you hard data. I've never heard of anyone even thinking of setting up a controlled study of vaccinating half the patients at the height of the chemotherapy suppression and the other half during the rebound.

UNKNOWN: I am thinking that Dr. Tseng and Dr. Harris should get together. Dr. Tseng will give cytoxan one hour before and 24 hours after surgery to achieve a therapeutic effect; and, it seems to me, from Dr. Harris' paper, the point of rebound is the time at which you might want to give immune stimulation. These are very important points clinically.

MAO TSENG: The reason we give cyclophosphamide 24 hours after surgery is because our studies showed that initial rapid tumor cell clearance usually became slower and steadier after 24 hours and therefore the time to treat. The reason we give cyclophosphamide one hour before tumor excision, in our mind, is that at the preoperative period the micrometastases and tumor volume is at a minimum.

DAVID SALKIN: Dr. Hanna, both experimentally and clinically the metastatic cell is very different from the parental cell. Are there any chemicals on the metastatic cell wall, as part of the cell wall, that have been discovered? I know some work has been done at the Salk Clinic where they felt they discovered sialic acid. Are there any other chemicals that are on the cell wall? Are some of those chemicals amenable to a penetration by other chemicals? I am thinking particularly of *coccidioides immitis* where amphotericin B is used; the use of tetracycline by itself has no effect but seems to augment the effect of the amphotericin B. Can we use something like amphotericin B or tetracycline plus some other agent to penetrate or damage that cell wall and get into the malignant cell?

HANNA: I think we have just recently with clones obtained the tools to study this thoroughly. I think, based on some of the studies of Garth Nicolson and Isaiah Fidler, we now have the armamentarium phenotypes to pursue this biochemically. The problem in the past has been that whenever we've tried to look at tumor cell surfaces for commonalities or differences from normal cell surfaces we've always been looking at a heterogeneous population of cells. We have to be very careful because many of these cell lines that are being cloned for high and low metastatic potential, phenotypic expressions and biological characterizations, are lines that have been passaged for a very long time in animal models. For all we know, they've changed from the original primary tumors. Recently, we began using ultraviolet radiation-induced tumors and fibrosarcomas and applying the same type of cloning procedures to them. We showed that a one generation transplant had the same heterogeneous nature in terms of high and low metastatic potential as the original. It encourages us to think this is general and, with good biochemistry of the surface components of these various lines, we may see some differences or similarities.

UNKNOWN: Recently, it has been seen in transformed sarcoma lines. The heterogeneity appears very quickly and that may be the hallmark of a very malignant population, the ability to spin off a variety of phenotypic variants. Then, sooner or later, variants will pop up which are highly successful in invading and metastasizing. We certainly know more now about the biochemistry of the cell surface; but you have to realize that even the structure of biological membranes was not known until about 1972. When you speak of certain chemical constituents at the cell surface, many of these such as sialic acid are on all cells that have been examined. A year or two ago, I reviewed all the biochemical cell surface data that I could find and my conclusion was that there was no generalized phenomena that changed the surface of the cell when it became transformed or more malignant. Each system tends to be different in terms of its cell surface properties and this probably reflects the fact that tumors arise from a wide variety of different cell types *in vivo* which have different properties. It is very hard to make generalizations from one system to another, from animal models to clinical situations, even from one patient to another patient. I think it is going to be a difficult problem to solve in the future.

HANNA: The interesting thing to think about is that the heterogeneity concept says that from any tumor there are various cell types, each with different biological properties. One that we can easily assess *in vivo* is metastatic potential. If you think about the genetics of any one tumor it means accepting that tumors originate from one cell and that during tumor development there is a lot of genetic alteration so you then have this array of phenotypes.

UNKNOWN: There does not even have to be genetic alteration going on to end up with many phenotypes. If you have an alteration in the controlling mechanism, then I think that would be all that would be necessary to spin off a large number of cell surface phenotypes. Without going into great detail, there have been a number of studies on cell surface antigens which indicate that the control of expression is under a very complex system of regulation. It's not so much that genes are altered during progression of tumors or during their selection *in vitro,* it's that their control seems to be altered. When you perform a series of fusions between cells which express high levels and cells which express low levels, you end up with a very wide variety of different types of lines. This suggests it's a controlling mechanism and not a gene-dosage effect that has to do with the display of these components on the cell surface.

Prognostic Indicators and Tumor Progression in Man

The Role of Polyamines as Predictors of Success and Failure in Cancer Chemotherapy

Brian G. M. Durie

Section of Hematology and Oncology, College of Medicine, University of Arizona, Tucson, Arizona

Summary

Polyamines are low molecular weight, highly charged organic cations ubiquitous in nature and intimately involved with cell growth. Intracellular levels of polyamines, primarily spermidine and putrescine, increase early and dramatically with growth, particularly in rapidly growing tissues. Increased levels of polyamines have been noted in both the blood and urine of patients with advanced cancer. Changes in polyamine levels in patients with early disease are insufficient to allow polyamines to be used effectively for diagnosis. However, changes in blood and urine levels in patients with known cancer would seem to reflect accurately both tumor burden and particularly, disease activity. The extracellular levels of polyamines have been correlated with the *in vitro* labeling index of tumor cells. Serial studies in patients with advanced cancer undergoing chemotherapy have shown statistically significant increases in both plasma and urine levels of spermidine in patients having substantial cell kill and responding to therapy. In contrast, the patients failing to respond to therapy do not have such significant elevations in extracellular levels. Initial studies in patients with several types of tumors indicate that this type of elevation in extracellular polyamine levels with successful chemotherapy may prove to be an excellent and early marker of tumor cell kill and response.

114

Introduction

In 1971 Russell reported the increased excretion of polyamines in the urine of patients with cancer.[1] This raised the possibility that measurement of polyamine levels in clinical fluid and tissue specimens could be useful in the diagnosis and evaluation of patients with cancer. Based upon animal studies of tumor growth and regression, both spontaneous and in response to radiation and chemotherapy, a model was proposed to summarize the potential role of polyamines as biochemical markers of human tumor cell growth and tumor cell death (Figure 1). This working hypothesis has simplified considerably the initial evaluation of the clinical role of polyamine determinations.

The difficulties and expense involved in measuring polyamine levels in clinical samples have required an early detailed analysis of what the potential applications might be. The results of studies to date indicate that the value of polyamine determinations will vary in the different areas of cancer diagnosis and treatment.[2] The conclusion of a recent conference on the question[2] was that, as for most currently available markers, the potential for using polyamine determinations in cancer screening is quite limited. However, there could well be considerable utility in predicting or monitoring the effectiveness of therapy.

Figure 1. Model of polyamines as biochemical markers of cancer.
Source: *Data reproduced with permission of Russell et al. and Lancet.*[16]

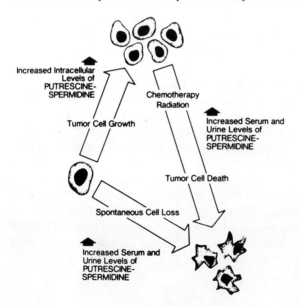

Polyamines and Cancer Screening

There are different criteria which can be used to define the utility of a specific test as a clinical laboratory tool. For cancer screening, as has been carefully outlined by Galen and Gambino,[3] there are at least four major parameters which include the sensitivity, specificity, predictive value and efficiency of the test(s) involved (Table 1). The value of polyamine determinations in cancer screening depends somewhat upon one's expectations in terms of accuracy for a single test or group of tests.

Unfortunately, no matter how one views it, both the sensitivity and specificity of polyamines and other markers in patients with cancer are considerably lower than one would hope. The sensitivity of polyamines ranges from 30–90 percent for patients with advanced cancer. However, this is not even the group of patients for whom the question of diagnosis arises. The overall sensitivity in patients with low tumor cell burden, as might be found in patients being screened for a possible early cancer, remains to be clarified. Data from several workers indicate that the percentage of patients with low tumor burden with abnormal polyamine levels is probably less than 30 percent. For example, Townsend et al.,[4] studying the pattern of urinary excretion of polyamines in patients with malignant melanoma, reported only four of 46 patients with Stage 1 malignant melanoma having elevations in two or more urinary polyamines (Table 2). However, Lipton et al.[5] and Sanford et al.[6] noted significant polyamine elevations in patients with localized cancer as did Fair et al.[7]

Table 1. Polyamines and Cancer Screening

Criteria for Clinical Laboratory Screening[a]	Meaning of Criteria	Value for Polyamines[b]
Sensitivity	Percentage of patients with documented cancer having positive result	30-90%[c]
Specificity	Percentage negative results in patients without cancer	Maximum probably 70-80%
Predictive Value	Percentage positive results that are true positives in comparison with both healthy and other disease subjects	Approximately 0.1%[d]
Efficiency	Percentage of all results in screened population which are true results	75%

[a] Galen and Gambino.[3]

[b] See text for discussion.

[c] Waalkes et al.[10]

[d] Based upon: average sensitivity of 75 percent; specificity of 75 percent; cancer incidence in screened population of 100,000 cases of 40/100,000.

Table 2. Number of Patients with Elevated Urinary Polyamines with Reference to the Number of Elevations Seen per Patient

Group	Number of Polyamines Elevated[a]			
	0	1	2 or 3	3
Stage I				
Active	1/5	3/5	1/5	0/5
Stable	22/41 (54%)	16/41 (39%)	3/41 (7%)	1/41 (2%)
Stage II				
Active.	3/6	0/6	3/6	2/6
Stable	9/13 (69%)	3/13 (23%)	1/13 (8%)	0/13
Stage III				
Active	2/23 (9%)	4/23 (17%)	17/23 (74%)	8/23 (35%)
Stable	2/3	0/3	1/3	0/3
Total Active	6/34 (18%)	7/34 (21%)	21/34 (62%)	10/34 (29%)
Total Stable	33/57 (58%)	19/57 (33%)	5/57 (9%)	1/57 (2%)

[a] Number of patients with number of elevations indicated per total number studied (percent elevated).

Source: Data reproduced with permission of Townsend, Banda, and Marton and Cancer.[4]

in patients with carcinoma of the prostate confined to the gland itself. In general, one must conclude that only a small percentage of patients can be expected to be detected on the basis of polyamine elevations at the time of early tumor growth. Elevations must be expected to be modest and potentially confused with other causes of polyamine elevations.

Extracellular elevations of polyamines occur with any significant cell growth and/or cell loss and this is perhaps the most troublesome facet of potential screening for cancer, as carefully outlined by Dreyfuss et al.[8] and subsequently by Waalkes et al.[9,10] Elevations of polyamines of a similar magnitude to those found in patients with cancer can be found in a wide variety of inflammatory and infectious disease processes. Elevations in two or more of the polyamines are clearly more specific for cancer as opposed to noncancer pathology. However, such elevations can still be found in at least 10–20 percent of patients with noncancer pathology. Requirements for an elevation of two or more polyamines also restrict the number of cancer patients who would be in this category. Thus, diagnostic specificity is obtained at the expense of a reduction in sensitivity. The best hope for improvement in specificity is from more sophisticated analysis of all polyamine levels (putrescine, spermidine, spermine) plus other disease markers which might be available in given tumor types could considerably improve the specificity. Woo et al.[11] have performed multiple correlations of various marker combinations with disease status of breast cancer patients and have found an R = 0.891 based on urinary polyamines, nucleosides and CEA. Polyamines and nucleosides together were excellent markers of disease status, R = 0.843. Alone, polyamines had an R = 0.594, nucleosides, R = 0.658, and CEA, R = 0.259.

Nishioka and Romsdahl,[12,13] evaluating patients with colon cancer, have looked at the diagnostic sensitivity and specificity of both polyamine and CEA determinations. Stage D patients had significantly more frequent polyamine elevations than B or C patients (p > 0.0025). Also, with the combined use of polyamines and CEA, the frequency of significant marker elevation increased overall by approximately 10 percent (from 65 to 75 percent).

The true predictive value of a clinical screening test is the usefulness in distinguishing cancer patients from other disease categories as well as control (normal) groups. Polyamines, particularly in patients with low tumor burden, have a very low predictive value. Thus, when used alone, polyamines have a very low overall efficiency in the detection of latent cancer. At present, the difficulty and expense of polyamine measurements in urine, plasma, cerebrospinal fluid, or other body compartments or fluids have resulted in a considerable lack of enthusiasm for the application of polyamine determinations in widespread cancer screening, even in high risk groups.

Polyamines and Cancer Staging

Over the past several years, it has become critically important to assess the stage or extent of cancer in an individual patient before deciding upon appropriate therapy. Patients with multiple myeloma, in whom tumor burden has been directly measured,[14] have provided especially good examples of the correlation between stage and extracellular polyamine levels (Table 3). Another example is outlined in Table 2 from the work of Townsend et al.[4] in which over 90 percent of patients with

Table 3. Pretreatment Urinary Spermidine Levels and Myeloma Cell Mass

Myeloma cell mass (Cells x 10^{12} / m^2)	Number of Patients	Urinary Spermidine (μg/mg Creatinine)	
		Mean	Range
High ($>$ 1.2)	20	3.41	1.36 – 4.93
Intermediate (0.60–1.2)	14	1.20	0.66 – 1.77
Low ($<$ 0.6)	10	0.32^a	0.20 – 0.55

^{a} P $<$ 0.01 for differences – high/intermediate/low.

active Stage III melanoma had significant elevations in polyamines as compared with a much smaller percentage in patients with Stage I disease. Since polyamine elevations are not always specific, the finding of polyamine elevations may only be used as supportive evidence for advanced stage disease. Polyamine determinations could be used in the same way liver function tests or lung tomograms are used as adjunctive staging measures.

Polyamines as Markers of Response to Cancer Therapy

Almost all the workers who have evaluated polyamine levels in patients with cancer have noted dramatic decreases toward normal values in patients who have undergone successful therapy—surgery, chemotherapy, immunotherapy or some other form of therapy. As noted originally by Denton et al.[15] and subsequently by Townsend et al.,[4] Russell et al.,[16] and in a recent large study by Durie et al.,[17] dramatic increases in extracellular polyamine levels occur concomitant with successful therapy. Figure 2 shows the comparison of polyamine levels in three groups of patients having complete, partial and no response to a given

Figure 2. Urinary spermidine level in patients receiving various cancer chemotherapeutic regimes. Time zero was prior to chemotherapy and Day one was the start of chemotherapy. Each point is the mean from 56 different patients with no response, partial response, or a complete response to therapy as judged by later standard clinical parameters.

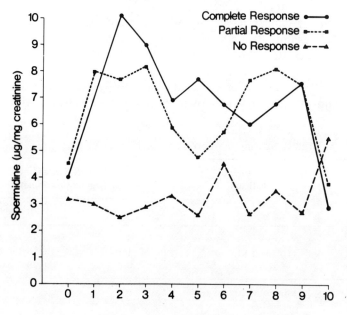

course of combination chemotherapy. There is a highly significant early rise in spermidine levels associated with a complete response to therapy. Other studies[18] and unpublished data have shown that comparable rises in plasma spermidine levels in the first 72 hours of initiation of therapy also correspond to excellent cell kill and subsequent response to therapy.

Although the early rise in extracellular spermidine levels associated with successful therapy has now been documented by several workers, much more work is necessary to clarify the details of the associated polyamine metabolism and clinical circumstances in which single or serial measurements of polyamines may be useful.

With respect to clinical applications, there can be no doubt that an early marker of tumor cell kill could be very useful. For example, in patients with solid tumors which have very few measurable lesions which can be used to evaluate response objectively, the early rises in plasma and/or urinary levels of spermidine and putrescine might be the only early markers of response available. The early rise in spermidine could precede by many weeks any change on X-ray or scanner.

Another area of potential application of polyamine information is in correlation with *in vitro* drug sensitivity testing. A stem cell assay system has been developed recently which enables *in vitro* culture (short term) and drug sensitivity testing of human tumor cells.[19] The combined evidence of *in vitro* sensitivity to a particular drug plus early evidence of tumor cell kill on treatment with the same drug (from determinations of polyamine levels) has already been useful in clinical decision making.

Another area of considerable importance with respect to quantitation of cell kill is in the adjuvant treatment of cancer. Polyamines are probably very insensitive for the detection of small amounts of residual disease after initial surgery and/or radiotherapy. However, with adjuvant chemotherapy following this initial debulking, it should be possible to quantitate the cell kill with specific adjuvant chemotherapy schedules. With this quantitative approach, it might well be possible to select an adjuvant program with the maximum cell kill capacity. The adjuvant breast chemotherapy protocol at the University of Arizona[20] is currently being tested in this way.

Polyamines and Tumor Kinetics

One exciting observation dealing with the clinical use of polyamines has been putrescine levels and the *in vitro* labeling index [(^{3}H)-thymidine] of tumors and other body tissues. A number of animal studies has shown a relationship between intracellular polyamines, particularly putrescine, and tumor growth rates. In the past several years, a number of human studies also have supported the concept of increased extracellular polyamines associated with rapid tumor growth. A specific, important observation is the correlation of urinary putrescine with the *in vitro* (^{3}H)-thymidine labeling of myeloma cells representing a direct correlation between apparent tumor growth fraction and urinary putrescine levels. This initial observation has been extended subsequently to include patients with other hematologic malignancies, including myelogenous leukemias and lymphomas. There is, therefore, the capacity to use urinary putrescine as a marker of tumor kinetics which could prove particularly valuable in the design of chemotherapy schedules.

Assessment of Remission or Relapse Status

Many observations that polyamine levels in body fluids, particularly urine, plasma and cerebrospinal fluid, return to normal levels during remission of a known cancerous process have stimulated the use of polyamine determinations in the evaluation of the remission or relapse of individual patients. It is clear that polyamine levels are frequently normal at the time of remission. However, evaluation of relapse status has been hampered by the specificity and sensitivity of polyamine determinations at low levels when tumor burden is small. Nonetheless, a number of studies[21,13] has now shown significant elevations associated with relapse as illustrated in Table 4. With adequate controls and clinical and laboratory evaluations for conditions which could give spurious elevations in polyamines, there is potential for the use of polyamine determinations in this way.

One of the more exciting possibilities in this area is the potential use of polyamine determinations in tissue specimens for evaluation of the presence or absence of malignant cells. The study of Rennert et al.,[22] summarized in Table 5, illustrates this role for polyamine determinations. Serial determinations of polyamines in bone marrow samples from patients, in this case children, with acute leukemia before treatment and at various stages thereafter, indicated that significant elevations were

Table 4. Urinary Putrescine Levels in Patients with Multiple Myeloma as a Function of Remission or Relapse

Disease Status	Number of Patients	Urinary Putrescine (μg/mg Creatinine)	
		Mean	Range
Remission	13	0.97	0.4–1.88
Relapse	20	6.4[a]	2.3–13.21

[a] P $<$ 0.01 for difference – remission/relapse.

Table 5. Free Polyamine Concentrations in Bone Marrow Cells in Patients with Acute Lymphocytic Leukemia[a]

	Putrescine	Spermidine (nmole/ml)	Spermine	Spermidine/ Spermine Ratio
Relapse	6.81	89.3	124.8	0.93
Remission	2.34	52.03	70.0	0.87

[a] Rennert et al.[22]

associated with the relapse state and that polyamine levels were substantially different with remission.

From this summary of the current and potential applications of polyamine determinations in the clinical setting, it is clear that much more work needs to be done. Probably the major requirement necessary to allow completion of the many conceived large clinical studies is a rapid, simple method for the measurement of polyamines in clinical samples. As discussed, it seems that development of the radioimmunoassay will be the best approach to this problem. When such a method becomes available, rapid progress in clarifying the many areas discussed can be anticipated.

References

1. Russell, DH: Increased polyamine concentrations in the urine of human cancer patients. *Nature* 233:144–145, 1971.

2. Cohen, SS: Conference on polyamines in cancer. *Cancer Res.* 37:939–944, 1977.

3. Galen, RS, Gambino, SR: *Beyond Normality: The Predictive Value and Efficiency of Medical Diagnosis,* pp. 1–237, John Wiley and Sons, Inc., New York, 1975.

4. Townsend, RM, Banda, PW, Marton, LJ: Polyamines in malignant melanoma. Urinary excretion and disease progress. *Cancer* 38:2088–2092, 1976.

5. Lipton, A, Sheehan, LM, Kessler, GF: Urinary polyamine levels in human cancer. *Cancer* 35:464–468, 1975.

6. Sanford, EJ, Drago, JR, Rohner, TJ et al.: Preliminary evaluation of urinary polyamines in the diagnosis of genitourinary tract malignancy. *J. Urology* 113:218–221, 1975.

7. Fair, WR, Wehner, N, Brorsson, U: Urinary polyamine levels in the diagnosis of carcinoma of the prostate. *J. Urology* 114:88–92, 1975.

8. Dreyfuss, F, Chayen, R, Dreyfuss, G et al.: Polyamine excretion in the urine of cancer patients. *Israel J. Med. Sci.* 11:785–795, 1975.

9. Waalkes, TP, Gehrke, CW, Bleyer, WA et al.: Potential biologic markers in Burkitt's lymphoma. *Cancer Chemother. Rep.* 59:721–727, 1975.

10. Waalkes, TP, Gehrke, CW, Tormey, DC et al.: Urinary excretion of polyamines by patients with advanced malignancy. *Cancer Chemother. Rep.* 59:1103–1116, 1975.

11. Woo, KB, Waalkes, TP, Ahmann, DL et al.: A quantitative approach to determining

disease status during therapy using multiple biologic markers: application to carcinoma of the breast. *Cancer* (in press).

12. Nishioka, K, Romsdahl, MM: Elevation of putrescine and spermidine in sera of patients with solid tumors. *Clin. Chim. Acta* 57:155–161, 1974.

13. Nishioka, K, Romsdahl, MM: Preliminary longitudinal studies of serum polyamines in patients with colorectal carcinoma. *Cancer Lett.* 3:197–202, 1977.

14. Durie, BGM, Salmon, SE: A clinical staging system for multiple myeloma. *Cancer* 36:842–854, 1975.

15. Denton, MD, Glazer, HS, Zellner, DC, Smith, FG: Gas-chromatographic measurement of urinary polyamines in cancer patients. *Clin. Chem.* 19:904–907, 1973.

16. Russell, DH, Durie, BGM, Salmon, SE: Polyamines as predictors of success and failure in cancer chemotherapy. *Lancet II:*797–799, 1975.

17. Durie, BGM, Salmon, SE, Russell, DH: Polyamines as markers of response and disease activity in cancer chemotherapy. *Cancer Res.* 37:214–221, 1977.

18. Russell, DH, Russell, SD: Relative usefulness of measuring polyamines in serum, plasma, and urine as biochemical markers of cancer. *Clin. Chem.* 21:860–863, 1975.

19. Hamburger, A, Salmon, SE: Primary bioassay of human myeloma stem cells. *J. Clin. Invest.* 60:846–854, 1977.

20. Hammond, N, Jones, SE, Salmon, SE et al.: Adjuvant treatment of breast cancer with adriamycin-cyclophosphamide with or without radiation therapy. In: Salmon, SE, Jones, SE, eds. *Adjuvant Therapy of Cancer,* pp. 153–160, Elsevier/North-Holland Biomedical Press, Amsterdam, 1977.

21. Miale, TD, Rennert, OM, Lawson, DL et al.: Bone marrow polyamines in children with acute leukemia as related to remission status, therapy, and cellularity of specimens. *Med. Pediatr. Oncol.* 3:209–230, 1977.

22. Rennert, O, Miale, T, Shukla, J et al.: Polyamine concentrations in bone marrow aspirates of children with leukemia and other malignancies. *Blood* 47:695–701, 1976.

Multivariate Analysis of Response and Survival of Patients with Advanced Prostate Cancer in a Combination Chemotherapy Program: Key Role of Serum LDH[a]

Edwin Cox, David Paulson, William Berry, John Laszlo

Department of Medicine and Department of Surgery, Duke University Medical Center, Durham, North Carolina

Summary

In 84 patients with estrogen refractory metastatic prostate cancer, we have found that a simple, nontoxic multiagent chemotherapy program is effective and have established objective response criteria. Multivariate analyses of survival and response were carried out to determine the contribution of various clinical factors to prognosis. Serum lactate dehydrogenase (LDH) level at study entry proved to be the single most important prognostic variable, both to response rate and survival duration. Lower values were associated with higher probability of response (p=0.0001) and longer survival (p=0.0001). LDH contributed to survival even when response had been accounted for. Other important prognostic factors disclosed were initial serum level of carcinoembryonic antigen and WBC nadir to response rate, degree of bone pain, serum acid phosphatase and age of presentation with regard to survival. Comparison of observed survival with that predicted from regression analysis indicates that the prolongation of survival in responders cannot be attributed solely to differences in underlying prognostic factors.

Metastatic prostate cancer has generally been treated like a redheaded stepchild by the oncologist for several obvious reasons. The disease

[a]These studies were supported in part by PHS Grant CA 14236 from the National Cancer Institute.

occurs in older men and, since it follows a fairly indolent course as compared with many other cancers we treat, patients frequently succumb to intercurrent disease. Metastatic prostate cancer is susceptible to estrogen therapy, which is simple to administer and often produces dramatic symptomatic improvement. Since bone is the predominant site of metastatic involvement, accurate objective measurement of disease extent is only occasionally possible. The published studies of chemotherapy, mostly with single agents, have not been particularly promising. Recently, a major review paper on prostate cancer depicted the role of chemotherapy as tentative and developmental, in contrast to its well-established role in the treatment of other solid tumors. We wish to provide a countercurrent to this prevailing trend by outlining a chemotherapy regimen, developed at the Duke Comprehensive Cancer Center, which is effective, relatively easy to administer and minimally toxic.[1,2] Factors prognostic to the attainment of response and length of survival will be explored with special emphasis on the central role of serum lactic dehydrogenase (LDH) and the contribution of chemotherapy responsiveness to survival.

In 1973, a study of multiagent chemotherapy was begun at the Duke Comprehensive Cancer Center by the collaboration of Dr. David Paulson, the head of urologic oncology, and Dr. John Laszlo, medical oncologist, the head of the clinical research program at the Center. The striking success of multiagent chemotherapy in treating metastatic breast carcinoma was becoming widely appreciated which contrasted with the previous modest results in treating that disease with single agent therapy. It was recognized that prostate cancer shares some important characteristics with breast cancer. Both are adenocarcinomas, and in each, there is endocrine modulation of the growth and development of the normal tissue from which the cancer arises, as well as hormonal receptors demonstrable on the tumors themselves in many cases. It was reasoned that if multiagent therapy were effective in breast cancer, then there was a reasonable probability that a similar type of therapy could be useful in prostate cancer as well. Breast cancer treatment, at the time, followed the Cooper regimen,[3] which included cyclophosphamide, methotrexate, fluorouracil, vincristine, and prednisone; a similar regimen was proposed for prostate cancer. It was thought that chemical cystitis, because of cyclophosphamide, might be a problem in these patients, many of whom had urinary obstruction, so melphalan was used as a substitute alkylating agent in the prostate cancer regimen (Table 1). The final objective was to keep the program simple and relatively nontoxic so that it could be used in a urology clinic where previous experience with the use of chemotherapy agents was limited.

All 88 patients had routine blood and chemistry surveys, measures of endocrine function and baseline radiologic and scintigraphic studies of

Table 1. Chemotherapy Regimen for Hormonally Refractory Metastatic
Prostate Cancer

Melphalan	2 mgm	p.o.	Daily	Continuous
Methotrexate	25 mgm	p.o.	Weekly	Continuous
5-FU	500 mgm	p.o.	Weekly	Continuous
Vincristine	1 mgm	IV	Weekly x 4 wk	Repeat 4 wk course every 4 mo
Prednisone	40 mgm	p.o.	Daily x 2 wk	Taper 5 mgm/wk to 10 mgm, then continuous

the skeleton. Most of these studies were repeated at intervals of one to three months, including bone scans and X-rays, to determine how the different serial measures of disease activity correlated. All patients entering the chemotherapy program previously had received either estrogen therapy, orchiectomy or both and all had failed or progressed on this treatment. Many patients who had responded previously to estrogens continued to have them during the course of chemotherapy.

It was apparent from the first group of patients who were treated that many of them were obtaining significant improvement from bone pain and, also, in their sense of well-being. Many patients who were cachectic from disease progression began to gain weight. Serial bone scans and X-rays often failed to show evidence of progression during treatment, but neither did they show resolution of lesions. What did change in the patients who seemed to be doing well were the levels of serum acid and alkaline phosphatase. There was usually a reversal of the trend to progressive rise in levels and reduction of these values into the normal range, even starting from markedly elevated levels. Although patients eventually relapsed and died, many of these remissions were of considerable duration and were accompanied by minimal toxicity from the chemotherapy.

To correlate degree of response of phosphatase levels with survival, we found that patients who had had a 50 percent or greater decline in elevated phosphatase levels, but had not declined into the normal range did not have any prolongation of survival compared with those who did not have any decline or less than 50 percent decline. The survival benefit was confined to those whose values became normal. A similar experience was noted for alkaline phosphatase. In our final definition of response, we have included only patients in whom the phosphatase values returned to the normal range. By comparison, many of the reported trials in prostate cancer accept stabilization, that is, lack of further progression in values, as part of the definition of response. Definition of partial responder in other studies has often included patients with a 50 percent or greater fall in phosphatase values. Our criteria for response are therefore stricter than the others generally used. The patients who did well generally gained weight during treatment. The increment in body weight exceeded 10 percent of their weights at initiation of treatment in most such patients. A few patients became edematous during treatment, but those who were not doing well otherwise had an overall weight gain because of fluid retention of less than 10 percent total body weight. Since approximately 15 percent of patients did not have acid or alkaline phosphatase abnormalities by which to gauge response, weight gain of 10 percent was added as a response criterion. The survival of patients having this degree of weight gain was significantly longer than that seen in patients not gaining at least 10 percent. Our final response criteria then were based on the presence of one or more of the following: the fall of an initially elevated acid phosphatase to normal; the fall of an initially elevated alkaline phosphatase to normal; or a weight gain of greater than 10 percent of the initial body weight. With these stringent criteria, the response rate of the chemotherapy program was 37 percent. This is an impressive result when compared with the published experience with chemotherapy in this disease, in which objective partial response rates are typically 10 percent.[4,5] The survival of responders, so defined, was 76 weeks median, compared with a median of 28 weeks for patients who failed to respond by this definition. The median survival for untreated hormonally refractory prostate cancer is in the range of 15–25 weeks.

At this point we became interested in identifying prognostic factors which would allow recognition of patients more likely to respond to treatment and survive longer. We wanted to know if the prolonged survival in the responders could be attributed to more favorable baseline prognostic factors in that group. The methods we used were logistic regression analysis for evaluating the factors contributing to response,[6] and Cox model regression for identifying factors contributing to survival.[7] The advantage of multivariate methods over comparisons in which the population is split into groups on the basis of a single criterion is that the multivariate methods allow the effect of a variable to be judged in the context of all other variables possibly contributing to the outcome. Multivariate analysis allows the exclusion of redundant variables. Finally, the effect of a variable may be obscured by covariance effects in simple analysis and may only become apparent once account has been taken of other variables. Tests of significance for variables added to the regression model were based on the resulting increment in log likelihood, which is distributed as half chi-square with degrees of freedom equal to the number of variables added to the model. A p-value of 0.10 or less was considered sufficient for inclusion in the models.

In the analysis of response (Table 2), our first finding was that the initial levels of acid and alkaline phosphatase were not predictive of

Table 2. Model of Prognostic Factors Relevant to Response and Comparison of Predicted and Observed Response Rates

$$\ln\left(\frac{p}{1-p}\right) = 11.747 - 2.12\,[\ln(LDH)] - 0.954\,[\ln(WBC\ nadir)] + 0.292\,[\ln(CEA)]$$

Predicted % Response	Number of Patients	Number of Responses Observed	Observed % Response
0- 20%	18	2	11.1
20- 40%	27	10	37.0
40- 60%	23	9	39.1
60- 80%	14	10	71.4
80-100%	2	2	100.0
Overall	84	33	37.0

response. This is comforting, since it indicates that returning to a normal value of phosphatase is not a reflection of merely having a minimally elevated level to begin with. The next finding was that only one of all the factors surveyed, serum LDH, was prominent regarding prognosis for response ($p = 0.0005$). Patients with normal or minimally elevated values had a higher probability of response than those with moderate or marked elevation. LDH was not simply a marker for tumor burden, since reductions in LDH were not often seen in patients considered to be responders by the criteria previously mentioned. There was no difference in survival in patients who had a fall in LDH level compared with those who did not. Only two other factors were found to make a contribution to understanding the variation in response rate. One was carcinoembryonic antigen (CEA) level for which a higher value was associated with higher response rate ($p=0.10$). The meaning of this relationship is unknown. The other factor was leukocyte nadir following treatment for which a lower nadir was associated with higher response rate ($p=0.04$). Since all agents were given in uniform dose without regard to patient weight or body surface area, it seems likely that leukocyte nadir was simply a functional assay for drug bioavailability, which could be expected to relate to response rate. Melphalan particularly has been shown to be highly variable in its rate of absorption when taken in oral form, as in this study. This finding would suggest that optimal use of the chemotherapy program might be obtained by adjusting dosages in each patient until some degree of granulocyte toxicity is seen.

The ability of this model to account for variability in response rate is confirmed by comparing observed response rates with those predicted by the model. Probability of response was predicted for each patient, and quintiles were formed in which the observed response rate was compared with the predicted response rate (Table 2). Patients are clearly separated into groups of high (greater than 60 percent), intermediate (20 to 40 percent), and low (less than 20 percent) probability of responding based on their covariate score. This multivariate prognostic score would be a excellent basis for stratification in prospective clinical trials.

In evaluating factors prognostic for survival (Table 3), initial LDH level again emerged as the most significant single factor (p=0.0006). Higher values were associated with shorter survival. Other factors found important were degree of bone pain (p=0.004), serum acid phosphatase level (p=0.02), and SGOT level. The information in SGOT was contained entirely in the other three variables, whereas each of the other three contained significant independent information, so SGOT was excluded from the model because of its redundancy.

Two striking results occurred when response was added as a variable to the survival regression model. Response was highly significant by itself. This was hardly surprising, since the response criteria were suggested from a consideration of changes in factors associated with prolonged survival. More important, when response was added to the model containing LDH, bone pain, and acid phosphatase, not only did response maintain its level of significance, which would not have been the case if our definition of response merely selected for patients with better underlying prognosis, but in addition the overall chi-square increased far more than could be accounted for by the simple additive effect of response, indicating that other variables had become more significant in the presence of response. These were bone pain, whose chi-square increased from 8.6 (p=0.004) to 16.9 (p=0.00007), and age (chi-square=3.8, p=0.05), which was not significant in the absence of response (chi-square=0.21).

We explored the intriguing question of why bone pain and age should

Table 3. Models of Prognostic Factors Relevant to Survival

Model 1 (Without response)

$\ln(\lambda_i/\lambda_0) = 0.629$ [ln(LDH) − 5.5] + 0.212 [ln(acid p'tase) −1.2] + 0.284 (bone pain − 2.7) + 0.0052 (age − 63.9)

$\chi^2 = 22.4$, d.f. = 4, p = 0.0002, N = 88

Model 2 (With response)

$\ln(\lambda_i/\lambda_0) = 0.391$ [ln(LDH) − 5.5] + 0.202 [ln(acid p'tase) − 1.3] + 0.421 (bone pain − 2.6) +0.0285 (age −63.5) − 0.467 (response − 0.8)

$\chi^2 = 41.8$, d.f. = 5, p $< 10^{-6}$, N = 84[a]

[a] Four patients not evaluable for response.

be so much more informative in the presence of response data by examining plots of log survival versus age and log survival versus bone pain in nonresponders and in responders. In nonresponders, the disease seems so uniformly and rapidly lethal that there is no opportunity for variation in the death rate with age, i.e., young men dying as rapidly as older men (Figure 1). Treatment response appears to attenuate the mortality from the cancer enough to partially restore the natural biological variation in death rate with age. Younger patients who respond survive longer than older patients who respond and have a three-fold increase in survival over their age-matched peers who do not respond to chemotherapy. In this context, the effect of age is probably a reflection of deaths caused by intercurrent disease. A comparable phenomenon is seen with respect to bone pain (Figure 2). In nonresponders, there is a gradient of increasing death rate with increasing degree of bone pain which fits in with the idea that bone pain is an indicator of tumor burden. The fact that this gradient is abolished in responders indicates that the effect of tumor burden on life expectancy has been levelled by the successful treatment.

Despite the fact that LDH has been recognized to be of diagnostic and prognostic value in prostate cancer since the work of Prout and his colleagues,[8] it has not received major attention in this disease. LDH

Figure 1. Regression of log survival on age in responders (R), nonresponders (NR), and overall group.

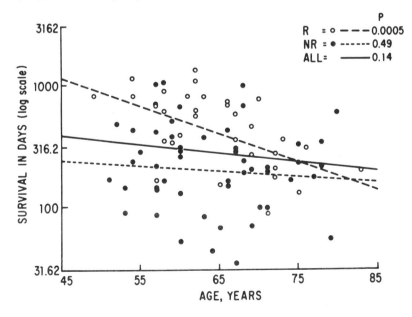

130

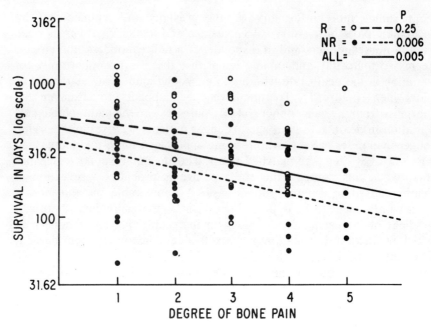

Figure 2. Regression of log survival on bone pain in responders (R), nonresponders (NR), and overall group.

isoenzymes IV and V are absent or barely detectable in prostate tissue, prostatic fluid or serum of normal individuals, but are prominently found from these sources in patients with prostate cancer.[9,10] Prout[8] noted a fall in isozyme V levels following orchiectomy or stilbestrol treatment, although its relationship to long term survival was not reported. Ishibe[11] reported that both total serum LDH and isoenzyme V prior to therapy were of prognostic significance to five-year survival in his patients with Stage C and D cancer. However he found that immediate changes in LDH V level in response to estrogen therapy or orchiectomy were of no prognostic value.

It is not known whether the source of LDH responsible for the elevated levels is the tumor itself or normal tissues compromised by the tumor. LDH isoenzymes IV and V are anaerobic dehydrogenases.[12] It is possible that an elevated level of this enzyme signals a switch to anaerobic metabolism when tumor vascularization fails to keep pace with tumor growth. Cells in poorly vascularized areas of the tumor may fail to receive exposure to cytocidal levels of chemotherapeutic agents, which could account for a lower response rate in this situation. However, LDH was found to contribute significant additional information regarding survival prognosis once response was accounted for, implying that its importance to survival is more than simply indicating which patients are likely to have a chemotherapy response.

In summary, we have defined an effective treatment regimen for metastatic endocrine refractory prostatic cancer and have defined rigorous response criteria which correlate well with survival prognosis. The role of serial bone X-rays and bone scans in evaluating response in prostate cancer is very limited. Multivariate analysis has identified LDH as the most prominent factor predicting chemotherapy responsiveness and subsequent duration of survival and it should be noted in analysis of similar studies of prostate cancer. This analysis indicates that response to treatment is associated with longer survival when the prognostic factors are considered.

References

1. Paulson, DF, Berry, WR, Cox, EB, Walker, A et al.: Treatment of metastatic endocrine-unresponsive carcinoma of the prostate with multiagent chemotherapy: indicators of response to therapy. *J. Nat. Cancer Instit.* (In press).

2. Berry, WR, Laszlo, J, Cox, E et al.: Prognostic factors in metastatic and hormonally unresponsive carcinoma of the prostate. *Cancer* 44:763-775, 1979.

3. Cooper, RG: Combination chemotherapy in hormone resistant breast cancer (Abstract). *Proc. Am. Assoc. Cancer Res.* 10:15, 1969.

4. Johnson, DE, Scott, WW, Gibbons, RP et al.: National randomized study of chemotherapeutic agents in advanced prostate carcinoma: a progress report. *Cancer Treatment Reports* 61:317-322, 1977.

5. Eagan, RT, Hahn, RG, Myers, RP: Adriamycin (NSC-123127) versus 5-fluorouracil (NSC-19893) and cyclophosphamide (NSC-26271) in the treatment of metastatic prostate cancer. *Cancer Treatment Reports* 60:115-117, 1976.

6. Cox, DR: Analysis of binary data. Methuen, London, 1970.

7. Cox, DR: Regression models and life tables. *J. Royal Statist. Soc.* B 34:187-220,1972

8. Prout, GR, Macalalag, EV, Denis, LJ, Preston, LW: Alterations in serum lactic dehydrogenase and its fourth and fifth isozymes in patients with prostatic carcinoma. *J. Urol.* 94:451-461, 1965.

9. Oliver, JA, El Hilali, MM, Belitsky, P, MacKinnon, KJ: LDH isoenzymes in benign and malignant prostate tissue.: the LDH V/I ratio as an index of malignancy. *Cancer* 25:863-866, 1970.

10. Grayhack, JT, Wendel, EF, Lee, C, Oliver, L, Cohen, E: Lactic dehydrogenase isoenzymes in human prostatic fluid: an aid in recognition of malignancy? *J. Urol.* 118:204-208, 1977.

11. Ishibe, T: Prognostic usefulness of serum lactic dehydrogenase and its fifth isoenzyme levels in carcinoma of the prostate. *Int. Urol. Neph.* 8:221-225, 1976.

12. Goldman, RD, Kaplan, NO, Hall, TC: Lactic dehydrogenase in human neoplastic tissues. *Cancer Res.* 24:389-399, 1964.

Prognostic Significance of Altered A, B, H Reactivity in Transitional Cell Carcinomas of the Urinary Bladder[a]

Catherine Limas, Paul Lange

Departments of Pathology and Urologic Surgery, Veterans Administration Medical Center, and the University of Minnesota, Minneapolis, Minnesota

Summary

Altered tissue reactivity for the blood group isoantigens A, B, and H has been reported in a number of neoplasms and attempts have been made to correlate this phenomenon with malignant potential. We examined A, B, H reactivity in papillary transitional cell carcinomas (TCCs) of the urinary bladder and correlated the results with the clinical course. Biopsies from noninvasive TCCs were tested for these antigens by the red cell adherence (RCA) method; 81 patients were followed for at least five years or until invasion was documented. Eighty-two percent of patients with tumors positive for the expected antigens did not progress to invasion, while 64 percent of those with negative tumors did so. Therefore, when the expected antigen(s) are retained, the prognosis is favorable while their absence denotes an aggressive potential. Testing for A, B, H antigens is particularly helpful for grade II TCCs the course of which is unpredictable. RCA-negative grade II TCCs became invasive in 69 percent of cases while 75 percent of the positive ones remained noninvasive. The reactivity of apparently positive tumors was found reduced when compared quantitatively to normal mucosa from the same patient. Therefore, "loss" of A, B, H antigens is a quantitative phenomenon. The absence of A or B antigen from tumors expected to be positive for these antigens was often associated with increased reactivity for H.

[a]Supported by Grant CA 22753 from the National Cancer Institute.

This is probably the result of changes in specific enzymes involved in the biosynthesis and/or degradation of blood group substances.

Introduction

Transitional cell carcinomas of the urinary bladder present, in the majority of patients, as low-grade noninvasive tumors which, in approximately 60 percent of cases, recur and in 30 percent, progress to invasion and metastasis.[1-2] Once the tumor becomes deeply invasive, currently available therapeutic modalities are largely ineffective.[3] Therefore, a major effort is made to control the disease in its early stages. This approach is hampered by the variability in the course of neoplasia and the limited prognostic value of morphologic criteria alone. Grade I tumors usually remain noninvasive while Grade III tumors are, in most instances, associated with evidence of invasion.[4] Grade II transitional cell carcinomas (TCCs) are unpredictable since approximately 50 percent of the cases become eventually invasive. The management of this group of patients is particularly problematic and would be improved by additional prognostic criteria.

Cell surface changes have been described in neoplasia[5-7] and may be relevant to the *in vivo* behavior of tumors. These changes affect the carbohydrate chains of glycolipids and glycoproteins and may thus interfere with the antigenic expression and the cell-to-cell interaction of the involved cells. The widely distributed A, B, H blood group antigens are of glycolipid and/or glycoprotein nature and could be altered as a consequence of the neoplastic process. Indeed, several investigators have reported that malignant tumors of various organs have reduced or absent reactivity for A, B, H antigens.[8-10]

Specifically for TCCs a study by Decenzo et al. suggested a correlation between the detectability of these antigens and the clinical course.[11] We explored this possibility further by focusing on patients who present at the noninvasive stages and would benefit most from additional prognostic criteria. Our results provide evidence that testing for A, B, H antigens is useful in assessing the prognosis of patients with bladder tumors.[12,13]

Changes in the detectability of A, B, H antigens in TCCs appear to result from specific defects in the biosynthesis of these substances.

Material and Methods

This study was designed to investigate three major aspects of the blood group antigen reactivity in transitional cell carcinomas (TCCs):

1. Reactivity of tumors presenting in invasive stages.
2. Reactivity of tumors presenting in noninvasive stages and its correlation with the subsequent clinical course.

3. Mechanisms involved in altering A, B, H reactivity in these tumors.

Pathological staging of tumors was accomplished according to Jewett and Strong.[14] Tumors limited to the mucosa (stages O and A) are hereforth referred to as "noninvasive" while higher stages are referred to as "invasive." The tumors were classified into Grades I-III according to previously published criteria.[15]

Staging and grading of tumors was performed on paraffin-processed tissue sections stained with H & E.

The A, B and H antigens were detected in tissue sections (paraffin-processed or fresh-frozen) with the Red Cell Adherence (RCA) method as described by Kovarik et al.[16] Briefly, 5μ thick tissue sections were placed on glass slides and incubated with the appropriate antiserum or Ulex extract at room temperature. Then the sections were washed thoroughly in Tris-buffered saline pH 7.4 and layered with a one percent suspension of indicator red blood cells (RBCs) (Blood group A, B or H depending on the antigen to be evaluated). The excess of RBC suspension was drained and the slides were gently inverted on applicator sticks in Petri-dishes containing buffered saline so that the tissue sections were touching the fluid. When left in this inverted position for 5-10 min, the nonadherent RBCs precipitated into the bottom of the dish while firmly adherent RBCs remain attached to the tissue. The sections were examined for adherent RBCs while inverted in the dish with the 10 and 20 × objectives of a Nikon microscope. A diagram of the principles of the RCA test is shown in Figure 1.

Anti-A and anti-B sera were purchased from Hyland Laboratory. The Ulex extract was prepared from the seeds of Ulex Europeus.[b] These reagents were titrated for their agglutinating strength against normal RBCs and used only whan a 4+ agglutination was obtained at dilutions 1:64 or 1:32. They were used undiluted routinely unless otherwise indicated.

Sections of normal bladder mucosa served as controls for quantitative and qualitative reproducibility every time the RCA test was performed. The vascular endothelium is positive for the expected BG antigen(s) and therefore it was a built-in control which assured that the tissue had been processed properly. The specificity of the Ulex reactions for L-α fucosyl groups (antigenically active groups of the H substance) was confirmed in each case by complete inhibition of the reactions by the addition of 0.4M L-α-fucose in the incubation medium. Each specimen was tested for each antigen in quadruplicate.

Figure 2 illustrates positive and negative reactions of normal bladder mucosa. Figures 3 and 4 illustrate positive and negative reactions on sections from TCCs. The results were semiquantitatively reported as:

[b]F.W. Schumacker Co., Sandwich, MA

136

RED CELL ADHERENCE (RCA) TEST

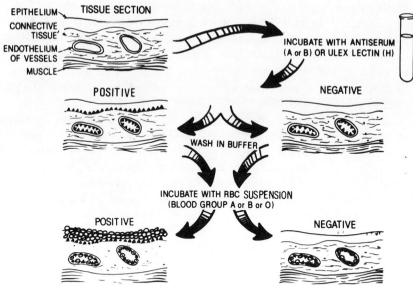

Figure 1. Diagramatic representation of the RCA test. In the first step the antiserum (▲) is adsorbed on the positive tissue elements and in the second step the indicator RBCs adhere on these elements. Note that the vascular endothelium is always positive for the antigen(s) corresponding to the blood group of the patient.

Figure 2. A. Positive RCA test on normal bladder mucosa with RBCs adherent on epithelium and vessels. The BG of the patient is A and the tissue has been incubated with anti-A serum and A RBCs.
B. Negative RCA test on the same tissue, which has been incubated with anti-A serum and O RBCs.

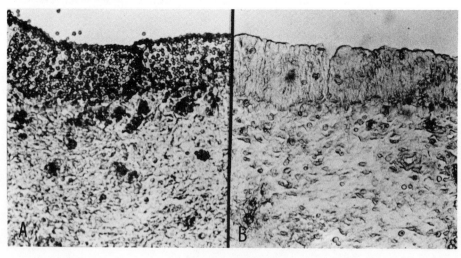

Strong positive: A sheet of overlapping RBCs covering the entire surface of tumor.

Positive: A one-cell-thick layer of RBCs covering at least 50 percent of tumor.

Weak positive: RBCs adherent on 30-50 percent of the tumor area.

Trace positive: Less than 30 percent of the tumor covered by RBCs.

Negative: No or rare RBCs on the tumor.

In the final tabulations of results, weak positive reactions were classified as positive and trace positive ones as negative.

1. A, B, H reactivity of transitional cell carcinomas presenting in stages B_1 or higher.

Sixteen patients who presented with biopsy-proven invasive TCCs were selected for this study. The initial biopsies and all subsequent tissue specimens were available in paraffin blocks and a record of the patient's blood group could be obtained. None of these patients had received any anti-tumor therapy prior to the initial diagnostic

Figure 3. Positive RCA test on a Grade II papillary TCC. The insert shows in detail the adherence of RBCs on the neoplastic epithelium and the vessels. The arrows point to vessels in the stalk of the papillary tumor.

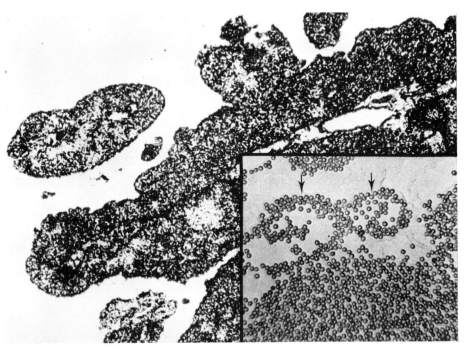

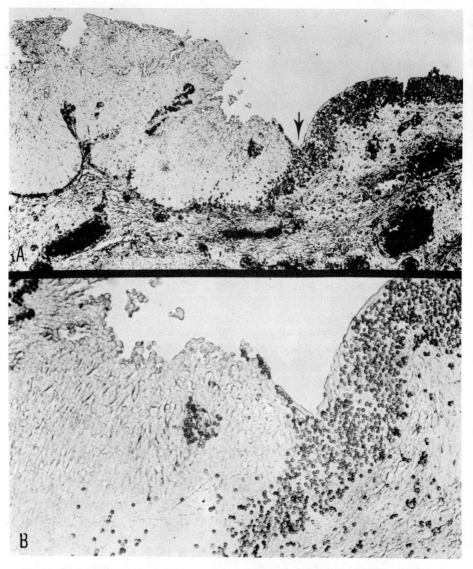

Figure 4. **A.** RCA test on tissue section containing both tumor *(left)* and normal mucosa *(right)*. RBCs are adherent on normal epithelium and vessels while the tumor is negative. The arrow points to the transition of normal to neoplastic epithelium, which is shown in detail in B.
B. Detail from A to show the abrupt change from positive reaction on the normal *(right)* to negative on the tumor *(left)*.

biopsy. This requirement eliminated the possibility of antigenic changes secondary to radiation and/or chemotherapy.

All but three of these patients had subsequent biopsies or cystectomies. Thus a total of 41 paraffin-processed tissue specimens were examined with routine histologic methods and 35 of these were evaluated for A, B, H reactivity.

2. A, B, H reactivity of transitional cell carcinomas presenting in stages O or A and correlation with the subsequent clinical course.

Eighty-one patients were selected according to the following criteria:

a) The initial biopsy had shown noninvasive TCC.

b) The patient was followed with cystoscopic examinations, cytology and, when indicated, biopsies for at least five years or until muscle invasion was demonstrated by biopsy, cystectomy or autopsy.

c) Adequate tissue and a record of the patient's blood group (BG) were available.

All biopsies, cystectomy specimens and autopsy material derived from these patients were studied using conventional histologic techniques. There was a total of 329 chronologically separate biopsies. The RCA test was performed on 252 sequential biopsies and on selected sections from the cystectomies and autopsies. All these tissue specimens had been processed in paraffin and stored in it for variable lengths of time.

3. Mechanisms of altered A, B, H reactivity in transitional cell carcinomas.

Tumor tissues from 35 patients were fresh-frozen and stored at $-70°C$ until used. Five μm thick sections were cut in a cryostat microtome, placed on glass slides and processed for the RCA test. For histologic evaluation, the first and last sections from each block were stained with H & E and examined microscopically. Each specimen was tested for the antigen(s) corresponding to the patient's blood group as well as for the H antigen. Quantitation of the tissue reactivity was attempted by using double-fold dilutions of the antisera and the Ulex extract on serial sections of fresh-frozen tissues and recording the results semiquantitatively for each dilution. Tissues to be quantitatively compared were processed simultaneously and each in quadruplicate.

Results and Discussion

Tumors from all 16 patients who presented in stages B_1 or higher were negative for the expected BG antigen(s) when initially biopsied. Tumor tissues obtained subsequently by biopsy or cystectomy remained negative in all but one patient. The exception was positive in one of two sequential biopsies and at cystectomy was found to have two distinct tumors in different locations: one invasive (Grade III) and one noninvasive (Grade II) corresponding to the sites of RCA-negative and -positive biopsies, respectively. Therefore, multiple urothelial tumors in the same individual may differ in their A, B, H reactivity as they may differ in their morphology and biological behavior.

It was noted repeatedly that necrotic and hemorrhagic areas of the tumor appeared positive by the RCA test, although the well preserved neoplastic tissue from the same specimen was negative. Careful evaluation of H & E stained sections is necessary in order to avoid erroneous interpretations caused by such secondary morphologic changes which are frequently encountered in high grade and invasive tumors.

These results indicate that most TCCs presenting in the invasion stages have no detectable reactivity for the antigen(s) that correspond to the patient's BG. No conclusions about the influence of cytologic grade on the A, B, H reactivity can be drawn since high grade cytologic abnormalities were noted at least in parts of all these invasive tumors.

Of the 81 patients who presented with noninvasive TCCs, 36(44%) progressed to stage B_1 or higher within the five years of followup. The tumors were classified into Grades I-III on the basis of the morphology in the initial biopsy; Table 1 shows the correlation of the grade with the subsequent clinical course. Invasive disease developed in only 8 percent of patients with initially Grade I TCCs while this occurred in 67 percent of those with Grade III lesions. The evolution of Grade II tumors was variable with 58 percent of patients advancing to high stages. These results point out that the morphologic grading has prognostic significance for the two extremes of the spectrum while patients presenting with intermediate grade tumors do not benefit from it. Since almost 50 percent of the patients did present with intermediate grade TCCs morphologic criteria are of limited value in assessing the prognosis of urothelial neoplasia prior to the occurrence of muscle invasion.

Table 1. Correlation of Tumor Grade in the Initial Biopsies with the Subsequent Clinical Course

Tumor Grade in Initial Biopsy	Number of Patients	Subsequent Course	
		Noninvasive	Invasive
I	25	23	2(8%)
II	41	17	24(58%)
III	15	5	10(67%)
Total	81	45	36(44%)

On the basis of the results of the RCA test in the initial diagnostic biopsy, tumors were classified as either positive or negative for the expected BG antigen(s). Table 2 shows the correlation of the RCA test results with the subsequent clinical course. Sixty-four percent of patients with negative tumors progressed to invasion, whereas only 18 percent of those with positive TCCs did so. The latter figure includes two patients who presented special problems: they had low-grade tumors in the bladder from which the initial positive biopsies derived; and at autopsy the bladder was free of tumor but invasive TCC was found in the renal pelvis.

In order to evaluate the relative significance of the morphologic grade and RCA test, the results of both approaches in the initial biopsies were correlated with the subsequent clinical course (Table 3). Of the 25 Grade I tumors, two progressed to invasion. One of these was negative for BG

Table 2. Correlation of the RCA Test Results in the Initial Biopsies with the Subsequent Clinical Course

Result of RCA Test in the Initial Biopsy	Number of Patients	Subsequent Course	
		Invasive	Noninvasive
Positive	34	6^a(18%)	28(82%)
Negative	47	30 (64%)	17(36%)
Total	81	36	45

^{a} Includes two patients with special problems as discussed in the text.

Table 3. Correlation of the Tumor Grade and the RCA Test Results in the Initial Biopsies with the Subsequent Clinical Course

Grades of Tumor	Initial Biopsy			Subsequent Course
	Number of Patients	Results of RCA test		Invasive/Total
I	25	Positive	16(64%)	1^a/16
		Negative	9(36%)	1/9
II	41	Positive	12(29%)	4^a/12
		Negative	29(71%)	20/29
III	15	Positive	6(40%)	1/6
		Negative	9(60%)	9/9

^{a} Includes two patients with special problems as discussed in the text (one Grade I and one Grade II).

antigen, the second is one of the two discrepancies discussed above, who had invasive tumor in the renal pelvis. Of the 41 Grade II tumors, 24 became invasive and 20 of them were RCA negative. Of the 15 Grade III neoplasms, 10 showed subsequent invasive course and nine of them had been negative for BG antigens. These results indicate that, within the same morphologic category, patients with aggressive course usually have RCA negative tumors. When both grade and RCA test results on the initial biopsy are taken into consideration, the prognostic assessment of Grade II and III tumors is significantly improved. Thus 69 percent of Grade II—RCA negative tumors and all of Grade III—RCA negative tumors became invasive.

Seventy of the 81 patients had recurrent tumors and the sequential biopsies obtained from their recurrences were analyzed for grade and A, B, or H reactivity. Twenty of the 39 initially Grade II tumors showed recurrent Grade III morphology in one or more of the subsequent biopsies. Three patients with initially Grade I lesions also showed more atypical changes in their recurrences. These 23 cases were classified as "variable grade." Patients presenting initially with Grade II noninvasive TCCs were analyzed in more detail to investigate the significance of the high frequency (51%) of increasing grade in the recurrences. Table 4 shows that 75 percent (18/24) of Grade II TCCs which became invasive had upgraded. Conversely, 90 percent (18/20) of upgraded tumors progressed to invasion. The RCA test showed that 17 of these morphologically changing tumors had been negative in the initial biopsy and remained so throughout the course.

The results of the analysis of sequential biopsies from recurrent TCCs are given in Table 5. The great majority (81%) of patients gave the same pattern of RCA reactivity in the initial biopsy and all subsequent recurrences. Only 12.5 percent of patients with consistently positive tumors progressed to stages B_1 or higher, while 68 percent of those with consistently negative neoplasms did so. Under "Variable" grade are classified patients whose tumors upgraded in the recurrences, mostly changing from Grade II to Grade III as described above and illustrated

Table 4. Evolution of TCCs Classified as Grade II in the Initial Biopsies

Grade	Number of Patients	Subsequent Clinical Course	
		Invasive	Noninvasive
Remained Grade II	19	6	13
Changed to Grade III	20	18	2
Total	39	24	15

Table 5. Correlation of the Tumor Grade and RCA Test Results of Multiple
Sequential Biopsies with the Clinical Course

Grade of Tumor	Number of Invasive/Total	Results of RCA Test		
		Always Positive	Always Negative	Variable
I	0/14	0/6	0/4	0/4
II	6/19	0/4	4/12	2/3
III	10/14	0/2	8/8	2/4
Variable	20/23	2/4	16/17	2/2
Total	46/70(66%)	2/16(12.5%)	28/41(68.3%) (invasive/total)	6/13(46%)

in Table 4. Under "Variable" RCA tests are classified patients whose TCCs changed their A, B or H reactivity from positive to negative or vice versa. Upgrading of tumor with conversion of positive to negative RCA test was noted in two cases. The reason for the variable RCA results in the remaining 11 cases is not certain. It is probable that these patients had multiple urothelial neoplasms which, although morphologically similar, differed in their A, B, H reactivity and possibly in their biological behavior. The effect of radiation and/or chemotherapy could explain these findings; so far, we have not observed any consistent change of the A, B, H reactivity in tumors treated with these modalities.

The group of variable grade, but consistently negative tumors, is particularly interesting. As mentioned above, 90 percent of the initially Grade II TCCs which changed into Grade III became invasive. Eighty-five percent of these upgrading tumors had been RCA negative in the initial biopsy, thus the antigenic abnormality became apparent prior to the appearance of malignant cytologic criteria and long before the demonstration of invasive growth.

The results of the study on the A, B, H reactivity of TCCs presenting in noninvasive stages are summarized as follows:

1. These tumors are heterogeneous in their A, B or H reactivity. Thus when paraffin-processed tissue is tested by the RCA method, 42 percent are positive and 58 percent are negative for the expected BG antigen(s).

2. There is a correlation between the A, B, H reactivity and the subsequent course: 82 percent of patients with positive tumors did not progress to invasion, while 64 percent of those with negative tumors did so.

3. In the majority of patients (81 percent), recurrent TCCs showed the same pattern of RCA reactivity as in the initial biopsy.

4. The heterogeneity of A, B, H reactivity also exists within the same morphologic grade; thus, tumors of any grade may be positive or negative. The majority of Grade I lesions are positive (64 percent) while the majority of Grade II and III TCCs are negative (71 percent and 60 percent, respectively).
5. The A, B, H reactivity of the tumor is prognostically significant for Grade II and Grade III tumors. Thus, RCA negative TCCs of these two grades are at high risk to become invasive and more radical surgical treatment may be indicated.
6. Testing for A, B, H reactivity is particularly helpful in assessing the clinical course of patients with Grade II tumors, which is unpredictable on the basis of morphologic criteria alone. Grade II tumors often upgrade their morphology prior to or simultaneously with the appearance of invasion; such tumors are usually negative for the expected BG antigen(s) in the initial biopsies long before they develop malignant morphologic changes.

Of the 35 patients, whose tumors were examined for A, B and H reactivity in the fresh-frozen state, 22 gave positive and 13 negative reactions for the expected BG antigen(s). These results confirmed that TCCs are heterogeneous in their reactivity for these antigens as was previously noted in the paraffin-processed tissues. The morphologically normal mucosa in 11 patients with TCCs was positive for the expected antigen(s).

To answer the question whether the tumor reactivity for the BG antigens is a quantitative or an "all or none" phenomenon, we quantitated the reactions of tumors and of morphologically normal bladder mucosa. Fresh-frozen tissues from tumors and mucosae which gave positive RCA results when tested with undiluted antisera and Ulex extract were tested with a series of double-fold dilutions of these reagents. It was concluded that the tumors in general had reduced reactivity for the antigen expected from the BG of the patient compared with the normal mucosa. This conclusion was based on the observation that the reactions of the tumors became negative at antiserum dilutions lower than those needed to eliminate the positive reactions of normal mucosa. The difference was usually two double-fold dilutions. For example, the tumor would become negative at a dilution of 1:4 while the mucosa remained positive up to a dilution of 1:16. Therefore, the "loss" of tumor reactivity for the BG antigen(s) appears to be a quantitative and not an "all or none" phenomenon. The obvious practical implication of this observation is that standardization of the reagents and the methodology used in the detection of BG antigens should be accomplished before testing for these antigens can have any clinical application.

Since the substance H is the required precursor substrate for the synthesis of A and B substances, it was thought that investigating the H reactivity of tumors from patients with BG other than O could help clarify the mechanisms involved in altering the reactivity of neoplastic tissues.

Twenty-six of the 35 patients had BG other than O; the results of the RCA test for the expected A or B antigen as well as for the H antigen are given in Table 6. In 15 cases, the tumors were A or B positive and of these, 11 were H positive when tested with full strength antiserum and Ulex extract. In 11 cases, the tumors were A or B negative and of these, 10 were H positive. Thus, only one of the 26 patients had a tumor negative for both the expected antigen(s) and for H. The normal bladder mucosa of patients with BG A or B gave positive or weakly positive reactions for H with undiluted Ulex extract. We, therefore, undertook to quantitate the reactions of tumors and normal mucosae for both the expected A or B antigen and the H. Representative results of the quantitative studies are shown in Table 7. It was noted that the tumors were less reactive for the expected antigen while they preserved and even enhanced the H reactivity compared to normal mucosa.

The simplified diagram of the biosynthetic interrelationship of the A,

Table 6. RCA Test Results in Fresh-Frozen Tumor Tissues from Patients Blood Group Other than 0

RCA Test Results for A and/or B Antigens	RCA Test Results for H Antigen (Ulex Europeus Lectin)	
	Positive	Negative
Positive	11	4
Negative	10	1
Total	21	5

Table 7. Quantitation of A, B, H Reactivity in Fresh-Frozen Tissues from Normal Mucosa and Tumors

Blood Group of Patient	Tissue	Antigen	Dilutions of Antiserum or Ulex Extract						
			1:1	1:2	1:4	1:8	1:16	1:32	1:64
A	Normal Mucosa	A	strong(+)	(+)	(+)	(+)	weak(+)	Trace(+)	–
		H	(+)	(+)	weak(+)	–	–	–	–
	Tumor	A	(+)	(+)	weak(+)	–	–	–	–
		H	(+)	(+)	(+)	(+)	weak(+)	–	–

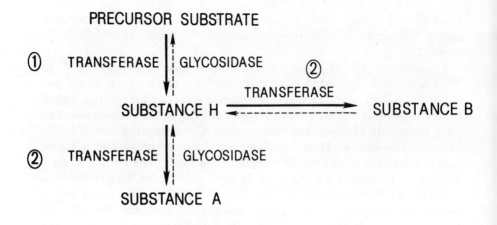

Figure 5. Simplified diagram of the biosynthesis of the A, B, and H blood group substances. Step 1 normally occurs in almost all individuals and depends on the presence of a fucosyl transferase. Step 2 occurs in individuals with BG other than O and depends on the presence of glycosyl transferase specific for substance A or B. Degradation of the A, B and H substances depends on the activities of glycosidases specific for each one of them.

B and H substances in Figure 5 helps understand why tumors from patients with BG A or B could have reduced A or B reactivity while exhibiting increased H. If defects exist in both steps 1 and 2, tumors from BG O patients could have reduced or absent H while the end result for patients BG other than O would depend on the relative activities of the enzymes involved in these two biosynthetic steps.

The nature of the biochemical abnormality has not been elucidated in TCCs. However, reduced activity of specific glycosyltransferases has been demonstrated in a variety of gastrointestinal carcinomas with decreased or absent BG antigens.[17,18] Our findings are consistent with a similar mechanism for reduced BG antigen in TCCs.

References

1. Marshall, VF: Current clinical problems regarding bladder tumors. *Cancer* 9:543-550, 1956.

2. Nichols, JA, Marshall, VF: Treatment of histologically benign papilloma of the urinary bladder by local excison and fulguration. *Cancer* 9:566-567, 1956.

3. Prout, GR Jr: The surgical management of bladder carcinoma. *Urol. Clin. North Amer.* 3:149-175, 1976.

4. Bergkvisk, A, Ljungqvist, A, Moberger, G: Classification of bladder tumors based on the cellular pattern. Preliminary report of a clinical-pathological study of 300 cases with a minimum followup of eight years. *Acta Chir. Scand.* 130:371-378, 1965.

5. Cumar, FA, Brady, EP, Kolodny, EH et al.: Enzymatic block in the synthesis of gangliosides in DNA virus-transformed tumorigenic mouse cell lives. *Proc. Natl. Acad. Sci. USA* 67:757-764, 1970.

6. Warren, L, Fuhrer, JP, Buck, CA: Surface glycoproteins of normal and transformed cells: a difference determined by sialic acid and a growth dependent sialyltransferase. *Proc. Natl. Acad. Sci. USA* 69:1838-1842, 1972.

7. Kim, US, Isaacs, R, Perdomo, JM: Alterations of membrane glycopeptides in human colonic adenocarcinoma. *Proc. Natl. Acad. Sci. USA* 71:4869-4873, 1974.

8. Davidson, I, Kovarik, S, Ni, L: Isoantigens A, B and H in benign and malignant lesions of the cervix. *Arch. Pathol.* 84:306-314, 1969.

9. Gupta, RK, Shuster, R: Isoantigens A, B and H in benign and malignant lesions of breast. *Amer. J. Pathol.* 72:253-257, 1973.

10. Dabelsteen, E, Pindborg, JH: Loss of epithelial blood group substance A in oral carcinomas. *Acta Pathol. Microbiol. Scand.* 81A:435-444, 1973.

11. Decenzo, JM, Howard, P, Irish, CE: Antigenic detection and prognosis of patients with stage A transitional cell bladder carcinoma. *J. Urol.* 144:874-878, 1975.

12. Lange, P, Limas, C, Fraley, EE: Tissue blood group antigens and prognosis in low-stage transitional cell carcinoma of the bladder. *J. Urol.* 119:52-55, 1978.

13. Limas, C, Lange, P, Fraley, EE, Vessela, RL: A, B, H antigens in transitional cell tumors of the urinary bladder: Correlation with the clinical course *Cancer* (in press).

14. Jewett, HJ, Strong, GH: Infiltrating carcinoma of the bladder relation to depth of penetration of the bladder wall to incidence of local extension and metastases. *J. Urol.* 55:366-372, 1946.

15. Koss, LG: Tumors of the urinary bladder. In: *Atlas of Tumor Pathology,* Fasc. 11, series 2, pp. 13-46. Armed Forces Institute of Pathology, Washington, D. C., 1975.

16. Kovarik, S, Davidsohn, I, Stejskal, R: ABO Antigens in Cancer. *Arch. Pathol.* 86:12-21, 1968.

17. Alroy, J, Teramura, K, Miller, AW et al.: Isoantigens A, B and H in urinary bladder carcinomas following radiotherapy. *Cancer* 41:1739-1745, 1978.

18. Stellner, K, Hakomori, S, Warner, GA: Enzymatic conversion of "H-glycolipid" to A or B-glycolipid and deficiency of these enzyme activities in adenocarcinoma. *Biochem. Biophys. Res. Commun.* 55:439-445, 1973.

An Analysis of the Metastatic Progression of Human Breast Cancers: The Breast Cancer Prognostic Study[a]

Philip Furmanski, Andrew B. Rudczynski,
Richard F. Mortensen, Michael J. Brennan,
Marvin A. Rich

Department of Biology, Department of Immunology, Laboratory of Cellular Immunology, Michigan Cancer Foundation, Detroit, Michigan

Summary

With the active participation of our clinical community, we organized the Breast Cancer Prognostic Study aimed at the detailed characterization of large numbers of human, primary breast tumors and their hosts and the identification of those factors associated with early recurrence and metastatic disease. Procedures for the acquisition of specimens, complete medical history and clinical findings have been developed. Maintenance of contact with the patient and her physicians for purposes of clinical followup and specimen collection have become part of a regularized system. We have established a system of assays to characterize both the tumors and their hosts with respect to their morphologic, endocrinologic and biochemical nature. These characteristics are being evaluated for their ability to predict recurrence of breast cancers and their association with metastatic behavior of cancer cells.

The long-term survival of the breast cancer patient is directly determined by the probability of metastatic spread and subsequent recurrence of the disease. This metastatic progression of a breast carcinoma likely is not the result of random colonization; the proliferation of a metastatic tumor, for example, requires a significant and complex inductive capacity to construct the requisite vascular and connective tissue frameworks which serve the neoplasm's survival and progression. In addition, the

[a]These studies were supported by Grant CA-16175 from the National Institutes of Health and an institutional grant from the United Foundation of Detroit.

processes probably are influenced by the immunologic and endocrinologic milieu of the host. It is likely, therefore, that the events associated with metastatic proliferation depend on specific and predeterminable characteristics of a patient and her tumor.

The Michigan Cancer Foundation Breast Cancer Prognostic Study was organized in 1975 to identify the characteristics of individual breast tumors and their hosts that are associated with early recurrence and patterns of development of metastatic disease. With the active participation of our clinical community, systems for entry of new patients, complete clinical work-up, histopathologic evaluation and patient follow-up were developed and implemented.

Tumors removed at primary surgery are segmented and the individual pieces sent to our laboratories for analysis of morphologic, biochemical, endocrinologic and immunologic cell surface and *in vitro* growth properties which might be related to metastatic behavior of the tumor and patient prognosis. In addition, blood and serum samples are collected preoperatively and at each followup visit. Complete histopathologic characterization of each tumor is carried out by a panel of five clinical pathologists. Statistical analysis and computerized data management are an integral component of the system and are maintained by a program unit dedicated to the purpose.

More than 300 clinical, pathologic and laboratory research data elements are collected for each tumor and host entered into the study. The application of this large series of laboratory and clinical tests to individual breast cancers is an important feature of the study. It allows not only for the correlation of these characteristics with disease recurrence and progression, but also for the identification of associations among different tumor properties.

In this report we describe the data obtained for two characteristics of breast cancer patients: serum C-reactive protein (CRP) and lymphoid cell infiltration of the tumor.

C-Reactive Protein

The acute phase serum proteins, exemplified by CRP, are generally elevated in patients with cancer.[1-3] Higher levels often are related to the presence of increased tumor burden or metastatic disease.[2,3]

To test the efficiency of CRP measurement as a prognostic indicator, preoperative serum CRP concentrations were measured in 299 patients entered into our study using radial immunodiffusion with a monospecific goat antiserum against CRP.[4] Serum CRP levels $\geq$ 10 μg/ml were considered elevated.

Twenty-four percent of the patients tested had elevated CRP levels. A significantly higher proportion of those patients with stage IV disease had elevated levels, compared with patients with stages I to III (p < 0.05, Table 1). Of thirteen patients with distant metastases at the time of surgery, ten (77 percent) had elevated levels of CRP.

In contrast to the association between CRP concentrations and stage or metastatic disease at the time of primary surgery, preoperative serum CRP levels did not predict recurrence behavior following surgery (Figure 1). Neither the incidence nor the mean time to recurrence were significantly different in patients with high or low serum CRP concentrations (27 versus 29 months; 20 percent versus 19 percent respectively).

Thus, while CRP levels appear to be related to tumor burden and the presence of metastatic disease, they do not predict prognosis following surgery for human breast cancer patients.

Lymphoid Cell Infiltration

The presence of a lymphocytic infiltrate in primary human breast cancers has been considered to be prognostically favorable.[5,6] Indeed, this observation has been used frequently to support the concept that cell-mediated anti-tumor immunity exists in breast cancer patients and is effective in control of the disease or the prevention of recurrences.

We examined stained sections of 373 breast cancers and found that 104 (28 percent) had marked lymphocytic infiltrates. The presence of the infiltrate occurred with equal frequency in patients that subsequently had recurrence of their cancer and those that remained disease-free (Table 2).

As reported by others,[5,7] two distinct patterns of lymphoid cell infiltrates were readily apparent in the breast cancers examined: a diffuse pattern; and a perivascular and/or periductal pattern. The incidence of recurrence differed in the patients with these different patterns of infiltration (Table 3); a diffuse pattern of lymphoid cell infiltration was associated with greater recurrence of the disease.

To further characterize the lymphocytic infiltrate in these tumors, the predominant lymphoid cell class in the tumor was determined. Antisera specific for human T lymphocytes were prepared by immunization of rabbits with the human T cell line, H-SB2, followed by extensive adsorption of the serum with the autologous B cell line, SB.[8,9] Similarly, specific anti-B cell antisera were obtained by extensive adsorption of anti-SB sera with H-SB2 cells. Cryostat sections of each tumor were tested for T and B cells using indirect immunofluorescence with these antisera. The results were confirmed using adsorbed anti-human thymocyte and anti-human IgM sera.

We found that the perivascular or periductal pattern of infiltrates most often consisted predominantly of T cells, whereas the diffuse infiltrates consisted predominantly of B cells in most cases (Table 4).

Table 1. Relationship of CRP Levels to Clinical Stage of Disease

Clinical Stage[a]	Number of Patients	Percent with Elevated CRP[b]
I	106	22
II	121	21
III	20	20
IV	52	38
Total	299	24

[a] Based on the American Joint Commission Classification for Staging of Cancer of the Breast, 1977.
[b] ≥ 10 μg CRP/ml.

Figure 1. Disease recurrence in patients with breast cancer. (-) indicates patients with serum CRP levels ≥ 10 μg/ml; (---) indicates patients with serum CRP levels < 10 μg/ml.

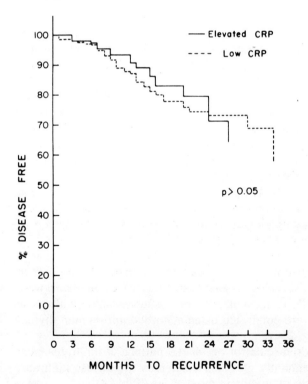

Table 2. Relationship Between the Presence of a Mononuclear Cell Infiltrate of Primary Human Breast Tumors and Recurrence of Disease

Disease Status	Mononuclear Cell Infiltrate	
	Present	Absent
Recurrent	25 (24%)	57 (21%)
Disease free	79 (76%)	212 (79%)
Total	104	269

Table 3. Distribution Pattern of the Lymphocytic Infiltrate in Primary Breast Tumors and Recurrence of the Disease

	Pattern of Infiltration	
Disease Status	Perivascular/Periductal	Diffuse
Recurrent	7 (13%)	18 (36%)
Disease free	47 (87%)	32 (64%)

$\chi^2 = 7.55$, p < 0.01.

Table 4. Distribution of T and B Lymphocytes in Primary Human Breast Tumors as Detected by Immunofluorescent Staining of Cryostat Sections with Specific Antisera to T Cells and B Cells

Predominant Cell Type Infiltrate	Perivascular/Periductal	Diffuse
T Cells	47 (87%)	12 (24%)
B Cells	5 (9%)	32 (64%)
Neither	2 (4%)	6 (12%)

Thus, while a lymphocytic infiltrate itself does not appear to affect the rate of disease recurrence in breast cancer patients, the pattern of infiltration, and perhaps more important, the lymphoid cell class in the infiltrate, does seem to be associated with patient prognosis. It is tempting to speculate that this difference in tumor behavior is related to the functional nature of the different lymphoid cell classes that infiltrate the tumor. Further studies will be required to confirm this association and determine its significance.

References

1. Claus, DR, Osmand, AP, Gewurz, H: Radioimmunoassay of human C-reactive protein and levels in normal sera. *J. Lab. Clin. Med.* 87:120–128, 1976.

2. Cowen, DM, Searle, F, Ward, AM et al.: Multivariate biochemical indicators of breast cancer: an evaluation of their potential in routine practice. *Europ. J. Cancer* 14:885–893, 1978.

3. Hedlund, P: Clinical experimental studies on C-reactive protein. *Acta Med.* (Suppl.) 361:35–61, 1961.

4. Osmand, AP, Mortensen, RF, Siegel, J, Gewurz, H: Interactions of C-reactive protein with the complement system. III. Complement dependent passive hemolysis initiated by CRP. *J. Exptl. Med.* 142:1065–1077, 1975.

5. Black, MM: Cellular and biological manifestations of immunogenicity to precancerous mastopathy. *Natl. Cancer Inst. Monogr.* 35:73–100, 1972.

6. Black, MM, Barclay, THC, Hankey, BF: Prognosis in breast cancer utilizing histological characteristics of the primary tumor. *Cancer* 36:2048–2060, 1975.

7. Hamlin, IME: Possible host resistance in carcinoma of the breast: a histological study. *Br. J. Cancer* 22:383–401, 1968.

8. Royston, IB, Smith, RW, Buell, DN et al.: Autologous human B and T lymphoblastoid cell lines. *Nature* 251:745–746, 1974.

9. Kaplan, J, Shope, TC, Peterson, WD: EB-virus negative human malignant T cell lines. *J. Expt. Med.* 139:1070–1076, 1974.

Quantitative Aspects of Monitoring Advanced Breast Cancer with Serial Plasma CEA Determinations

J. Lokich

Division of Medical Oncology, Department of Medicine, New England Deaconess Hospital, Harvard Medical School, Boston, Massachusetts

Summary

The usefulness of serial monitoring of plasma CEA levels in patients receiving therapy for metastatic breast cancer is determined by: the frequency of abnormal CEA levels in the patient population, the quantitative relationship of circulating CEA to host tumor burden, the reliability of the assay particularly at super elevated levels, the physiologic variability of circulating plasma CEA, and the ability of plasma CEA to predict (rather than be coincident with) clinical response. It is evident that 50 to 70 percent of patients have abnormal elevated plasma CEA levels and osseous metastases are more frequently associated with elevated CEA levels than with other metastatic sites. Plasma CEA levels do not consistently correlate directly with tumor burden, but at levels greater than 50 mg/ml (Hansen assay) the correlation is clinically consistent and useful. The reliability of the assay at the higher levels has not been evaluated but the standard error probably does not exceed 10–15 percent. With few exceptions serial plasma CEA levels anticipate subsequent tumor growth or regression by 6–12 weeks and discordant alterations in CEA levels are rare. The minimal criteria for significance in evaluating changing CEA levels are 20 percent. The importance of monitoring plasma CEA levels lies in the ability to adjust therapy early, thus permitting less toxicity of an inactive treatment and a greater likelihood of response to alternative treatments.

The clinical usefulness of serial plasma CEA levels as a monitor of host tumor burden is a controversial issue. O'Connel et al. have challenged the application and particularly, the cost effectiveness of CEA relative to standard biochemical tests (alkaline phosphatase) for monitoring gastrointestinal cancer.[1] In addition, critical quantitative criteria for determining the significance of alterations in the plasma CEA levels have not been developed. Finally, it is apparent that not all tumors produce CEA and that a direct quantitative relationship between circulating CEA levels and tumor burden does not necessarily exist. In spite of these limitations, however, serial plasma CEA levels have been a helpful monitor of therapy in metastatic breast cancer with a single exception.[2-9]

Breast cancer is particularly adaptable to an analysis of the usefulness of sequential monitoring by CEA levels in that it is an exquisitely responsive tumor to a variety of therapeutic modalities. Moreover, breast cancer is a tumor for which the most common metastatic site (osseous structures) is extremely difficult to quantitate objectively with regard to an anti-tumor effect so that CEA could provide a handle on this metastatic site. A characteristic of studies which evaluate plasma CEA in relationship to the extent of disease has been the lack of quantitative criteria for changes in plasma CEA levels. The majority of such studies focus on the *direction* of change in relationship to the clinical circumstances and emphasize the concordancy of serial plasma CEA levels in relationship to the clinical extent of disease in response to therapy.

This paper will review the literature on previous studies which correlate plasma CEA levels with disease distribution and growth and regression in relationship to therapy and will update the expanded study at the New England Deaconess Hospital of patients monitored with serial plasma CEA levels. The goal of these studies has been to develop quantitative criteria for significant changes in plasma CEA. The importance of such studies for clinical trials is to provide identification of ineffective treatment at an early point in time permitting discontinuation of toxic therapy and the introduction of an alternative therapy which is more likely to be effective with the lesser tumor burden and less depleted host reserve. In addition, sequential CEA determinations may identify responses in lesions which are occult or difficult to measure, e.g., bone lesions.

Review of the Literature

Tormey et al. in three consecutive publications from 1975 through 1977 evaluated CEA in relationship to other biological markers including HCG and polyamines.[2-4] They observed elevated CEA levels in 70.9 percent (83/117) of patients with metastatic disease and found that hepatic and osseous metastases were more commonly associated with elevated levels than with pulmonary or soft tissue disease sites. Only 25 patients with an elevated CEA were evaluated sequentially and the sequential measurement always paralleled the clinical course of the disease. Tormey further suggested that response rates and response duration correlated with CEA levels, in that higher levels of CEA were associated with the lower responses and shorter duration of response. In these studies no quantitative criteria of significance for CEA level alterations were indicated. Stewart et al. evaluated serum CEA in 69 patients of whom 47 had metastatic disease.[5] Seventy-nine percent had elevated levels when the criteria for abnormal was greater than 2.5 ng/ml. In 14 patients serially monitored, the serum CEA level correlated with response to chemotherapy or hormone treatment. Hagensen et al. studied 216 patients with metastatic breast cancer and again determined elevated levels to be present in almost 40 percent of patients with visceral metastasis and 50 percent of patients with osseous metastasis.[6] In patients with levels greater than 10 ng/ml, monitoring of hormone treatment correlated with patient response and the time course for change was observed over two to six weeks. Borthwick studied a small group of patients with advanced disease treated with antiestrogens and the correlation with response appeared erratic.[7] Similarly, Chu and Namoto in 136 patients, 83 of whom had metastasis identified elevated CEA levels in 68 percent of patients.[8] In 32 patients undergoing treatment, serial CEA was not considered an adequate marker. Meyers et al. analyzed 260 patients with advanced (UICC) clinical Stage IV disease, 73 percent of whom had elevated levels, but sequential analysis and quantitation were not determined.[9] In 1977 a symposium on the clinical application of CEA assays was held and three studies of plasma CEA in breast cancer were presented and are applicable to this discussion.[10–12] Haegele et al. found elevated levels in 76 percent of patients with metastatic breast cancer while employing a different method for the CEA assays.[10] Osseous metastasis had elevated levels in 96 percent of the patients. Namer et al. studied 67 patients and 11 apparently demonstrated discordant shifts of CEA levels in relationship to the clinical behavior of the disease, but in all such patients a precise analysis of the graph suggested that the discordancy occurred in the borderline CEA level.[11] Finally, Chatel studied a small group of patients with metastases, 80 percent of whom had elevated CEA levels and no discordant observations were noted.[12] Beatty et al. studied 567 patients with malignant disease of whom 115 had breast carcinoma. The quantitative level of CEA was directly related to the stage of disease but 31 percent had elevated levels.[13]

In all of the studies indicated quantitative criteria are not addressed in terms of monitoring the extent of disease, but rather the focus is on the qualitative direction of change. In only two studies do the authors direct attention to the issue of predictability of CEA in determining and evaluating response as opposed to a mere coincidental observation.

Updated Quantitative CEA Study

Our original study[14] analyzed sequential plasma CEA determination in 42 patients with metastatic breast cancer treated with chemotherapy (either standard CMF/cyclophosphamide, methotrexate, 5-fluorouracil, or combinations of alkylating agents and adriamycin). Standard criteria for response were employed in the evaluation of the anti-tumor effect. Partial response was defined as a minimum reduction of 50 percent in the area of all measurable tumor lesions as determined by the product of the perpendicular diameters of the lesions. Complete response was defined as the complete regression of all demonstrable lesions with improvement in symptoms. Responses must be maintained for a minimum of one month and were measured from the time of initiation of response.

Patients were evaluated for response at monthly intervals and plasma CEA was determined at either monthly intervals or coincident with chemotherapy. The Hansen assay was employed; the indirect assay with perchloric acid extraction applied for plasma CEA levels up to 20 ng/ml and the direct assay for CEA levels greater than 20 ng/ml.

Three arbitrary groups were established. Patients with plasma CEA levels less than 5 ng/ml in the presence of metastases were designated as having normal levels. In this group of patients, plasma CEA levels did not rise with subsequent progression of disease and therefore were not a monitor of the disease which implied that in such patients the tumor did not produce CEA. This group comprised approximately 50 percent of the study population. The second group had CEA levels between 5 and 20 ng/ml and were designated as the group in whom CEA was not an accurate predictor. Although discordant responses were not observed, shifts in plasma CEA levels were not meaningful quantitatively and were generally within the standard error of the method. This group comprised approximately 15 percent of the overall group of patients with metastatic breast cancer. The remaining 35 percent of patients had CEA levels greater than 20 ng/ml and in all patients serial monitoring was a precise and effective means of predicting response and adjusting therapy.

Approximately 75 percent of patients with elevated plasma CEA levels beyond 5 mg/ml responded to systemic therapy with regression of the disease. The response rate in patients who did not demonstrate elevated levels of plasma CEA was comparable with approximately 55 percent complete plus partial response. The difference is not significant for the heterogeneous patient population monitored.

The objectives of our study were: to determine if sequential plasma

CEA levels correlated with the clinical course of the disease, to propose or develop quantitative guidelines for monitoring plasma CEA levels, and to determine if plasma CEA levels could be serially monitored for all sites of metastatic disease and most particularly for the difficult-to-measure disease sites such as osseous metastasis and pleural effusions.

The frequency of elevated plasma CEA levels correlates crudely with the sites of metastasis (Table 1). Cutaneous lesions which are easily monitored and measurable were least likely to be associated with significant elevations of plasma CEA in our study as well as other reports. Osseous and liver metastasis, however, had significant elevations of plasma CEA in more than half of the patients. This observation is particularly relevant in that these sites of disease are difficult to monitor because of slow healing in both sites and the confusion with osteoblastic tumor in osseous metastasis. Quantitatively, the osseous and liver metastases are associated with comparable levels. Of those patients with levels greater than 100 mg/ml (Hansen assay), one half had dominant disease in the bone and one third in the liver.

This study focuses on the clinical course of disease in patients with elevated levels of CEA. Of the 22 patients with elevated levels, 17 responded to therapy. Fourteen of the 17 (82%) demonstrated a fall in the plasma CEA level consistent with the clinical determination of response. In the three patients in whom response was observed and CEA did not decrease, pre-treatment CEA levels varied from 6.7 to 11 mg/ml and there was no discordant elevation of the CEA but instead the level remained stable within the error of the method for CEA determination.

Five of the initial 22 patients were nonresponders to therapy and five of the initial responders subsequently relapsed clinically. In the total of 10 clinical events of progressive disease by clinical parameters, eight developed rising plasma CEA levels and in two patients the CEA levels remained stable again within the 10 percent standard error of the methodology. In no instance was there a discordant observation. Thus,

Table 1. Correlation of Elevated Plasma CEA Levels with Sites of Metastases

Study	Dominant Site of Metastases[a]			
	Liver	Cutaneous	Bone	Lung
Present Report	100%	25%	55%	66%
Chu & Nemoto[8]	93	41	64	83
Waalkes & Tormey[2-4]	82	52	79	61
Haagensen et al.[6]	–	34	61	–

[a] Percent elevated.

CEA was a reliable and consistent parameter precisely reflecting the clinical course and activity of the disease. Furthermore, in every instance in which CEA paralleled the course of the disease, the alteration in CEA levels predicted the subsequent clinical evidence of response by a minimum of eight weeks.

The quantitative considerations in monitoring CEA levels is related to the pre-treatment absolute level, the variation in plasma CEA levels under physiologic circumstances (that is without alteration in the tumor status), and the variability relative to the methodology of the assay. Three groups of patients with elevated CEA levels were separable. Of the group with levels between 5 and 20 ng/ml, the correlation of response with sequential CEA levels were imperfect. At levels between 30–50 ng/ml the use of either direct or indirect assay system must be consistent in order to monitor accurately CEA in relationship to clinical disease. At levels greater than 50 ng/ml CEA was a precise and reliable predictor of tumor activity.

The determination of a significant quantitative alteration in plasma CEA level requires an understanding of the reliability of the assay and the normal variability under physiologic circumstances for circulating plasma CEA. The standard error of the assay is 10 percent irrespective of the absolute level of plasma CEA. In patients monitored with daily or every other day CEA levels, variation in levels did not exceed 20 percent in the absence of an alteration in clinical status. Therefore the minimum criteria for significant alteration in plasma CEA level are 20% of the pre-treatment level.

The rate of change of plasma CEA has been studied in patients with both regressing and progressing disease. A composite of the patients initially treated with chemotherapy and elevated plasma CEA level is illustrated by Figure 1. There is a precipitous decline in 86 percent of the responding patients and the rate of decline was related to the circulating CEA pool at a rate of 1–5 ng/ml day. In the sub-group of patients who developed progressive disease primarily or who progressed after response (10 patients), the rate of increase in plasma CEA level was 3–6 mg/ml day. In a small proportion of patients, plasma CEA levels rose paradoxically in patients who demonstrated clinical response subsequently. The rise observed was four to six weeks and was followed immediately by a precipitous fall in plasma CEA levels predicting the subsequent clinical response.

A patient example will serve to illustrate the clinical and quantitative features of CEA monitoring:

A 60-year old woman presented with advanced breast cancer metastatic to the bone as well as the pleural surface, neither of which represented immeasurable lesion but the patient was symptomatic with bone pain. At the

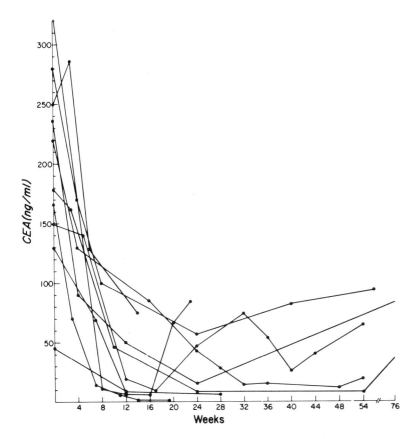

Figure 1. Graphic display of sequential plasma CEA levels in advanced breast cancer responding to therapy.

time of initiation of combination chemotherapy, the plasma CEA level was 360 mg/ml. She received therapy at four-week intervals and by eight weeks the plasma CEA level had fallen to 60 mg/ml and the bone pain had disappeared. Healing of the bone lesions, however, by radiograph was not demonstrated. At week 16, the patient developed CNS metastasis but the plasma CEA level had not risen. These lesions were treated by radiation therapy with resolution of the CNS syndrome. Subsequently, the CEA level rose but no evidence of visceral metastasis was demonstrable. At postmortem, however, there was complete replacement of the liver by metastasis.

The case example illustrates the ability of plasma CEA to predict response, particularly in patients with difficult-to-measure lesions. Furthermore, the case illustrates the fact that CNS lesions do not apparently secrete or produce CEA into the circulation (Figure 2).

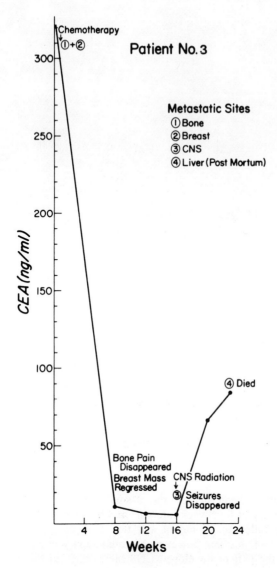

Figure 2. Sequential plasma CEA levels in a patient undergoing systemic chemotherapy for advanced breast cancer metastatic to multiple sites.

Discussion

The usefulness of serial determinations of plasma CEA in monitoring the effectiveness of treatment for advanced breast cancer has been established in the present study as well as in previous reports from other institutions. The importance of specific quantitative criteria to evaluate significant alterations in plasma CEA levels is crucial and the present

Table 2. General Guidelines for Quantitative Significance to Serial Plasma CEA Determinations

1. CEA levels <5 ng/ml in the presence of advanced metastatic breast cancer do not rise with progressive disease.
2. CEA levels >5 <20 ng/ml are unreliable and inconsistent predictors of response.
3. CEA levels >20 <50 ng/ml are potentially useful if the assay (direct or indirect Hansen) is consistent.
4. CEA levels >50 ng/ml are consistent predictors of response without discordant rises.
5. A parodoxical but transient rise in plasma CEA levels may be observed in less than 15 percent of responding patients.

study suggests some general guidelines. A summary of the general guidelines is detailed in Table 2.

Future studies will expand the present experience to confirm the consistency of plasma CEA as a predictor of response. In addition, studies on the variability of plasma CEA in relationship to absolute levels are ongoing. Finally, the ability to correlate the rate of change in plasma CEA levels with quantitative degree of response and prognosis are potentially fruitful areas of clinical investigation.

References

1. O'Connell, M et al.: Carcinoembryonic antigen and monitoring of metastatic colorectal carcinoma. *Annals of Int. Med.* 89:573, 1978.
2. Tormey, DC, Waalkes, TP: Clinical correlation between CEA and breast cancer. *Cancer* (Supp.) 42:1507, 1978.
3. Tormey, DC, Waalkes, TP, Ahmann, D et al.: Biological markers in breast carcinoma. *Cancer* 35:1095–1100, 1975.
4. Tormey, DC, Waalkes, TP, Snyder, J, Simon, RM: Biological markers in breast carcinoma. *Cancer* 39:2397–2404, 1977.
5. Steward, AM, Nixon, D, Zamchek, N, Aisenberg, A: Carcinoembryonic antigen in breast cancer patients: serum levels and disease progress. *Cancer* 33:1246–1252, 1974.
6. Haagensen, DE, Kister, SJ, Vandevoorde, JP et al.: Evaluation of carcinoembryonic antigen as a plasma monitor for human breast carcinoma. *Cancer* (Supp.) 42:1513, 1978.
7. Borthwick, NM, Wilson, DW, Bell, PA: Carcinoembryonic antigen (CEA) in patients with breast cancer. *Europ. J. Cancer* 13:171, 1977.
8. Chu, TM, Nemoto, T: Evaluation of carcinoembryonic antigen in human mammary carcinoma. *Jour. National Cancer Inst.* 51:4, 1973.
9. Myers, RE, Sutherland, DJ, Meakin, JW et al.: Carcinoembryonic antigen in breast cancer. *Cancer* (Supp.) 42:1520–1526, 1978.
10. Haegele et al.: Symposium Nice Clinical Applied of CEA Assay. Oct. 7–9, 1977. Krebs, BP, Lalaime, CM, Schneider, M. eds. *Pub-Excerpta Medica 1978.*
11. Namer et al.: Symposium Nice Clinical Applied of CEA Assay Oct. 7–9, 1977. Krebs, BP, Lalaime, CM, Schneider, M. eds. *Pub-Excerpta Medica 1978.*

12. Chatel et al.: Symposium Nice Clinical Applied of CEA Assay Oct. 7–9, 1977. Krebs, BP, Lalaime, CM, Schneider, M. eds. *Pub-Excerpta Medica 1978.*

13. Beatty, JD, Romero, C, Brown, PW et al.: Clinical value of carcinoembryonic antigen: diagnosis, prognosis, and followup of patients with cancer. *Arch. Surg.* 114:563, 1979.

14. Lokich, JJ, Zamcheck, MD, Lowenstein, M.: Sequential carcinoembryonic antigen levels in the therapy of metastatic breast cancer: a predictor and monitor of response and relapse. *Annals Int. Med.* 89:902–906, 1978.

Skin Window Studies as Improved *in Vivo* Prognostic Factors in Lung Cancer Patients[a]

Brian F. Issell, Jerri Arnett, Manuel Valdivieso, Evan M. Hersh, Gerald P. Bodey

Department of Developmental Therapeutics, The University of Texas System Cancer Center, M.D. Anderson Hospital and Tumor Institute, Houston, Texas

Summary

Delayed hypersensitivity skin reactivity to various recall antigens has been shown to predict for survival in lung cancer patients. The skin window technique was examined and compared with delayed hypersensitivity skin reactivity in an effort to identify more sensitive and readily measurable prognostic characteristics. Forty-eight patients with inoperable nonsmall cell lung cancer who were to receive chemotherapy were studied. The total number of neutrophils at three and one half hours and mononuclear cells at seven hours migrating onto a sterile glass coverslip placed over a 0.5 cm² abraded skin area were measured. Increased neutrophil and mononuclear cell migrations were more sensitive predictors of longer survival than was increased delayed hypersensitivity skin reactivity. The difference in survival between patients with neutrophil migrations > 300 and those with < 300 total cells was significant at $p = 0.0003$. Mononuclear cell migration at the 75 cell level was also significant at $p = 0.006$. In contrast, delayed hypersensitivity skin reactivity to dermatophyton, candida, mumps and Varidase even at the most significant levels of induration did not significantly predict for survival ($p = 0.16$ at 10 mm induration for dermatophyton, $p = 0.27$ at 10 mm for candida, $p = 0.29$ at 5 mm for mumps and $p = 0.19$ at 20 mm for Varidase). These data suggest new *in vivo* prognostic factors with

[a]Supported by Contract NO1-CM-57042 from the Division of Cancer Treatment, National Cancer Institute, National Institutes of Health, Department of Health, Education, and Welfare.

increased sensitivity and clinical utility. Further studies in larger patient populations seem indicated.

Introduction

Skin sensitivity to various recall antigens and hypersensitivity to primary antigenic stimulation have been shown to predict for survival in patients with various malignancies including lung cancer.[1] Furthermore, in a group of patients with nonsmall cell lung cancer, where a logistic regressional analysis of multiple prognostic characteristics was undertaken, skin test reactivity to dermatophyton was found to be the second most important independent characteristic determining survival.[2] However, published data are confusing as to which antigenic skin test or battery of tests is the most appropriate. Considerable variability has been reported both between and within tumor cell types.[3] The effect of prior antigenic testing on subsequent skin tests with the same antigen also questions the validity of serial recall antigen skin testing.

The technique of skin test measurement questions this test as a sensitive objective parameter. The maximum induration at one or two days following antigen inoculation is usually considered as an appropriate measurement. However, the interpretation of induration is subjective and may vary between observers. For the sake of convenience, patients are often asked to record these measurements themselves and this may result in further inconsistency. The question of which exudative component of induration is the most relevant, in terms of prognosis, is also important and the inability to measure these individual components with regular antigenic skin testing may, in part, account for the lack of specificity demonstrated.

There is, thus, the need for a simple, more easily reproducible and sensitive test of immunocompetence. The skin window technique which directly measures the cellular exudative response to trauma and is not dependent on specific exogenous antigen was examined as a test with the potential for improved clinical utilization.

Materials and Methods

The exudation of neutrophils and mononuclear cells using a modification of the skin window technique originally described by Rebuck and Crowley[4] was examined as a prognostic characteristic and compared with a battery of delayed hypersensitivity skin test reactions in 48 patients with metastatic nonsmall cell lung cancer. Testing was carried out prior to the administration of any myelosuppressive or immunosuppressive therapy and the peripheral white blood cell count was within the normal range for all patients.

For each patient tested, the volar surface of the left forearm was shaved as necessary and cleaned with Betadine® followed by alcohol and allowed to dry. Figure 1 illustrates the method of abrasion. By using firm, constant pressure and a side-to-side scraping motion with a sterilized scalpel, the epithelium was slowly removed until the papillary layer of the corium was reached. A lesion of approximately 5 mm² was made. A small amount of capillary oozing was noticed when the proper depth was reached. Increased bleeding meant that the lesion was too deep. A sterile round glass coverslip was applied immediately to the abraded area. A flat piece of cork cut slightly larger than the coverslip was placed over the coverslip and taped down firmly so that the edges of the cork were covered with tape as illustrated in Figure 2. The exudative cells adhered to the underside of the coverslip and the coverslip could be removed at any time and replaced with another. After removal, the coverslip was mounted on a glass slide with Permount® leaving the cell side exposed for easy handling and staining. The slide was air dried and stained with Wright-Giesma. After the final coverslip was removed, antiseptic ointment and a Bandaid® were applied to the abrasion.

An estimate of the total number of cells on the coverslip was made using the 10× microscope objective. The approximate number of cells per field was multiplied by the total number of cell-containing fields. The percentage of neutrophils and mononuclear cells was then obtained by counting 10 representative fields with the 40× objective. This allowed

Figure 1. Abrading the volar forearm skin with a sterilized scalpel until the papillary level of the corium is reached.

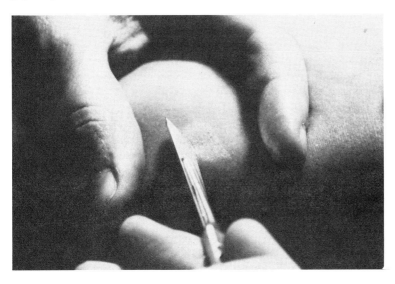

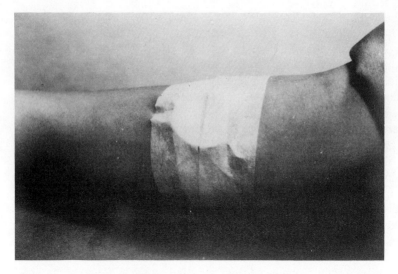

Figure 2. A sterile coverslip is placed over the abrasion which is in turn covered by a circular flat piece of cork taped securely in place.

the calculation of the total amount of neutrophils and mononuclear cells adhering to the coverslip.

We had previously examined changing the coverslip at various intervals over the 24-hour period following skin abrasion. The selection of the neutrophil response over the first three and one half hours following abrasion and the mononuclear cell response between three and one half and seven hours following abrasion were based on the consistency and quality of our readings at these times, combined with minimal patient inconvenience. Delayed hypersensitivity skin tests to recall antigens dermatophyton, Varidase, candida and mumps were placed intradermally according to the technique of Hersh et al. [5] Induration was measured at 24 and 48 hours, respectively. The data recorded were the average of two right-angle measurements of the induration at the time it was the largest.

Survival calculations were determined from the day of skin testing by the method of Kaplan and Meier.[6] The differences between survival curves were evaluated by the two-tailed generalized Wilcoxan test according to Gehan.[7]

Results

The qualitative kinetics of the cellular skin window responses in our patients were essentially the same as those originally described in detail by Rebuck and Crowley.[4] Over the first three and one half hours, the cellular response was at its maximum and consisted almost entirely of neutrophils. Over the next three and one half hours the response slowed and mononuclear cells appeared. Examples of these responses are illustrated in Figure 3.

The median total neutrophil response at three and one half hours was 443 cells with a range of 43–990, while the median total mononuclear cell

Figure 3. (A) Over the first three and one-half hr, and initial brisk neutrophil response is usually observed.
(B) From three and one-half to seven hr, the start of a slower mononuclear cell response is usually observed.

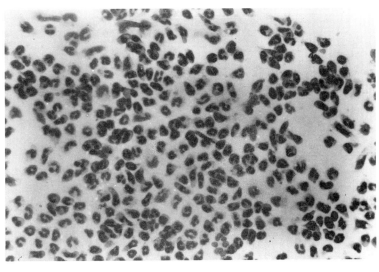

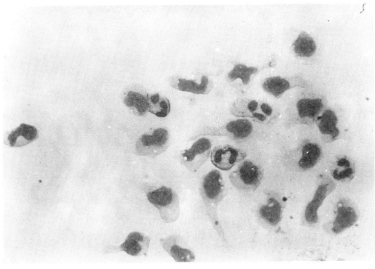

response at seven hours was 85 (range 0–520). The examination of survival at several levels of neutrophil and mononuclear cell response led to the selection of a neutrophil response of 300 cells at three and one half hours and a mononuclear response of 75 cells at seven hours as the most sensitive levels affecting survival. Similarly, delayed hypersensitivity skin test induration at several levels for all antigens tested were examined and the response to dermatophyton at the 10 mm level was found to be the most sensitive affecting survival.

The survival curves for patients with >300 neutrophils migrating at three and one half hours and those with <300 neutrophils at the same time are shown in Figure 4. The difference in survival is significant at p = 0.0003 and favors those patients with an increased neutrophil response. Similarly, a significant survival advantage was demonstrated for those patients with a mononuclear cell response >75 at seven hours (Figure 5), but this characteristic (p = 0.006) was less sensitive than the neutrophil response. In comparison, the delayed hypersensitivity skin reactivity to dermatophyton, candida, mumps and Varidase, even at the most sensitive levels of induration, did not significantly predict for survival as shown in Table 1.

The skin window technique was extremely well tolerated by all

Figure 4. Survival of patients related to the neutrophil response over the first three and one-half hr.

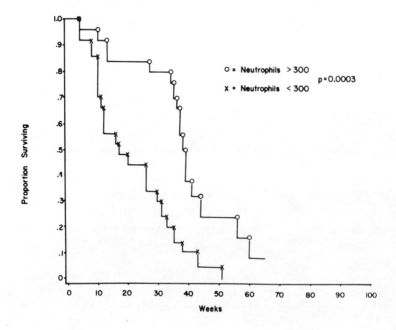

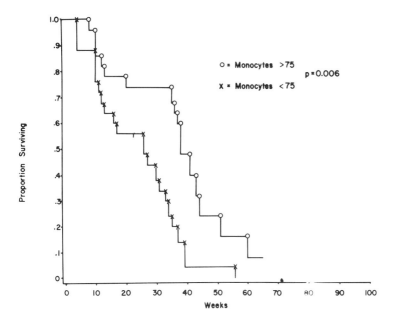

Figure 5. Survival of patients related to the mononuclear cell response between three and one-half and seven hr.

patients. It appeared to be a pain-free procedure in our hands and there were no cases of abrasion infection. The change of coverslip at three and one half and seven hours, respectively, after the initial placement on arrival to clinic in the morning caused little inconvenience to both patients and staff.

Discussion

The identification of more sensitive prognostic factors so that cancer patient populations can be better defined is urgently needed. Many cancer therapy studies suggest advantages for one treatment over another based on either historical or prospective randomized control studies. However, even in prospective randomized studies, unless patients in both groups can be proven to be prognostically equivalent, little meaning can be attached to modest survival advantages.

Using a modification of the Rebuck skin window technique described above, the migration of neutrophils and mononuclear cells both appear to be more sensitive predictors of survival than recall antigen skin testing in the patients of this study. These data, together with excellent patient tolerance and only minor inconvenience, suggest that further studies of this technique in larger patient populations are indicated.

Table 1. Effect of *in vivo* Skin Studies on Survival

Test	Level	Significanc
Skin Window		
Neutrophil migration at 3½ hr	300 cells	p = 0.0003
Mononuclear migration at 7 hr	75	p = 0.006
Recall Antigen Skin Reactivity		
Dermatophyton	10 mm Induration	p = 0.16
Varidase	20 mm	p = 0.19
Candida	10 mm	p = 0.27
Mumps	5 mm	p = 0.19

The skin window response may have further utilization in cancer patients. Fortuny et al. described this technique as a possible predictor of infectious complications in 21 neutropenic cancer patients.[8] Therefore, further studies should also examine serial testing in patients throughout therapy administration.

References

1. Hersh, EM, Mavligit, GM, Gutterman, JU: Immunodeficiency in cancer and the importance of immune evaluation of the cancer patient. *Med. Clin. N. Am.* 60(3):623–639, 1976.

2. Issell, BF, Valdivieso, M, Hersh, EM et al.: Combination chemoimmunotherapy for extensive non-oat cell lung cancer. *Can. Treat. Rep.* 62(7):1059–1063, 1978.

3. Bolton, PM, Mander, AM, Davidson, JM et al.: Cellular immunity in cancer: comparison of delayed hypersensitivity skin tests in three common cancers. *Brit. Med. J.* 3:18–20, 1975.

4. Rebuck, JW, Crowley JH: A method of studying leukocytic functions *in vivo. Ann. NY. Acad. Sci.* 59:757–805, 1955.

5. Hersh, EM, Gutterman, JU, Mavligit, GM et al.: Immunocompetence, immunodeficiency, and prognosis in cancer. *Ann. NY. Acad. Sci.* 276:386–406, 1976.

6. Kaplan, EL, Meier, P: Nonparametric estimation from incomplete observations. *J. Am. Stat. Assoc.* 53:457–481, 1958.

7. Gehan, EA: A generalized Wilcoxan test for comparing arbitrarily singly-censored samples. *Biometrika* 52:203–223, 1965.

8. Fortuny, IE, Deinard, A, Theologides, A: The Rebuck skin window as a guide in cancer chemotherapy. *Can. Treat. Rep.* 60(7):903–906, 1976.

Panel Discussion

DALE RANK: Dr. Issell, have you had an opportunity to evaluate neutrophil migration in patients on lithium?

BRIAN ISSELL: No sir, I haven't. That's a further point.

BRIAN DURIE: Have you looked at the difference in chemotherapy tolerance in the two groups? As was mentioned earlier, changes in the white count reflected the amount of chemotherapy given.

ISSELL: Yes, I looked at this according to dosage and there wasn't a correlation. We need larger patient numbers. We gave the doses of chemotherapy according to their tolerance and we adjusted it according to the nadir. The number of patients and the number of observations are not sufficient to give you a ready answer; but I could not find a correlation.

UNKNOWN: In what way did neutrophil migration correlate with zinc levels; high zinc or low zinc levels?

ISSELL: Yes, high zinc levels correlated with a good neutrophil response.

UNKNOWN: All your patients were lung patients with relatively high tumor burden. Have you tried this test in patients with modest tumor burdens or in patients with other types of cancer?

ISSELL: No, we've only done it in metastatic non-small cell lung cancer patients. That would be a good thing to do.

UNKNOWN: Did you do the test in patients before and after giving them levamisole?

ISSELL: No, I didn't.

CARL PINSKY: I have a question that relates, I think, to the CEA presentation of Dr. Lokich, but I think it has a more general application as well. How are some of the assays, which have been described, related to more commonly performed assays and their prognostic ability? About seven years ago we did one CEA assay in over a thousand patients with cancer, including several hundred with breast cancer. The test was not done serially so it couldn't be used for serial monitoring. It was done to see if the CEA level could be useful in staging the patients and in reflecting the clinical and pathologic stage we already had. We were not able with CEA or any other measure to differentiate those with or without nodes in surgical patients. But, it was very good, in fact, many different assays were good, in picking up patients with disseminated disease and differentiating them from earlier patients. Not only were CEAs done but also the whole battery of tests including the entire SMA battery, blood counts and so forth. It turned out that the best discriminant of disseminated disease was the combination of albumin and alkaline phosphatase. CEA in breast cancer didn't add anything to what we already could tell from these very commonly performed tests. What can you tell us about what you've done in multivariate analyses including those common tests as hemaglobin, liver chemistry and so forth?

JOSEPH LOKICH: I'll comment on the relationship to CEA. Dr. Pinsky has pointed out a very important distinction here between using any one of the determinants as a prognostic indicator versus using it as a monitor for therapy. I focused on monitoring for therapy. In my series of patients, CEA was a predictor consistently six to eight weeks prior to the patient having a clinical response, whether one was using alkaline phosphatase or any other measurement. Now, Mike O'Connell at the Mayo Clinic has made a major case for alkaline phosphatase in metastatic G.I. cancer being equivalent to and certainly in a cost effective way much better than CEA. However, it is clear that alkaline phosphatase is merely an enzyme. It doesn't directly relate to the host tumor but merely relates to an impact on whatever organ happens to be involved, the liver or the bone. CEA is clearly directly identifiable on the tumor. When we're affecting the tumor cells, we see these changes immediately in the CEA which is unlike these other parameters which are very much nonspecific.

PINSKY: I am aware that the example I gave used staging procedure and that you used serial testing. But nonetheless, I think it is still a valid question to ask you, did you do other more commonly applied tests, which are more cost effective as you pointed out, in your study and was CEA superior to these others used serially?

LOKICH: Yes, we did use them and CEA was the only test that would predict response in patients with bone lesions. What I was trying to emphasize was that CEA is the first test that does change and that CEA is the only test that we use that is tumor-specific.

DURIE: I can perhaps comment. I have tried to use polyamines as predictors of response and survival in patients with myeloma. In myeloma patients there are a number of ways to evaluate cell mass, stage and response using the serum component. You can get a very accurate handle on extent of disease and on the response to treatment by monitoring the serum M component. Using the component is relatively cheap and I have actually carried out a multivariant regression analysis using Cox's model system. At the time of initial diagnosis, polyamines drop out as a significant factor. All you really need are the more commonly used lab tests such as hemoglobin, calcium, and serum creatinine. I tried to indicate, as far as staging and initial prognosis go, that polyamines are very expensive and really don't add to the information that you already have. In terms of monitoring patients serially, in myeloma the serum marker is very useful. In patients who have stable disease, however, it can be hard to know if early relapse is occurring. Although I haven't done a multivariant regression analysis in the remission phase yet, it seems that polyamines may add some information in terms of indicating a early relapse. I think that it is very important to emphasize that you have to compare that information with information that you already have but may not have analyzed. Does anyone else wish to comment?

EDWIN COX: I think that is a very critical point. All the patients in our study undergo rather extensive and complete clinical work-up. In fact, my purpose in showing the lymph node slide in relation to the Con A was to make the point that one does have to compare the efficacy of various prognostic indicators. In our case multivariant analysis is now just starting and indeed will be a major component of the study.

DURIE: You showed one slide where the survival in patients with ER negative and ER positive biopsies seemed to converge; that would seem to be a group where maybe multivariant analysis would pick up populations.

COX: Absolutely. In relation to another question that was asked, and that is the difference in pre- and post-menopausal patients with respect to the efficacy of estrogen receptor as a prognostic indicator. Indeed they do differ in that the convergence patterns are different. They are not the same population.

UNKNOWN: I'm not so sure that we should be worrying about cost effectiveness when we are talking about diagnostic tests for cancer. We don't have the best available test yet. As a result I think that all studies that are done, obviously with some sort of thought to them, should be considered worthwhile. The concept that it's going to cost a patient $18 or $30 should not play a part right now. That's my own opinion. One of the other things that I consider in my own patients with metastatic breast cancer is following them, even though the literature may dictate against it, with a liver scan, with a bone scan, and perhaps even a brain scan if you believe in the systemic concept of the disease. We think that, perhaps now, we have chemotherapeutic agents that are sensitive to the disease if treated early. Continuing on the subject, I would like to ask Dr. Furmanski if he would add these tests to his group approach at the risk of cost? Also, I would like to know, what are your treatment modalities for these patients you are following? For instance, you are treating early lesions; I believe some of them are Stage II breast cancers. Are all these patients on adjuvant therapy protocols? Is this going to be part of your analytical schema when you come to some conclusions with your data?

PHILIP FURMANSKI: Let me point out that when this program was set up it was decided to go to the community hospitals to access patients into the study. One reason is that in our area it is the only way to enter large numbers of patients into a study. Also, the patient population that appears at the academically affiliated institutions is not representative of the total population of breast cancer patients. Unfortunately, that means we don't have full control over the patient population. Most of the physicians have agreed to follow a fairly strict protocol. But, if we introduce elements like multiple liver scans or bone scans, it is not just our notion of cost effectiveness that has to be taken into account; it is the notion of cost effectiveness in each of 14 community hospitals that has to be considered. The way we have gotten around this is that we have convinced many of the participants of the importance of a study of this type and tell them the cost effectiveness of these tests. One really doesn't know how efficacious bone scans are on a wide range of breast cancer patients in the community hospitals in terms of picking up metastases and in terms of how often they should be done. Specifically, we are doing bone scans in our Stage I and Stage II patients. Now, your other question about treatment. Most of our patients are Stage I and II and the vast majority of them are treated only by surgery. They don't receive adjuvant chemotherapy. There is a sub-population that does receive adjuvant chemotherapy and it varies from hospital to hospital and we are keeping records. In most instances we segregate out the untreated patient population until recurrence occurs. In our area the standard treatment is modified radical mastectomy and no further treatment until recurrence is observed, unless the patient comes in with frank metastases.

UNKNOWN: My question is to Drs. Furmanski and Lokich. Early Memorial Sloan-Kettering studies show some correlation with CEA and ER positivity in breast tissue, both normal and malignant. My question, Dr. Lokich, is did you do a CEA test and tests for ERP on your patients and was there a correlation?

LOKICH: We did not do a correlation with ERP on our patients with metastatic disease. That would be an interesting thing to go back and look at. I don't know about the correlation of CEA. There have been at least two studies, one by Wyan and one by Borthwick, which have looked at CEA as a correlate of prognosis of patients with primary disease. I think the correlation is difficult to establish because, predominantly, these patients have CEA levels in the normal range from zero to not greater than 5.

I'd like to go back to the previous comment about cost effectiveness. I think we have to prove first that early disease is, in fact, more responsive disease. I don't think we know that, in a definitive way, and the routine application of liver scans, bone scans, and brain scans on a regular basis for patients with early disease could be catastrophic to a nation. I certainly would not advocate it. I think many clinicians would suggest that patients who get metastatic disease basically are getting incurable disease. You treat patients who are symptomatic from their disease and, therefore, you wait until the symptom declares itself before you do the scan. The scan and other tests are means for measuring and determining the effectiveness of our treatment.

UNKNOWN: May I comment on that? Basically, I agree. I don't think that you can make a general statement about what to do in every patient. But, on the other hand, if you are at a medical center and if you do randomized perspective trials and if part of those trials in studying breast cancer happens to be the evaluation of not only diagnosis but surgery and then adjuvant therapy afterward, then I think every issue should be questioned. There is no doubt, and I see it at my center, that we've changed operations based on preoperative scanning. We've diagnosed advanced breast cancer when, indeed, all we had was a primary tumor in the breast and the surgeon had already determined that a modified radical or radical mastectomy was going to be done to not only further stage the patient but eliminate "all disease." Maybe we are dealing, as many people espouse, with systemic disease and these studies may be worthwhile until we find a good screening agent. I'm not saying every cancer should do this; but this is something we are committed to and to determine what the answers are. Then, you go to what is cost effective; it's not cost effective from that standpoint. The point is if you learn from one patient or two patients and you stage them out of a more radical procedure as the result of these studies, then the studies are worthwhile.

UNKNOWN: I think you basically made the distinction then between care in the community and care in the center on a study and I think certainly all of us would agree with that.

DURIE: Perhaps I could say something beyond that. Obviously you should identify a study setting where you are doing a lot of tests. To get correlations, even within that setting, you should consider whether something is useful and once it is established, whether it is going to be reasonable. If you've got a test that costs $500, it may be very good but that still is not going to be a reasonable test to do once a week.

UNKNOWN: I would like to address a question to Dr. Limas regarding ABH antigens and blood group antigens in cancer. I think you are probably aware that Philip Levine described back in the 1940's a patient with stomach cancer that had a modified antigen, I think it was TJA antigen. This patient became sensitized to this particular variant blood group antigen during the time of transfusion and then went on to live another 20 years. Davidsohn, here in Chicago, and many others have looked at ABH and cervical cancer and Springer at Northwestern University in Evanston has been looking at MN variants in terms of some types of cancers. You mentioned that in bladder cancers there were some changes in the ABH groups; but you didn't say what the changes were. In other words, if you had A, is that changing to O? Many of the reports of stomach cancers have had Os. In fact, I think there are six reports of Os changing to As which has always surprised me. I could understand the reverse. Also, you correlated these ABH groups with their potential for invasiveness, as if they were indicating a poor differentiated cell. Did you find any correlation once there was invasiveness with A, B or H? In other words, was the ABH of positive cell more aggressive in terms of its invasiveness?

CATHERINE LIMAS: I will start with the last question first because I remember it best. All the invasive tumors that we started were negative.

UNKNOWN: What do you mean negative?

LIMAS: Negative for the antigen that corresponds to the patient's blood group. When I say that the tumor is negative I mean for the antigen that you would expect according to the patient's ABO group.

UNKNOWN: So, if they were A, then did they go to O?

LIMAS: Yes, that was the point of the last two slides that I showed. You expect the blood group A patient will have his normal mucosa, a strong A reactivity and a week H reactivity simply because there is always some H reactivity in the residual that has not been transformed into a substance. However, the tumors showed just the reverse relationship. The reactivity for A substance, I didn't actually measure levels of A substance, was reduced compared to the patient's normal mucosa and the reactivity for H substance as detected with the Ulex lectin was increasing. This tells you that there is H that has not been transformed into A. There is one more comment about the Ulex. The Ulex extract has two lectins, one that is the specific for the L-α-fucosyl groups of the H substance and one that doesn't have anything to do with the H substance. In all the cases where we are detecting excessive H, we put into the reaction medium L-α-fucosyl to demonstrate that we are really detecting L-α-fucosyl groups that are related to the H substance. However, the detection of L-α-fucosyl groups is not 100% specific for H substance. Dr. Hakomori has written many papers on the subject and he has found that there is an excess of L-α-fucosyl groups, but not necessarily the real substance H. I believe that is the point you wanted me to clarify. Are they really the H antigens ready to be made into A and B antigens or are they precursors and more proximal to the biosynthesis of this substance? One way we have approached this problem is by using the Lewis antigens, because the Lewis antigens have also fucosyl groups as their final determinants and we are in the process of finalizing the results. It seems to be specific for H. Now, your other question, regarding changing from one group to the other, from A to B or B to A? There are published papers, one of them from Hakomori's group. They found A-like, they don't call it A, it's A-like reactivity and this A-like reactivity has something to do with the CEA reactivity. There is an overlapping of their reactivity. I have not done any studies in that direction to demonstrate a whole change. To find excess H on someone that is A or B is not a change in the enzymatic system, it is a defect, and not a new gene coming in. If you demonstrate a B patient getting it that way, it is a different gene and a different situation. In all our studies, the effects presented were on tumors that are in Stage O or A that have no muscle invasion and could not be detected by blood substance or anything like that. I tried to demonstrate especially for the grade II patients that the grading system does not have any predictive value in half of the patients. To our knowledge invasive tumors were all negative. Dr. Alroy has reported in *Cancer*, 1978, that if you irradiate the tumors, you may have a reappearance of the blood group antigens. I have not seen it myself. I didn't systematically look at that. I have simply irradiated tumors and they continued to be negative. I think the desire to irradiate a tumor is difficult morphologically because you have a lot of tumor degeneration and tumor necrosis. In the areas where the cells have degenerated, you get a nonspecific positive reactivity because of nonspecific absorption of serum. We have done serial experiments and you have to evaluate the results on well preserved cells and not on degenerating or necrotic cells.

MYLES CUNNINGHAM: I can not help but respond to the spirited discussion on serial monitoring and staging of the various biological and biochemical markers. We reported data to the SSO a year ago on bone scans and Dr. Edward Scanlon, of our group, just reported the same data on recurrence to the national ACS Conference. Our bone scan data not only were not helpful in staging patients but were frequently confusing. It tended to exclude occasionally patients, who did not have metastatic bone cancer from breast and who often had benign disorders as a cause for positive bone scans. Furthermore, we are going on record as saying that frequent laboratory investigations as followup for these patients is not only useless but terribly expensive. The single best criteria in identifying early recurrence is very frequent physical examination. The number of asymptomatic recurrences identified on laboratory testing was infinitesimally small. The number of symptomatic recurrences vastly exceeded asymptomatic and were generally easily confirmed only when patients became symptomatic. The physical exam was our very best tool. One might argue that this is not terribly cost effective because it requires a lot of patient time and physician time and is tedious, but it does work.

DURIE: I think it is a very important point and there have been studies exploring it. For example, I remember a melanoma study which looked at all the different bone scans and liver scans and the conclusion was that a physical examination and a chest X-ray were really all that were necessary.

UNKNOWN: Just a comment. The data which I presented were serial measurements at the time of diagnosis, but other serial measurements which we have done would essentially confirm that statement.

DURIE: I have a question for Dr. Helson, who presented data on the use of the immune complexes with respect to prognosis and staging in neuroblastoma. Is this data useful in making a treatment decision?

LAWRENCE HELSON: At this time, I think it is too early to utilize this information to make treatment decisions. The one thing I have tried to emphasize is that tumor burden is probably the major discriminant in terms of prognosis and not in measuring disease. The tumor burden at diagnosis is the major factor in determining the overall survival of patients. Unless you can distinguish other factors from the burden, per se, I think there are a lot of studies being done that are not really productive in the long run. I indicated that the immune complex is probably going to be worthless if you cannot isolate tumor burden per se from the immune complexes which depend upon it. Certain tumors, which are responsive and which we might find in these assays *in vitro* may be a more predictive discriminant to look at in terms of what the ultimate prognosis will be in spite of the tumor volume the patient has at diagnosis.

Chemotherapy of Clinical Metastases

Chemotherapy of Advanced Lung Cancer: The Memorial-Sloan Kettering Experience, 1974–1979 [a]

R.E. Wittes, R.J. Gralla, E.S. Casper,
D.P. Kelsen, E. Cvitkovic, R. Natale, J. Sierocki,
B. Hilaris, R.B. Golbey

Solid Tumor and Developmental Chemotherapy Services, Department of Medicine, and the Department of Radiation Therapy, Memorial Sloan-Kettering Cancer Center, New York, New York

Summary

For the past five years, clinical investigation in the chemotherapy of advanced lung cancer has proceeded along several lines. In nonsmall cell lung cancer, the failure of four combinations active in other neoplasms to show any significant anti-tumor effect in bronchogenic carcinoma led us to abandon efforts in this direction and to concentrate instead on the identification of active new agents from the roster of experimental drugs. From these Phase II trials, vindesine has emerged as the most active agent with a response rate of 33 percent in previously untreated patients with good performance status. Vindesine has been combined with cis-dichlorodiammineplatinum (II) (DDP), the latter given in both low and high dose. Although response rate of the combination appears to be independent of DDP dose, response durations are significantly longer with high dose treatment.

In small cell carcinoma, since many conventional agents show significant activity, we have been concentrating on the construction of new combinations of agents, adding experimental drugs where appropriate and radiotherapy for the control of specific sites. During this period, the complete response rate has risen dramatically and survival of the treated population has increased as well. It is, however, too early to say whether

[a]Supported in part by Grants CA-08748 and CA-08526 from the National Cancer Institute, National Institutes of Health, Bethesda, Maryland.

the most recent treatment plans have resulted in an increased rate of continuous disease-free survival, but an increased cure rate seems probable for a substantial fraction of the population with limited disease.

Introduction

As the leading cancer-related cause of death in the United States, bronchogenic carcinoma is certainly one of the most difficult and pressing problems in cancer therapy. Numerous studies dealing with the natural history of the disease and the failure of local treatment modalities[1-3] serve to emphasize that all histologic types of bronchogenic carcinoma are likely to be widespread at the time of presentation. Thus the need for effective systemic therapy with manageable toxicity is obvious.

Table 1 shows the estimates of activity of the various conventional agents in the histologic subtypes of lung cancer. These figures have been gathered by pooling data from many studies which, in the case of the older drugs, were often performed before criteria of response became standardized. In addition to varying criteria of response, the dose and schedule of the agents often varied widely from study to study. Perhaps most important, however, the criteria of patient selection were not uniform so that, for example, variables of great prognostic importance such as age, performance status and extent of disease, might differ in important and unspecified ways from one study to another. Not surpris-

Table 1. Percent of Patients Responding to Treatment with Single Agents by Cell Type[a]

	Epidermoid	Adenocarcinoma	Large Cell	Small Cell
Methotrexate	25	32	12	39
Dibromodulcitol	23	–	–	–
Mechlorethamine	21	28	26	39
Cyclophosphamide	20	21	23	31
Adriamycin	19	15	25	25
CCNU	17	13	17	19
Vinblastine	16	–	–	–
Bleomycin	13	13	–	0
Procarbazine	13	–	–	25
Hexamethylmelamine	12	15	18	26
Busulfan	7	4	–	–
BCNU	6	0	9	–
Methyl-CCNU	6	13	17	–
Mitomycin C	0	–	–	–
VP-16	–	–	–	36
Vincristine	–	–	–	30

[a] Data from References 31, 32.

ingly, therefore, response rates to individual agents commonly vary a good deal among studies and estimates such as those shown in Table 1 are often imprecise and, particularly in the case of the older agents, overly optimistic.

Discussion

For the nonsmall cell lung cancers (NSCLC), therapy with single agents has been disappointing because the available agents induce remissions at a very low frequency. With small cell lung cancer (SCLC), however, many of the agents in current use can induce tumor regression with fair frequency. Despite the relative chemosensitivity of SCLC, however, the responses achieved with single agents are generally only partial; hence, although prolongation of survival in the treated population is often seen in single-agent studies of SCLC, durable long term remissions are almost never achieved. Because of the difference in chemosensitivity of the small cell and nonsmall cell subtypes of lung cancer, we have evolved quite distinct approaches to the therapy of each and shall therefore discuss each class separately.

Nonsmall Cell Lung Cancer—Combination Chemotherapy

The success in the late 1960s of combination chemotherapy in Hodgkin's disease and the acute leukemias engendered a similar optimism for the treatment of many of the common solid tumors, including lung cancer. A large number of clinical trials have identified a few combinations of conventional agents with response rates in the 30–50 percent range.[4–8] Whether based on kinetic considerations, biochemical factors or simple empiricism, most protocols have ended up including an alkylating agent, Adriamycin, and methotrexate. In two cases,[6,7] although initial response rates appeared promising, subsequent multi-institutional randomized trials revealed that the actual activity, as assessed in a cooperative group setting, was much lower (5–21 percent). Survival medians ranged from two and one half to seven months, with the previously mentioned prognostic variables probably playing a role in the differences observed among the combinations.

Several years ago at the Memorial Sloan-Kettering Cancer Center (MSKCC), we attempted to employ combinations of drugs active in other solid tumors in the treatment of lung cancer. These included the vinblastine–actinomycin D–bleomycin combination designed for germ cell tumors of the testis; the mitomycin C–5FU–arabinosylcytosine combination designed for gastric cancer; methyl-CCNU–Adriamycin–vincristine for soft-tissue sarcomas, and cyclophosphamide-Adriamycin-5FU-methotrexate, which had been used in breast cancer. Each of these combinations had shown activity in the disorder for which it was designed and yet no major response was seen in any patient with NSCLC. Although an accumulation of patients with poor prognostic features may have been important in some of these trials, we became disillustioned with the potential utility of these drugs in NSCLC. Despite the lack of significant responses to any of these combinations, however, the median survival in these trials was two and one half to six months—comparable with the survival experience in other institutions which have employed protocols with an ostensibly higher response rate. Although comparison of results across institutions is hazardous, the comparability of survival suggests that the reported responses may not produce sufficient tumor cell kill to alter significantly the natural history of the disease. Alternatively, the response rates may simply not be high enough to effect the median survival of the treated population as a whole, since in even the most optimistic trials fewer than 50 percent of patients have shown a significant objective response.

Nonsmall Cell Lung Cancer—Phase II Studies

With the poor results observed in the combination studies at MSKCC, we concluded that the use of conventional agents was unlikely to improve results significantly in the treatment of NSCLC. We therefore turned to more intensive trials of experimental drugs. Recently, several new agents have been tested (Table 2) including: pyrazofurin, an orotidylate decarboxylase inhibitor;[9] vindesine, a new vinca alkaloid;[10] chlorozotocin, a water-soluble nitrosourea;[11] phosphonacetyl-1-aspartate (PALA), an inhibitor of de novo pyrimidine synthesis,[12] and m-AMSA, an intercalating agent.[13] As shown in Table 2, only vindesine showed enough activity to warrant further study. This agent was active in both epidermoid and adenocarcinoma with only mild toxicity (peripheral neuropathy and leukopenia) and with a median duration of response of five months. While an overall response rate of 22 percent was observed with vindesine, patients with no prior chemotherapy had a 33 percent response rate, compared with 12 percent for those previously treated.[10]

Recent trials of cis-dichlorodiammineplatinum (II) (DDP) in patients who have not received prior chemotherapy have been encouraging. At

Table 2. Phase II Studies in Nonsmall Cell Lung Cancer at MSKCC 1976-1979

Agent	Patients	PR	MR	PR Rate (percent)
Pyrazofurin	27	0	3	0
Vindesine	46	10	7	22
Chlorozotocin	27	2	3	7
AMSA	21	0	1	0
PALA	28	0	4	0

several institutions,[14-17] trials have shown response rates ranging from 10–21 percent, with a combined 17 percent partial response rate in 63 patients. currently, studies with the antifol metoprine and the immuno-modulator interferon are in progress at MSKCC.

For the past two years the combination chemotherapy of NSCLC at MSKCC has been based on the introduction of new agents into initial treatment. DDP has been an attractive agent for combination in that it represents a new class of alkylating agent, is associated with only mild myelosuppression and has some degree of activity in lung cancer. Several centers have tested protocols which involved cyclophosphamide, Adria-mycin and DDP (CAP). Response rates have ranged from 18–38 per-cent[18,19] in trials which involved these three drugs in a variety of doses and schedules. In the study at MSKCC (Table 3),[20] an overall major response rate of 28 percent was observed in 46 patients; in those with no prior chemotherapy, however, the rate was 35 percent and greater toxicity occurred in the previously treated group. No patient with a performance status of less than 60 experienced a major response. Median duration of partial responses was 8.5 months and responding patients showed a clear survival advantage (13 months versus four months for nonresponders). We believe that DDP has played a significant role in the therapeutic activity of this combination and that the toxicity, primarily leukopenia, has been largely secondary to the cyclophosphamide and Adriamycin.

Thus, both DDP and vindesine appeared to be agents with useful activity in lung cancer and the two drugs exhibited differing toxicities. Patients with poor performance status or a history of prior chemotherapy experienced greater toxicity and lower response rates. From the results with the various CAP protocols, it was not clear whether high doses of DDP offered an advantage over more modest doses. Thus a study was initiated in which previously untreated patients with performance status 60 or greater were given vindesine (3 mg/m^2 IV weekly for seven weeks and every other week thereafter) and were randomized to receive simultaneously either low-dose or high-dose DDP (60 mg/m^2 IV versus 120 mg/m^2 IV with a mannitol-induced diuresis, given initially and repeated once at four weeks and every six weeks thereafter). To date 60 patients with measurable, inoperable NSCLC have been treated with this combination.[21] Toxicity has been managed easily with a median platelet nadir of 190,000 and a WBC nadir of 2900. Significant azotemia and peripheral neuropathy were observed in 12 percent and 4 percent of patients respectively. Twenty-six patients have experienced complete or partial responses for a 43 percent major response rate. Response rates were similar for epidermoid and adenocarcinoma and for those treated with high- or low-dose DDP. The duration of response, however, has been significantly greater (p < 0.05) for patients receiving high-dose DDP

Table 3. Combination Chemotherapy in Nonsmall Cell Lung Cancer at MSKCC 1977-1979

Regimen	Patients	PR	MR	PR Rate (percent)
Cyclophosphamide DDP Adriamycin	46	13	7	28
Vindesine DDP	60	26	6	43

(9+ months versus 5.5 months for those treated with low-dose DDP). While it is too early to comment on survival in the two treatment groups, we expect the improvement in response duration to lead to an advantage in survival.

In summary, NSCLC is a disease for which a "state of the art" treatment does not exist. Recent improvements in response rates and durations have been encouraging. In the experience at MSKCC, these improvements have been the result of the implementation of new active agents in initial therapy. Current combinations which appear useful represent a starting point for further investigation. We plan to continue the testing of new agents and the incorporating of those which are found active into initial treatment programs.

Small Cell Lung Cancer

As noted previously, in SCLC the clinical challenge has been not only the discovery of new active agents, but also the optimal use of existing tools. In common with most investigators, therefore, we have been exploring the potential of combination chemotherapy, often integrated into a combined modality approach along with radiation. From July, 1974, to March, 1978, a total of 101 patients were treated on three protocols designed for SCLC (Table 4). Our initial regimen (COMA) was based on the encouraging preliminary report from the Dartmouth-Hitchcock Medical Center[22] on the activity of vincristine and methotrexate in combination with high doses of cyclophosphamide; we cut the dose of the alkylating agent and added Adriamycin. Radiation therapy to the primary complex was employed in most patients with limited disease. Although the regimen yielded a respectable response rate (Table 5), the complete response rate was only 17 percent.[23] From the original population of 30 adequately treated patients, only one has remained continuously free of disease; she is currently four years from start of treatment and has been off all therapy for two years. Analysis of the patterns of relapse revealed that the use of radiation to the primary complex did not prevent treatment failure at that site; in fact, of a total of 23 patients who

Table 4. Regimens for Small Cell Carcinoma at MSKCC 1974-1978[a]

	COMA	CAV-BMP[b]	PVP-CAV[c]
	Dates: 7/74-12/75	Dates: 12/75-3/77	Dates: 4/77-3/78
Cyclophosphamide	1000 d 1 q29d	1000 d 1,22	1000 d 43,64,85,106
Adriamycin	30 d 1 q 29d	30 d 1,22	40 d 43,64,85,106
Vincristine	1.4 d 1 q 29d	1.4 d 1,22	1.4 d 43,64,85,106
BCNU	–	100 d 43,44	–
Methotrexate	30 d 22 q29d	30 d 50,64	–
Procarbazine	–	100 po d 51-64	–
DDP	–	–	60 d 1,22
VP-16	–	–	120 d 4,6,8 & 25,27,29
1° RT	3000 rads/10 fx[d]	–	–
Brain RT	–	–	3000 rads/10 fx

[a] All drug doses are mg/m^2 IV unless otherwise specified.
[b] On day 85, recycle with CAV.
[c] On day 127, recycle with PVP.
[d] Limited disease patients only.

had received primary complex irradiation at some time in their course, seven developed their initial sign of uncontrolled disease at that site. Viewed differently, of 26 relapsing sites in 19 patients available for analysis, 10 relapsed initially in the chest.

We also learned that the delivery of mediastinal radiation in close temporal proximity to chemotherapy could be hazardous; four of 13

Table 5. Results with Regimens for Small Cell Carcinoma

	COMA	CAV-BMP	PVP-CAV
Total adequate	30	33	38
Percent limited disease	48%	67%	55%
PS[a] (median)	70 (50-90)	80 (40-100)	90 (60-100)
Percent male	50%	76%	71%
Age (median)	62 (44-74)	59 (40-78)	58 (36-84)
CR (%)	17%	16%	47%
PR (%)	63%	55%	47%
Total Response Rate	80%	71%	94%
Continuous NED[b] as of 8/79	1 (48+)	1 (42+)	4 (27+, 21+, 21+, 18+)

[a] Karnofsky scale.
[b] Durations in parentheses are in months.

patients so treated developed severe esophagitis which necessitated hospitalization and parenteral fluid support. One of these patients developed a late esophageal stricture[24] prior to her death.

In order to increase the complete response rate, we altered this regimen by adding BCNU and procarbazine to the four agents in the COMA regimen; we also rescheduled the drugs to form two independent three-drug regimens to be administered sequentially. Radiation therapy was reserved for the local treatment of relapse and was not given as part of the primary treatment.

The results of this regimen were disappointing in several respects.[25] Neither the total response rate nor the complete response rate was significantly different from those obtained with the COMA regimen. Moreover, all responses appeared to be maximal within the first six weeks of treatment with CAV; in other words, BMP did not seem to add any measurable anti-tumor effect to that already achieved with CAV. This result surprised us. Since the three drugs in the BMP combination were each active in SCLC and did not share a common mechanism of action with the components of CAV, we had expected to see additional tumor shrinkage with BMP administration. Since we did not, however, we were not surprised to find that the survival characteristics of the treated population were not very different from that treated with COMA (Figures 1, 2). At present, two patients treated on this protocol remain alive, but only one of these has been continuously disease-free since starting treatment (currently 42+ months, off treatment for 18 months). Interestingly, this patient presented with extensive disease (mediastinum with superior vena caval syndrome, pleural effusion) and never received radiation therapy.

In this protocol, intrathoracic relapse constituted a larger percentage of relapsing sites than in the COMA experience, probably because radiation was not routinely given to the primary complex as part of initial treatment. In the 26 patients analyzed for relapse as of January, 1978, 22 of the 34 relapsing sites were intrathoracic. Despite the inclusion of a lipid-soluble nitrosourea, central nervous system recurrences occurred at about the same rate as before (15–20 percent of initial relapses).

By this time the activity of VP-16 in SCLC had been well established.[26,27] Since we had not been able to increase our CR rate to 20 percent or more with chemotherapy regimens based on cyclophosphamide, Adriamycin and vincristine, and since we had failed to increase the CR rate by using BMP after remission induction with CAV, we believed that the early use of new agents was justified. Since the CR rate with VP-16 alone was presumably quite low,[26,27] we preferred to use this agent in combination. Despite the lack of information on the activity of DDP in SCLC, we decided that this drug represented a reasonable one for combination with VP-16. Since DDP is only mildly myelosup-

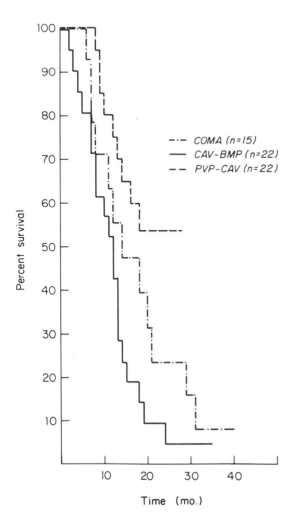

Figure 1. Small cell lung cancer: Survival of limited disease patients for each of the three protocols described in the text.

pressive, it can be used in good doses in combination with VP-16. In addition, its relatively broad spectrum of anti-tumor activity made us sanguine about its potential utility in the initial combination therapy of SCLC.

We should note that in certain tumor types such as SCLC and carcinoma of the breast, investigators in clinical oncology often face a vexing problem in deciding on a strategy for incorporating new agents into initial therapy. Traditionally, new agents are tested for anti-tumor activity in patients who have already failed primary therapy; in the case

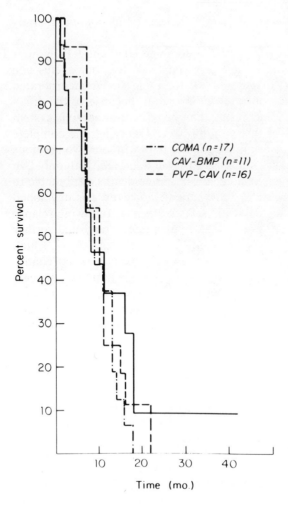

Figure 2. Small cell lung cancer: Survival of extensive disease patients for each protocol.

of SCLC or breast cancer, this usually implies failure to several cytotoxic agents. Such patients may have widely disseminated disease, a poor performance status and severely impaired marrow reserve. Under such circumstances, the activity of a new agent may not reflect what the same agent could achieve as primary therapy. Since the "response rate" of a drug is surely a function of the host factors just outlined, we were unwilling to assume that a traditional Phase II study of DDP in SCLC would be an accurate mirror of the agent's potential as primary treatment. We were also unwilling to use it as a single agent in previously untreated patients, since we did not want to deprive these patients of initial therapy of known effectiveness.

For these reasons, then, we elected to combine DDP and VP-16; after two such cycles, the patients then received CAV for four cycles and then were switched back to DDP and VP-16 (Table 4). We incorporated prophylactic cranial irradiation into this program, because of the effectiveness of this modality in decreasing the rate of central nervous system relapse. The early results of this program were gratifying; the complete response rate (47 percent) was notably higher than with our two previous regimens (Table 5). The chemotherapy was well tolerated, with only two hospitalizations for treatment-related sepsis and no deaths attributable to the acute effects of treatment.[28] One patient, however, has developed a hematologic picture consistent with aplastic anemia; following relapse on the present protocol, he was treated with radiotherapy and further chemotherapy with CCNU, methotrexate and procarbazine, of which after two cycles he developed refractory pancytopenia which has continued for several months. Survival on the PVP-CAV protocol appears somewhat better for the limited disease group than with our previous protocols. The median survival has not yet been reached, but will exceed 18 months (Figure 1). Only four patients, however, have been continuously free of disease since the start of therapy; these patients have been at risk for 18, 21, 21, and 27 months, respectively. Since it is reasonable to assume that they represent the only possible candidates for long survival among the total group of survivors, it is clear that ample room for improvement still exists. It is also obvious that the survival of the extensive disease group has not been altered by any of the manipulations in therapy that we have tried thus far (Figure 2).

A rather striking feature of our experience with alternating sequences of combinations (both the CAV-BMP and the PVP-CAV regimens) was that all responses were maximal by the end of the first six weeks of treatment. That is, in no case did the use of BMP in the CAV-BMP regimen, or the CAV in the PVP-CAV regimen improve any of the responses already induced. Moreover, the survival characteristics of the population of patients divided by response category (Figure 3) reinforced our opinion that the achievement of a complete response was the only immediate end point of real interest. We therefore concluded that the first 6 weeks were a critical period in the therapy and the efficacy of treatment during this time would determine whether the patient achieved CR status or not. Accordingly, we modified the PVP-CAV regimen[29] as shown in Table 6. Aside from a change in the sequencing of the two combinations and a slight increase in the dose of the CAV portion, the major modification was the abandonment of fixed time intervals for recycling treatment; instead, treatment is repeated as soon as each patient's pattern of toxicity allows. We suspected that the more drugs

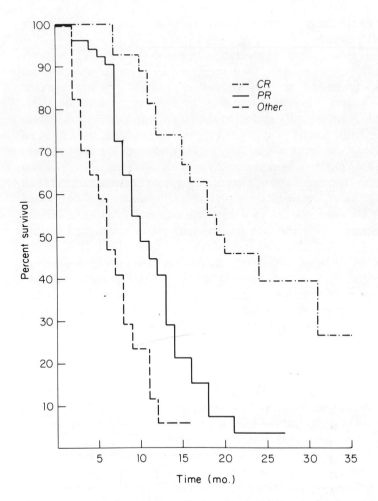

Figure 3. Small cell carcinoma of lung: Survival by response category. All three protocols have been combined for calculation of these curves. Although the CR group clearly enjoys a survival advantage over the other groups, the CR group remains at risk for relapse for the entire time period shown.

the patient could receive during the induction period, the more likely was attainment of a CR. In addition, we decided to re-introduce radiation therapy to the primary complex in limited disease, since it seemed likely that at least some patients might be converted from PR to CR by such treatment. Because of our disappointing experience with such radiation in the COMA protocol, and because a dose-response curve for radiation probably exists in SCLC,[30] we decided to increase the dose of radiation delivered to the target volume to 4500 rads via a three-field technique.

Table 6. Current Regimen for Small Cell Carcinoma at MSKCC 1978-1979

A. Induction
   (i)   Cycles 1 and 3
         Cyclophosphamide 1200 mg/m^2
         Adriamycin 50 mg/m^2
         Vincristine 1.4 mg/m^2
   (ii) Cycles 2 and 4
         DDP 60 mg/m^2 d 1
         VP-16 120 mg/m^2 d 4,6,8

B. Radiotherapy (to begin when induction is completed)
   (i)   Prophylactic brain
   (ii) Primary complex (limited disease only), 4500 rads via three-field technique
   (iii) Cyclophosphamide 600 mg/m^2 and vincristine 1.4 mg/m^2 IV on days 1 and 14 of the
         radiation course

C. Maintenance
   (i)   Limited disease patients who have attained CR on (A) and (B) above are given no
         maintenance therapy
   (ii) All others are maintained with alternating cycles of:
         (1) CCNU, methotrexate, procarbazine
         (2) Cyclophosphamide, vincristine, Adriamycin
         (3) DDP, VP-16
         for a total duration of therapy of one year in the absence of relapse

The preliminary results of this induction program look very encouraging. Of 43 patients treated thus far, the CR rate from the chemotherapy induction is 62 percent. The limited disease group (24 patients) has a CR rate of 67 percent after induction chemotherapy; after conclusion of radiation, 83 percent are in CR. Nothing significant can be said about duration of response or survival, since followup is too short. As might be anticipated, the toxicity of this regimen is significantly greater than that of our previous programs; although the regimen is designed to be given entirely to outpatients, about one third of patients have to be admitted to the hospital for fever in the presence of neutropenia. This increased rate of morbidity will be justifiable only if the therapeutic results are strikingly better than we have seen in the past.

References

1. Lanzotti, VJ, Thomas, OR, Boyle, LE et al.: Survival with inoperable lung cancer. *Cancer* 39:303–313, 1977.
2. Green, N, Kurohara, SS, George, FW: Cancer of the lung: an in-depth analysis of prognostic factors. *Cancer* 28:1229–1233, 1971.
3. Mittman, C, Bruderman, I: Lung cancer: to operate or not? *Am. Rev. Resp. Dis.* 116:447–496, 1977.

4. Bitran, JD, Desser, RK, DeMeester, TR et al.: Cyclophosphamide, Adriamycin, methotrexate, and procarbazine (CAMP)—effective four-drug combination chemotherapy for metastatic non oat cell bronchogenic carcinoma. *Cancer Treatment Rep.* 60:1225–1230, 1976.

5. Chahinian, AP, Mandel, EM, Holland, JF et al.: MACC (methotrexate, Adriamycin, cyclophosphamide, and CCNU) in advanced lung cancer. *Cancer* 43:1590–1597, 1979.

6. Livingston, RB, Heilbrun, L, Lehane, D et al.: Comparative trial of combination chemotherapy in extensive squamous carcinoma of the lung: a Southwest Oncology Group study. *Cancer Treatment Rep.* 61:1623–1629, 1977.

7. Bodey, GP, Lagakos, SW, Gutierrez, AC et al.: Therapy of advanced squamous carcinoma of the lung. *Cancer* 39:1026–1031, 1977.

8. Butler, TP, MacDonald, JS, Smith, FP et al.: 5-fluorouracil, Adriamycin, and mitomycin-C (FAM) chemotherapy for adenocarcinoma of the lung. *Cancer* 43:1183–1188, 1979.

9. Gralla, RJ, Currie, VE, Wittes, RE et al.: Phase II evaluation of pyrazofurin in patients with carcinoma of the lung. *Cancer Treatment Rep.* 62:451–452, 1978.

10. Gralla, RJ, Raphael, BG, Golbey, RB et al.: Phase II evaluation of vindesine in patients with nonsmall cell carcinoma of the lung. *Cancer Treatment Rep.* (in press).

11. Casper, ES, Gralla, RJ: Phase II evaluation of chlorozotocin in patients with nonsmall cell carcinoma of the lung. *Cancer Treatment Rep.* 63:549–550, 1979.

12. Casper, ES, Gralla, RJ, Kelsen, DP et al.: Phase II evaluation of PALA (N-Phosphonacetyl-1-aspartate) in patients with nonsmall cell carcinoma of the lung. (submitted for publication).

13. Casper, ES, Gralla, RJ, Kelsen, DP et al.: m-AMSA, 4-(9-acridinylamino)-methanesulfon-m-anisilide: a Phase II evaluation in patients with nonsmall cell lung cancer. (submitted for publication).

14. Casper, ES, Gralla, RJ, Kelsen, DP et al.: Phase II study of high-dose cis-diamminedichloroplatinum (II) in the treatment of nonsmall cell lung cancer. *Cancer Treatment Rep.* (in press).

15. Rossof, AH, Bearden, JD, Coltman, CA Jr.: Phase II evaluation of cis-diamminedichloroplatinum (II) in lung cancer. *Cancer Treatment Rep.* 60:1679–1680, 1978.

16. Longeval, E, DeJager, R, Libert, P et al.: Phase II clinical trial of high-dose cis-diamminedichloroplatinum (II) with mannitol-induced diuresis in advanced bronchogenic carcinoma. (personal communication).

17. Britell, JC, Eagen, RT, Ingle, JN et al.: Cis-dichlorodiammineplatinum (II) alone followed by Adriamycin plus cyclophosphamide at progression versus cis-dichlorodiammineplatium (II), Adriamycin, and cyclophosphamide in combination for adenocarcinoma of the lung. *Cancer Treatment Rep.* 62:1207–1210, 1978.

18. Eagan, RT, Ingle, JN, Frytak, S et al.: Platinum-based polychemotherapy versus dianhydrogalactitol in advanced nonsmall cell lung cancer. *Cancer Treatment Rep.* 61:1339–1345, 1977.

19. Bjornsson, S, Takita, H, Kuberka, N et al.: Combination chemotherapy plus methanol extracted residue of Bacillus Calmette-Guérin or *Corynebacterium Parvum* in Stage III Lung Cancer. *Cancer Treatment Rep.* 62:505–510, 1978.

20. Gralla, RJ, Cvitkovic, E, Golbey, RB: Cis-diamminedichloroplatinum (II) in nonsmall cell carcinoma of the lung. *Cancer Treatment Rep.* (in press).

21. Casper, ES, Gralla, RJ, Golbey, RB: Vindesine and cis-dichlorodiammineplatinum (II) combination chemotherapy in nonsmall cell lung cancer. *Proc. Am. Soc. Clin. Oncol.* 20:337, 1979.

22. Eagan, RT, Maurer, LH, Forcier, RJ, Tulloh, M: Small cell carcinoma of the lung—staging, paraneoplastic syndromes, treatment, and survival. *Cancer* 33:527–532, 1974.

23. Wittes, RE, Hopfan, S, Hilaris, B et al.: Oat cell carcinoma of the lung: combination treatment with radiotherapy and cyclophosphamide, Adriamycin, vincristine, and methotrexate. *Cancer* 40:653–659, 1977.

24. Chabora, BM, Hopfan, S, Wittes, RE: Esophageal complications in the treatment of oat cell carcinoma with combined radiation and chemotherapy. *Radiology* 123:185–187, 1977.

25. Sierocki, JS, Hilaris, B, Hopfan, S et al.: Small cell carcinoma of the lung—experience with a six-drug regimen. *Cancer* (in press).

26. Eagan, RT, Frytak, S, Rubin, J: VP-16 vs polychemotherapy in small cell lung cancer. *Proc. Am. Soc. Clin. Oncol.* 17:243, 1976.

27. Dombernowsky, P, Hansen, HH, Nissen, NI: Treatment of small cell anaplastic carcinoma of the lung with an oral solution of VP 16-213—a phase II trial. *Proc. Am. Soc. Clin. Oncol.* 17:129, 1976.

28. Sierocki, JS, Hilaris, BS, Hopfan, S et al.: Cis-dichlorodiammineplatinum (II) and VP-16: an active induction regimen for small cell carcinoma of the lung. *Cancer Treatment Rep.* (in press).

29. Natale, R, Hilaris, B, Golbey, RB, Wittes, RE: Induction chemotherapy in small cell carcinoma of the lung. *Proc. Am. Soc. Clin. Oncol.* 20:343, 1979.

30. Choi, CW, Carey, RW: Small cell anaplastic carcinoma of the lung. *Cancer* 37:2651–2657, 1976.

31. Muggia, FM, Rozencweig, M, eds. *Lung Cancer: Progress in Therapeutic Research; Progress in Cancer Research and Therapy,* Volume 11, p. 614, Raven Press, New York, 1979.

32. Selawry, OS: On chemotherapy of lung cancer. In: Muggia, FM, Rozencweig, M, eds. *Lung Cancer: Progress in Therapeutic Research; Progress in Cancer Research and Therapy,* Volume 11, Raven Press, New York, 1979.

The Treatment of Advanced Diffuse "Histiocytic" Lymphoma[a]

Donald L. Sweet, Harvey M. Golomb

The Department of Medicine and The Cancer Research Center,
The University of Chicago, Chicago, Illinois

Summary

A program of combination sequential chemotherapy using high dose cyclophosphamide, Oncovin®, methotrexate with leucovorin rescue and cytosine arabinoside (COMLA) was administered to 42 previously untreated patients with advanced diffuse histiocytic lymphoma (DHL). Twenty-three patients (55 percent) achieved a complete remission. The observed median duration of survival for the complete responders is in excess of 33 months. Eight patients (19 percent) achieved a partial response, with a median survival in excess of 21 months. Eleven patients (25 percent) showed no response, with a median survival of five months. Toxicity was acceptable. There was no difference in response rates between patients with stage III or IV lymphoma or between asymptomatic ("A") or symptomatic ("B") patients. None of the responders has shown central nervous system relapse. The COMLA regimen was administered also to 14 previously treated patients with advanced DHL; only two (14 percent) achieved a complete remission. The COMLA program produces a high rate of complete remissions and may prevent central nervous system relapse.

[a]This study was supported in part by The Joanne Heppes Fund, The Goldblatt Brothers Employees Nathan Goldblatt Cancer Research Fund, The Kathy Shaheen Fund and The Jean Heiman Fund.

Introduction

Prior to 1972, patients with advanced diffuse histiocytic lymphoma (DHL; as defined by Rappaport)[1] were often treated with single agent therapy. Complete remission rates were less than 10 percent and median survivals were less than one year. In 1972 and 1975 Leavitt et al. reported on six of eight patients with DHL who achieved a complete remission after treatment with a combination sequential chemotherapy program of cyclophosphamide, Oncovin® (vincristine), methotrexate and leucovorin rescue and cytosine arabinoside; median survivals were in excess of one year.[2]

Since 1972, the efficacy of several combination chemothereapy programs has been reported including C-MOPP (Cyclosphophamide, Oncovin®, Procarbazine, and Prednisone);[3] BACOP (Bleomycin, Adriamycin, Cyclophosphamide, Oncovin®, and Prednisone);[4] CHOP/HOP (Cyclophosphamide, Hydroxydaunomycin [Adriamycin], Oncovin®, and Prednisone/Hydroxydaunomycin, Oncovin®, and Prednisone);[5] and COPA (Cyclophosphamide, Oncovin®, Prednisone, and Adriamycin). These programs have resulted in improved complete remission rates (14 percent to 68 percent) and disease-free survivals. These programs are limited to toxicity related to Adriamycin, bleomycin or prednisone. Some centers using these regimens have reported a number of central nervous system (CNS) relapses in patients achieving a complete remission which is reminiscent of acute lymphoblastic leukemia of childhood.

In 1974 we initiated a prospective study of COMLA (the acronym includes "L" to describe more accurately the regimen) for patients with advanced DHL. The following is a summary of our results.

Methods

Characteristics of the Patient Population

Between March, 1974, and March, 1979, 42 previous untreated patients with stage III or IV DHL were treated with the COMLA regimen. There were 21 males and 21 females and the median age was 52 years (range 18 to 75 years). An additional 14 patients with advanced DHL who failed prior chemotherapy, radiation therapy or both were also treated with COMLA. Of these patients, four had received chemotherapy, six, radiation therapy and four, chemotherapy, as well as radiation therapy. All hematopathologic material was classified according to the criteria of Rappaport.[1] Patients with nodular histiocytic, mixed-cell type, or two histologies are not included in this study.

Staging Evaluation

Staging criteria were those as suggested by the Ann Arbor Conference of Hodgkin's Disease.[6] Staging evaluation included four bilateral posterior iliac crest bone core biopsies and a percutaneous liver biopsy if appropriate. Patients with two parameters for abdominal involvement (CS III) were not subjected to laparotomy. Most patients with bone marrow involvement had a lumbar puncture for cytologic examination. Two patients with clinical stage IV (lung) were too ill to undergo surgical biopsy. Thirty-eight of the 42 patients had their stage pathologically documented.

COMLA Regimen

The COMLA regimen (Figure 1) consists of high dose cyclophosphamide, 1.5 g/m², on Day one, and vincristine, 1.4 mg/m², on Days one, eight, and 15. Methotrexate, 120 mg/m² and cytosine arabinoside, 300 mg/m² are then administered for eight consecutive weeks, on Days 22, 29, 36, 43, 50, 57, 64 and 71. A two-week rest period is given and the cycle is repeated. Three total cycles are administered. All of the agents are administered intravenously with the exception of the leucovorin rescue, which is given *per os*, 25 mg/m², beginning 24 hours after the methotrexate infusion for four doses, six hours apart. The dosage of myelosuppressive agents was reduced according to a sliding scale (Table 1).

Figure 1. Graph showing time sequence and drug dosages of a single cycle of combination sequential chemotherapy.

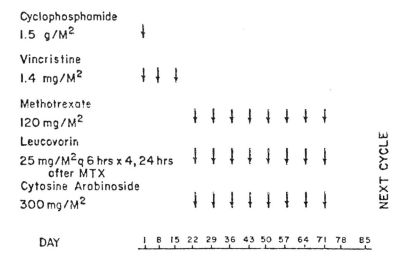

Table 1. Dosage Reduction Schedule for Bone Marrow Depression

If neutrophil count on day of therapy was:	If platelet count on day of therapy was:	Dose to be given:
> 4000/mm³	> 100,000/mm³	100 percent all drugs
3000-3999/mm³	75-100,000/mm³	100 percent cyclophosphamide, vincristine, methotrexate; 75 percent cytosine arabinoside
2000-2999/mm³	50-74,999/mm³	100 percent vincristine, methotrexate; 75 percent cyclophosphamide; 50 percent cytosine arabinoside
< 2000/mm³	< 50,000/mm³	None[a]

[a] If cytopenia(s) are due to bone marrow replacement, 100 percent dose is given. For severe nausea or vomiting, cytosine arabinoside was reduced up to 50 percent.

Patients who received at least four weeks of chemotherapy were eligible for study.

One month after the completion of the third COMLA cycle, all patients felt to be in complete remission clinically were reevaluated. Residual or suspicious lymphadenopathy was biopsied. Two patients underwent a repeat laparotomy in order to document equivocal data generated during the restaging procedure. If all evidence of disease had disappeared, the term "complete remission" was employed and no further therapy was given. Such patients were followed at two-month intervals thereafter. For this study, a "partial remission" (PR) indicates a 50 percent or greater reduction in a measurable tumor mass lasting for more than two months. The majority of these patients was given BACOP or other chemotherapy.

Survival was calculated from the date of diagnosis. Remission duration was determined from the date of first objective CR to relapse. The data were analyzed by the life-table method,[7] and subgroup evaluation was made with 2×2 contingency tables employing the Yates correction method.[8]

Results

Response to Therapy

Twenty-three or 55 percent of the 42 previously untreated patients achieved a complete remission (CR). The median disease-free survival was more than 21 months. The observed median survival of the complete responders was in excess of 36 months (range six to 63 months). Three patients relapsed at 12, 16 and 31 months, respectively, but all three achieved a second CR with COMLA.

Eight patients, or 19 percent, achieved a partial response (PR). All of these patients demonstrated objective progression of disease during the subsequent course of therapy after their initial response. The median survival of the PR group was in excess of 21 months (range six to 42 months).

Eleven patients, or 26 percent, showed no response to chemotherapy. The median survival was five months (range three to 19 months). Eight of 10 patients who failed COMLA were advanced to BACOP.[4] One achieved a CR with a long unmaintained disease-free survival; seven patients showed a PR or NR.

There was no difference in response rates between the patients in Stage III and those in stage IV. None of the patients who achieved a CR or PR has demonstrated a central nervous system relapse.

Nine of the 42 patients demonstrated significant sclerosis in their tumor histology. Of these patients, two (22 percent) achieved a CR, three a PR (33 percent), four (44 percent) showed NR. The median survival differences between the CR group and the sclerosis subgroup approach, but do not achieve statistical significance in results with COMLA ($.1 > p > .05$).

Of the entire group, the median survival interval has not yet been reached, and currently is in excess of 28 months. There have been a total of 15 deaths, but only one patient who achieved a CR has relapsed and died.

Previously Treated Patients

Fourteen patients who had received prior radiation therapy, chemotherapy or both received COMLA. Two patients (14 percent) achieved a CR, three patients (21 percent) had a PR and nine patients (64 percent) showed no response to COMLA. The two complete responders are currently alive and disease-free at 18 and 21 months, respectively, since completing COMLA therapy. The median survival of the 14 patients from the initiation of COMLA therapy was six months (range one to 26 months).

Toxicity

Table 2 summarizes the hematoxicity of our patients for each cycle.

Three patients developed sepsis. There were no significant hemorrhagic phenomena and no transfusions were needed. There were no drug related deaths. All patients complained of nausea or vomiting related to the chemotherapy, occasionally requiring dosage reduction of the cytosine arabinoside.

There was no difference between the complete responders and the

Table 2. Summary of Hematotoxicity in Previously Untreated Patients Treated with COMLA[a]

Nadir Blood Counts	Cycle I	Cycle II	Cycle III
WBC[b] $\leqslant 2,500/mm^3$	62	62	50
WBC $\leqslant 500/mm^3$	9	7	0
Platelets $\leqslant 100,000/mm^3$	18	24	20
Platelets $\leqslant 50,000/mm^3$	3	10	5
Hematocrit $\leqslant 30$ percent	38	52	40
Hematocrit $\leqslant 25$ percent	12	7	0

[a] Data indicates percentage of patients developing a cytopenia during a given cycle of chemotherapy.

[b]WBC = White blood cell count.

partial or nonresponders in the mean percent of ideal drug dose received during cycle 1.

Discussion

The outlook for patients with DHL has improved considerably during the last 10 years. Fifty percent response rates and significant disease-free remissions are now reported with C-MOPP, BACOP and CHOP/HOP. We now demonstrate a similar remission rate and long unmaintained disease-free remissions with COMLA. The program does not use Adriamycin, bleomycin or prednisone, agents common to other successful DHL treatment regimens. In our study, median survival has not been reached, with a median followup of 28 months. We suspect that the complete responders will have long term survivals. These patients have had their tumor burden reduced to a very few or no malignant cells and may be cured of their disease.

The effectiveness of COMLA is probably the result of using high dose cyclophosphamide, a cell-cycle active agent which follows first order log kill kinetics in a tumor which has a doubling time of about 17 days (range 12–23). [9] The three most successful programs for advanced DHL, COMLA, BACOP, CHOP/HOP, all incorporate an intensive inductive phase, using very high dose cyclophosphamide or high dose cyclophosphamide plus Adriamycin.

Of concern, has been the observation of central nervous system (CNS) relapse by patients with DHL, after successful therapy with BACOP or CHOP/HOP.[10] None of our patients successfully treated with COMLA has developed a CNS relapse (although six of 42 patients had bone marrow or bone involvement and were at very high risk for this complication). McKelvey has noted the rarity of CNS relapse in patients with DHL maintained with OAP (Oncovin®, Cytosine arabinoside,

Prednisone) compared to those maintained with COP.[11] The difference in these results may be the result of using cytosine arabinoside in the maintenance regimes. Methotrexate and cytosine arabinoside both penetrate the blood brain barrier. The long term induction and consolidation nature of the COMLA regime may prevent CNS relapse in DHL. Systemically administered cytosine arabinoside is efficacious in mice with intracranially transplanted L1210 tumors.[12] A randomized trial between COMLA and other successful regimens may obviate the need for prophylactic CNS irradiation as suggested by some authors.[10,14]

The presence of sclerosis is not part of the Rappaport classification. Once thought to be of favorable prognostic significance, Miller et al.[13] have shown that sclerosis may be a distinct histologic subtype of DHL with a poor prognosis. Only two, or 22 percent, of our patients with sclerosis achieved a CR.

The toxicity of the COMLA program is acceptable. Leukopenia and an underproduction anemia are common but transient and transfusions are not required. Thrombocytopenia is infrequent and no hemorrhagic phenomena because of it occurred.

We have shown that patients previously treated but failing significant radiation therapy, chemotherapy other than COMLA, or both, are unlikely to respond to COMLA. Our observation is similar to Schein et al. who observed a low response with BACOP in previously treated patients demonstrating relapse, or progressive disease.[4] It appears that patients failing a chemotherapy regimen are unlikely to respond to second-line therapies.

The COMLA regimen is a unique form of sequential chemotherapy for patients with DHL, producing a high rate of durable complete remissions. The COMLA program lacks the toxicity of Adriamycin, bleomycin and prednisone and may be useful for patients in whom one or more of these drugs may be contraindicated. The COMLA regimen appears to protect the responders from central nervous system relapses and thus obviates the need for prophylactic therapy. These observations warrant the use of the COMLA regimen as the initial form of therapy in previously untreated patients with advanced DHL without sclerosis.

References

1. Rappaport, H: Tumors of the hematopoietic system. In: *Atlas of Tumor Pathology.* Section 3, Fascicle 8, Armed Forces Institute of Pathology, Washington, D.C. 1966.

2. Levitt, M, Marsh, JC, DeConti, RC et al.: Combination sequential chemotherapy in advanced reticulum cell sarcoma. *Cancer* 29:630–636, 1972.

3. DeVita, VT Jr, Canellos, GP, Chabner, B et al.: Advanced diffuse histiocytic lymphoma, a potentially curable disease. Results with combination chemotherapy. *Lancet* i:248–250, 1975.

4. Schein, PS, DeVita, VT, Hubbard: S et al.: Bleomycin, Adriamycin, cyclophospha-mide, vincristine and prednisone (BACOP) combination chemotherapy in the treatment of advanced diffuse histiocytic lymphoma. *Ann. Int. Med.* 85:417–422, 1976.

5. McKelvey, EG, Gottlieb, JA, Wilson, HE, Haut, A et al.: Hydrodaunomycin (Adria-mycin) combination chemotherapy in malignant lymphoma. *Cancer* 38:1484–1493, 1976.

6. Carbone, PP, Kaplan, HS, Musshoff, K et al.: Report of the committee of Hodgkin's disease staging classification. *Cancer Res.* 31:1860–1861, 1971.

7. Hill, AB: *Principles of Medical Statistics*, Oxford University Press, New York, 1961.

8. Colton, T: *Statistics in Medicine*, Little, Brown and Co., Boston, 1974

9. Skipper, HE: Combination therapy. Booklet 2, Southern Research Institute, 1975.

10. Bunn, PA, Schein, PS, Banks, PM, DeVita, VT: Central nervous system complications in patients with diffuse histiocytic and undifferentiated lymphoma: leukemia revisited. *Blood* 47:3–10, 1976.

11. McKelvey, EM: Cyclophosphamide vs. arabinosyl cytosine combination maintenance chemotherapy in malignant lymphoma. *Am. Soc. Clin. Oncol.* C99:261, 1976.

12. Kline, I, Vendetti, JM: Chemotherapy of leukemia L1210 in mice with 1-β-D-arabino-furanosyl cytosine hydrocholoride. *Cancer Res.* 26:1931–1935, 1966.

13. Miller, JB, Variakojis, D, Bitran, JD, Sweet, DL et al.: Diffuse histiocytic lymphoma with sclerosis: a clinicopathologic entity with frequent occurrence of superior vena caval syndrome. *Blood* 52 (Suppl 1): No. 567, 1978.

14. Cabanillas, F, Litam, JP, Bodey, GP, Freireich, EJ: Central nervous system relapse in malignant lymphoma other than Hodgkin's disease: risk factors and implications for prophylaxis. *Proc. of Am. Soc. Clin. Oncol.* (Abstract) C-54, 1979.

Adriamycin-Vincristine-Prednisone Combination in Adult Acute Leukemia[a]

Michael T. Shaw, L. Elias

University of New Mexico, Albuquerque, New Mexico

Summary

The anthracycline antibiotic Adriamycin has been found to be effective in successful induction therapy for acute leukemia. In an attempt to improve remissions and survivals in such patients, we treated 25 adults with previously untreated acute lymphoblastic leukemia (ALL) and 29 previously treated adults—10 with ALL, 18 with acute myeloblastic leukemia (AML) and one with acute unclassifiable leukemia (AUL) who were in relapse. The induction regimen included Adriamycin 75 mg/m² IV Days 1 and 15, vincristine 1.4 mg/M² (max 2 mg) IV q week × 4, and prednisone 40 mg/M² PO q d × 28 (AVP). Patients in complete remission (CR) were maintained with 6 mercaptopurine, 75 mg/M² PO daily and methotrexate 15 mg/M² PO weekly. Patients with ALL also received reinforcement with prednisone and vincristine every four weeks. Eighteen (72%) of the 25 previously untreated ALL patients entered CR with a median duration of 10.2 months and a median survival of 24 months. Six of these patients remain in CR at 15, 30, 43, 51, 53, and 55 months. Five CRs (45%) and 1 partial response (PR) were noted among previously treated ALL and AUL patients. Of the AML patients, five entered CR (28%) and one PR. Responses of AML patients were confined to those 10 with one prior induction attempt, and responding AML patients were younger than nonresponders. Actuarial median duration of CR for

[a]This investigation was supported in part by Public Health Service Grants CA 16957 and CA 19980 awarded by the Cancer Institute, National Institutes of Health, DHEW.

previously treated patients was 15 weeks with no difference between ALL and AML patients. Responders had longer actuarial survival (median 30 weeks) than nonresponders (9 weeks, p < .01). AVP is a useful combination for remission induction in adult ALL and reinduction in adult ALL and AML.

Introduction

The treatment of adult acute leukemia has centered around the drug cytosine arabinoside for acute myeloblastic leukemia (AML), and the combination of prednisone and vincristine for acute lymphocytic leukemia (ALL). In recent years, the anthracycline antibiotics Adriamycin and daunorubicin which are active in the treatment of acute leukemia[1,2] have been combined with these drugs. Adriamycin has been particularly favored by the Southwest Oncology Group.[3]

There are two fundamental problems to be faced in the treatment of adult acute leukemia. The first is that despite the fact patients with ALL more easily enter complete remission (CR), long term survivors from this disease even with successful reinductions are exceptionally rare, whereas a proportion (albeit a very small one) of patients with AML do have long term CRs and may in some cases even have been cured.[4] Nevertheless, those large numbers of patients with AML who do relapse are often resistant to second line drugs.[5,6]

The purpose of our studies with an Adriamycin, vincristine, prednisone combination in adult acute leukemia was two-fold: to evaluate the efficacy of producing CR in previously untreated adult ALL while assessing its effect on remission duration and survival; and to test the effectiveness of this combination in reinduction therapy in previously treated patients with AML and ALL.

Materials and Methods

Twenty-five previously untreated evaluable patients with ALL were entered into this study. Relevant clinical and hematologic data are presented in Table 1. Previously treated patients consisted of 18 with AML and 11 with ALL (one of these patients had acute undifferentiated leukemia, but is included with the ALL patients in this report). Characteristics of these patients, with details of previous therapy, are shown in Table 2.

Induction therapy consisted of Adriamycin 75 mg/M² IV on Days 1 and 15, vincristine 1.4 mg/M² (maximum dose 2 mg) IV on Days 1, 8, 15, and 22, prednisone 40 mg/M² per day P.O. for 28 days. CR was defined by the following criteria: no symptoms ascribable to leukemia, no evidence of leukemic infiltration on physical examination; hemoglobin

Table 1. Initial Clinical Features of Previously Untreated Patients

| Number of males | 20 | |
| Number of females | 5 | |

	Median	Range
Age (years)	21	15 - 69
Hgb (g/100ml)	9.3	4.4- 13.5
WBC (x $10^3/\mu$l)	11.6	2.2-180
Percent blasts	97	48 -100
Platelets (x $10^3/\mu$l)	31	1 -174

>11 g/100 ml, circulating granulocyte levels in excess of 1000 per mm³, and bone marrow aspirates with a blast count of 5 percent or less of the total nucleated cells, 40 percent or less of lymphocytes, and normal appearing granulopoiesis, erythropoiesis and thrombopoiesis, qualitatively and quantitatively, except for morphologic changes definitely attributed to medication. Partial remission (PR) met the above requirements with the exception that bone marrow blast count was 6-25 percent of the total nucleated cells.

Bone marrow aspiration was performed on Day 28 and patients not entering CR received further Adriamycin 75 mg/M² IV on Day 29, vincristine 1 mg/M² IV on Days 29 and 36, and prednisone 40 mg/M² per day orally until Day 42, after which a further bone marrow aspiration was performed.

Patients entering CR received the following maintenance regimen: 6 mercaptopurine (6-MP) 75 mg/M² per day P.O. in a single dose plus methotrexate (MTX) 15 mg/M² P.O. once per week as a single dose. If the blood urea nitrogen was ≥ 20 mg %, MTX was omitted until a value of < 20 mg % was observed. Reinforcement therapy with prednisone 40 mg/M² per day P.O. for seven days and vincristine 1.4 mg/M² (maximum 2 mg) IV once only was administered to ALL patients every four weeks. If moderately severe oral ulceration or any diarrhea or infection supervened, MTX was discontinued until symptoms abated. If the WBC count fell to < 1000/mm³ or the platelet count was less than 100,000/mm³, both drugs were omitted and resumed at full doses when the WBC count ≥ 4000/mm³, and the platelet count ≥ 50,000/mm³. If the WBC count was 1000-2000/mm³, half doses of 6-MP and MTX were given. Four patients with previously untreated ALL received cranial irradiation and intrathecal MTX on attaining CR.

Statistical methods used included the Wilcoxon rank sum test for comparison of means,[7] the modified Wilcoxon test for comparison of remission duration and survival[8] and the Fisher exact test for compari-

Table 2. Characteristics of Previously Untreated Patients

	ALL	AML
Age, $\bar{X} \pm SD$	29.7 ± 12.26 ——— p < 0.02 ———	46.81 ± 17.55
(and range)	(17 – 47)	(21 – 71)
Males:Females	6: 5	7:11
Prior disease duration:	36	55
(weeks), median (range)	(19 – 154)	(14 – 154)
Prior induction attempts:		
1	8	10
> 1	3	8
Prior chemotherapy[a]:		
OAP	3	10
COAP	2	4
V+P	8	0
Hx/Ara-C	0	4
Ara-C/6TG	1	2
AdOAP	0	1
6MP	5	1
Mtx	4	0
Mtx-Asp	1	0
AzaC	0	1
Other combinations[b]	4	2
Peripheral blood counts:		
$\bar{X} \pm SD$ (x $10^{-3}/mm^3$)		
Blasts	13.8 ± 32.18	5.2 ± 11.06
Neutrophils	3.3 ± 2.98	1.4 ± 2.06
Platelets	98.6 ± 59.70	136.2 ± 133.09

[a] Abbreviations: V = vincristine; A, AraC = cytosine arabinoside; P = prednisone; C = cyclophosphamide; Hx = hydroxyurea; 6TG = thioguanine; Ad = adriamycin; 6MP = 6-mercaptopurine; Mtx = methotrexate; Asp = L-asparaginase; AzaC = azacytidine.

[b] Other combinations including above agents other than adriamycin.

son of proportions.[7] Actuarial survival and remission duration curves were plotted by the method of Kaplan and Meier;[9] all p values cited are two-tailed.

Results

Of the 25 evaluable previously untreated patients with ALL, 18 (72%) entered CR, one had a PR. There were six with no response, including one early death after seven days of therapy. One patient (a nonresponder) was removed from the study after two weeks because he developed premature ventricular contractions confirmed by ECG. Of twelve patients in the 15-20 age group, there were 11 CRs and one PR. The latter occurred in a patient who had presented initially with bone marrow plus meningeal leukemia; the PR lasted four weeks. In the 21-30 age group, there were 6 CRs in eight patients. In patients over the age of 30, there was one CR in five patients. Of the 18 CRs, 16 patients achieved this status by the 28th day and two by the 42nd day of induction therapy. The median duration of remission was 10.2 months, as previously described.[10] The median survival was 24 months and the survival curve is shown in Figure 1. Six patients are still alive and in complete remission, at 15, 30, 43, 51, 53, and 55 months, following initiation of induction. Three of 14 patients who relapsed did so in the meninges, one had a combined bone marrow-meningeal relapse. Of four patients who had prophylactic precranial irradiation and intrathecal methotrexate, none developed meningeal leukemia and the longest survivor at the present time did receive central nervous system prophylactic therapy.

In the 29 previously treated patients, there were 10 CRs and 2 PRs (41%). ALL patients responded more frequently (5 CRs, 1 PR, 60%) than those with AML (5 CRs, 1 PR, 33%), but this difference is not significant. Responses in AML patients were confined to those with one prior induction attempt (Table 3). The AML patients with CR included one with the PH' abnormality and one with erythroblastic leukemia. Actuarial median duration of CR was 15 weeks (Figure 2) and was identical for AML and ALL patients. Actuarial median duration of survival was 13 weeks, and was also the same for AML and ALL patients (Figure 3). Responders survived longer than nonresponders (P < .02). Among patients with acute leukemia of all cytologies with only one prior

Figure 1. Survival of previously untreated ALL patients.

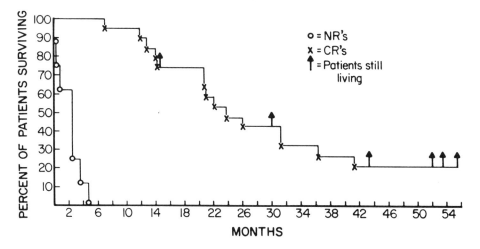

Table 3. Comparison of Patients with One and More than One Prior Induction Attempt

	ALL		AML	
Prior Induction Attempts	1	>1	1	>1
Number of Patients	8	3	10	8
Age (years), $\bar{X} \pm SD$	30.4 ± 11.62	28.0 ± 16.52 $p < 0.01$	53.3 ± 18.71	38.6 ± 12.68 $p = .075$
Blasts/mm³ x 10³, $X \pm SD$	14.0 ± 37.98	13.1 ± 11.26	7.8 ± 14.58 $p < 0.02$	2.1 ± 1.74
Neutrophils/mm³ x 10³, $\bar{X} \pm SD$	3.7 ± 3.01	2.2 ± 3.21	2.0 ± 2.63	0.66 ± 0.49
Platelets/mm³ x 10³, $\bar{X} \pm SD$	89.9 ± 68.98	121.7 ± 8.14 $p = 0.084$	197.0 ± 150.41 $p = 0.067$	60.3 ± 45.40 $p < 0.05$
CR/PR	3/1	2/0	5/1	0/0 $p < 0.05$

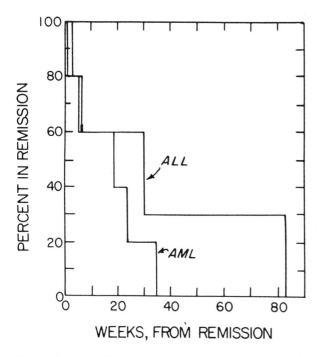

Figure 2. Actuarial duration of complete remission of previously treated AML and ALL patients. A single patient who was lost to followup during remission is indicated as a censored point at six weeks.

induction attempt, patients with CR had lower numbers of peripheral blood blasts (Table 4). This difference was reflected in better survival of patients with low blast counts (P < .05, Figure 4).

Toxicity

Details of toxicity in 54 both previously untreated and previously treated patients are shown in Table 5. It should be noted that all patients had alopecia and hematologic toxicity and that only one developed electro-cardiographic abnormality, presumably related to Adriamycin administration.

Discussion

In the patients treated with ALL in our series, the CR rate of 72 percent is similar to the CR rate in other series in which an anthracycline antibiotic has been used in the induction therapy of adult ALL.[11] It seems to be superior to the 50 percent CR rate achieved by prednisone and vincristine alone.[12] However, it is necessary to point out that no

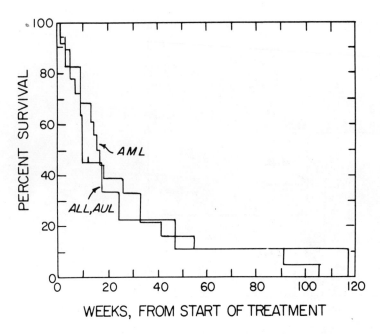

Figure 3. Actuarial duration of survival of AML as compared with ALL in previously treated patients. There is no significant difference. A single patient who was lost to followup is indicated as a censored point at 12 weeks.

satisfactory randomized study has been carried out, largely because of the paucity of patients with this disease as compared with AML. Furthermore, immunologic heterogeneity is now known to exist in the leukemic cells found in patients with a diagnosis of ALL. Some patients have a Ph' chromosome.[13] Maintenance therapy with 6-MP and MTX,

Table 4. Comparison of Patients with Complete Remission to those with Partial Remission or No Response

	Patients with One Prior Induction Attempt		
	CR	PR, NR	P
ALL/AML	3/5	5/5	NS[b]
Age[a]	35.9 ± 17.43	48.9 ± 19.87	NS
Blasts x 10^{-3}/mm^3	1.3 ± 2.66	18.0 ± 34.80	0.05
PMN x 10^{-3}/mm^3	1.8 ± 2.04	4.3 ± 3.32	NS
Platelets x 10^{-3}/mm^3	177.3 ±131.11	115.9 ±137.60	NS

[a] Among patients with AML only there is a significant difference in age between responders and nonresponders (see text).

[b] Not significant.

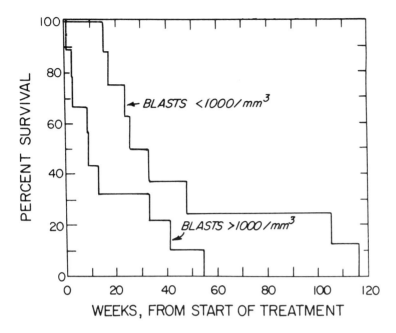

Figure 4. Actuarial duration of survival of patients with one prior induction attempt. Patients with peripheral blood blasts $> 1000/mm^3$ compared to those with $< 1000/mm^3$; $p < 0.05$.

plus periodic reinforcement with prednisone and vincristine, produced disappointingly short remission durations. As we have pointed out previously, we are now of the opinion that central nervous system prophylaxis should be instituted after successful induction in adult patients with ALL.[10]

The longest remission durations reported in adult ALL have been described by Gee and Clarkson, following use of their L-2 protocol[14] and it may be that various multi-drug combinations and cyclic chemotherapy should be used. A similar study is now being developed by the Southwest Oncology Group.

Few data have been presented previously regarding relapsed adult acute leukemic patients following previous therapy, except for those involving single new agents. Our study indicates that second remissions can be obtained in a number of patients with Adriamycin, vincristine and prednisone. Surprisingly, response to this combination was found to depend on factors other than the cytological type (Table 4). Among patients with AML, responses occurred more frequently in patients undergoing their second induction attempt than in those with multiple prior induction attempts (Table 3). These results either could be caused by differences in prior drug exposure and consequent drug resistance, or

Table 5. Toxicity of Induction Regimen

Toxicity	No. of Patients
Hematologic	All
Alopecia	All
Mucositis	10
Peripheral neuropathy	9
Infections	14
Cardiac arrhythmia	1

to the tendency toward lower neutrophil and platelet counts in the latter patients (Table 3) which might be expected to increase the risk of therapy. As has been noted in several previous studies of first inductions, older patients with AML did not respond frequently.[3,15-17] Patients with AML and one prior induction attempt were older than those with multiple prior inductions (Table 3), perhaps reflecting preferential loss of older patients in the course of multiple induction attempts or case selection in favor of younger patients. Numbers of circulating blasts were also found to influence the response rate (Table 4). Patients with AML in this series tended to have lower blast counts than those with ALL (Tables 2 and 3), and the influence of blast counts on response and survival (Figure 4) was not found to be confined to a particular cytological type. Blast counts have been noted to influence prognosis in few other adult leukemia series.[16,17] Its emergence as a prognostic factor in this study could be the result of the relatively low dosages of myelosuppressive drugs used, which, in turn, could favor patients with lower tumor burdens or less explosive disease.

Among previously treated patients with ALL, the response rate (CR = 50%) noted here was not surprisingly high when the known single agent response rate for the drugs used is considered. The CR rate in previously treated patients was slightly, but not significantly, lower than noted with the identical regimen in previously untreated ALL patients, presumably caused in part by prior exposure to regimens including vincristine and prednisone (Table 2) and consequent drug resistance. The response rate of AML patients, particularly the group with one prior induction attempt, is perhaps slightly higher than might be expected from the single agent response to anthracyclines.[1,2,18,19] Although vincristine and prednisone have little single agent activity in AML,[19] it is possible that they add some efficacy to combinations. The durations of response and survival were disappointingly short in this series (Figures 2 and 3) and were identical for AML and ALL patients. Survival was slightly superior for responders compared with nonresponders, in patients with one prior induction attempt and in those with low blast counts (Figure 4).

Although the results of the study of previously treated patients are encouraging insofar as they reveal the activity of Adriamycin, vincristine and prednisone in successful reinduction of adult acute leukemic patients, optimism is curbed by the short duration of remission. The latter emphasizes the need to develop regimens which will prolong first remission duration. There are already indications that the addition of Adriamycin to cytosine arabinoside, vincristine and prednisone may to a large extent achieve this aim.[3] Clearly, there is a need also for the development of better reinduction and maintenance therapy for these patients when they relapse.

References

1. Dreyfus, B, Sultan, C, Borion, M et al.: Sur le traitement d'attaque par la rubidomycine de 19 cas de leucémia aigue myéloblastique. *Presse Med.* 76:55-57, 1968.

2. Mathé, G, Amiel, JL, Haya, JM et al.: Essai de l'adriamycine dans le traitement des leucémies aigue. *Presse Med.* 78:1997-1999, 1970.

3. Freireich, EJ, Keating, MJ, Gehan, EA et al.: Therapy of acute myelogenous leukemia. *Cancer* 42:874-882, 1978.

4. Coltman, CA, Freireich, EJ, Savage, EA et al.: Long term survival of adults with acute leukemia. *Proc. Am. Soc. Clin. Oncol.* 20:389, 1979.

5. Rodriguez, V, Bodey, GP, McCredie, KB et al.: Combination 6-mercaptopurine-Adriamycin in refractory adult acute leukemia. *Clin. Pharm. Therap.* 18:462-466, 1975.

6. Embury, SH, Elias, L, Heller, PA et al.: Remission maintenance therapy on acute myelogenous leukemia. *West. J. Med.* 126:267-272, 1977.

7. Armitage, P: *Statistical Methods in Medical Research,* John Wiley & Sons, New York, 1971.

8 Gehan, EA: A generalized Wilcoxon test for comparing arbitrarily singly censored samples. *Biometrika* 52:203-223, 1965.

9. Kaplan, HS, Meier, P: Non-parametric estimations from incomplete observation. *Am. Stat. Assoc. J.* 53:457-480, 1958.

10. Shaw, MT, Raab, SO: Adriamycin in combination chemotherapy of adult acute lymphoblastic leukemia: a Southwest Oncology Group study. *Med. Ped. Onc.* 3:261-266, 1977.

11. Woodruff, R: The management of adult acute lymphoblastic leukemia. *Cancer Treat. Rev.* 5(2):95-113, 1978.

12. Clarkson, BD, Dowling, MD, Gee, TS et al.: Treatment of acute leukemia in adults. *Cancer* 36:775-795, 1975.

13. Peterson, LC, Bloomfield, CD, Brunning, RD: Blast crisis as an initial or terminal manifestation of chronic myeloid leukemia. *Amer. J. Med.* 60:209-220, 1976.

14. Humphrey, GB, Lankford, J: Acute leukemia: use of surface markers in classification. *Sem. Onc.* 3:243-252, 1976.

15. Whitecar, JP, Body, GP, Freireich, EJ et al.: Cyclophosphamide (NSC 26271), vincristine (NSC 67574), cytosine arabinoside (NSC 63878) and prednisone (NSC 10023) (COAP) combination chemotherapy for acute leukemia in adults. *Cancer Chem. Repts.* 56:543-550, 1972.

16. Bloomfield, CD, Theologides, A: Acute granulocytic leukemia in elderly patients, *JAMA* 226:1190-1193, 1973.

17. Report of the Medical Research Council's Working Party on leukemia in adults: treatment of acute myeloid leukemia with daunorubicin, cytosine arabinoside, mercaptopurine, L-asparaginase, prednisone and thioguanine: results of treatment with five multiple drug schedules. *Brit. J. Haemat.* 27:373-389, 1974.

18. VonHoff, DD, Rozenczweig, M, Slavik, M: Daunomycin: an anthracycline antibiotic effective in acute leukemia. *Adv. Pharm. Chem.* 15:1-50, 1978.

19. Henderson, ED: Acute myelogenous leukemia, Chapter 92, pp. 830-840. In: Williams, WJ, Beutller, E, Erslev, AJ, Rundles, RW, eds. *Hematology,* 2nd ed., McGraw-Hill, New York, 1977.

Levamisole and Chemotherapy for Disseminated Melanoma[a]

Muhyi Al-Sarraf, John J. Costanzi, Dennis O. Dixon

School of Medicine, Wayne State University, Detroit, Michigan; University of Texas Medical Branch, Galveston, Texas; M.D. Anderson Tumor Institute, University of Texas, Houston, Texas

Summary

Patients with disseminated malignant melanoma were randomized, with stratification according to age, performance status, normal or impaired bone marrow and liver and brain involvement to receive BCNU, Hydrea and DTIC (BHD), BHD plus levamisole or DTIC and actinomycin-D. The overall response rate (CR+PR) was 31 percent, 32 percent with BHD, 31 percent with BHD+levamisole and 29 percent with DTIC+actino−D. No difference in duration of the response was found. There is some evidence that survival for patients treated with DTIC+actinomycin−D is better than that for patients who received other therapy. The superiority seems most prominent among patients in the poor prognosis groups.

Introduction

In the treatment of patients with disseminated malignant melanoma, DTIC appears to be the single agent of choice, producing a response rate of 12 percent to 25 percent.[1−3] The addition of other agents such as nitrosoureas, vincristine, procarbazine and actinomycin-D has not substantially improved these results.[4] In a previous study, the response rate to the combination of BCNU, hydroxyurea and DTIC (BHD) were 31 percent.[5]

[a]This investigation was supported by Grant Nos.: CA 14028, CA 03096-22, CA 17701-05 and CA 12014 awarded by the National Cancer Institute, DHEW.

In most studies DTIC was given as a single daily dose intravenously for five days with subsequent courses given at 21–28 day intervals. Cowan and Bergsagel[3] reported that intermittent single dose administrations of DTIC could be given safely without sacrificing anti-tumor effect.

Actinomycin-D has been found to be effective in the treatment of patients with disseminated melanoma.[6] Benjamin et al.[7] have reported the use of actinomycin-D in an intermittent schedule in patients with malignant melanoma. The response rate was 9 percent and an additional 27 percent of patients demonstrated stabilization of their disease.

The combination of single dose DTIC and actinomycin-D in an intermittent dose schedule has been evaluated and reported by Samson et al.[8] with good results and tolerable toxicities.

In melanoma patients, levamisole increased pre-existing specific and humoral and cellular anti-tumor immunity.[9] It also prolonged specific immunity induced by a tumor cell vaccine and potentiated the immune response to sub-optimal and normally ineffective doses of the vaccine. Levamisole and BCG seem to be additive in their effects.[9]

Wilkins and Olkowski[10] reported on effect of levamisole on immune competence in patients with malignant melanoma who had surgical resection for complete removal of the tumor. Eight of the nine patients who responded well clinically showed increased levels of T lymphocytes and increased c-AMP levels.

This study was designed to determine if the addition of levamisole to the combination of BHD increases its effectiveness, also to determine if high dose DTIC+actinomycin−D is effective as compared with the other two groups of therapy.

Materials and Methods

Patients with histologically proven disseminated malignant melanoma with measurable lesion(s) who have not been treated previously with BCNU hydroxyurea, DTIC, levamisole or actinomyin-D were included in this study. All patients must have adequate renal and hepatic function and estimated survival of at least two months. The patients must have recovered from toxic effects of prior chemotherapy and it must be at least two weeks since the completion of radiotherapy to the bone marrow bearing areas.

Initial pre-study workup included: complete blood count, platelet count, urinalysis, BUN, creatinine, bilirubin, SGOT, alkaline phosphatase, bone marrow biopsy, EEG, brain scan, liver scan, chest X-rays and bone X-rays. History and physical were performed and tumor measurement and performance status were recorded.

CBC and platelets were performed weekly during the first four courses and then before the start of subsequent courses. Tumor measurements and performance status and the rest of the blood tests were done before each subsequent course and recorded. Bone marrow biopsy, EEG, brain scan, liver scan and X-rays were repeated as indicated or to document completeness of a sustained remission.

Patients were stratified according to age, performance status and normal or impaired bone marrow, then were randomized to either arm of therapy (Table 1). Those with impaired bone marrow received reduced doses of BCNU, DTIC and actinomycin−D. Subsequent dose schedules were adjusted in relation to the nadir white blood counts and/or platelet counts. The randomization ratio to BHD, BHD+levamisole and actinomycin−D+DTIC were 1:2:2 because of previous experience of the Southwest Oncology Group Study with the results of BHD therapy.

Patients with brain metastases were treated first with Decadron 8–12 mg/day for three days then tapered. On the third day, whole brain irradiation was started for a total dose of 4,000 rads over a two-week period. During the second week of radiotherapy these patients were randomized as above.

Patients with massive liver involvement defined as a liver span of at least 16 cm at the mid-clavicular line, 12 cm at the anterior axillary line and 4 cm below the xyphoid area with diffuse involvement in both lobes by liver scan will be randomized separately. These patients were recommended to have hepatic artery infusion with DTIC 200 mg/m²/day over 24 hours for five days. After five to seven days post-therapy, these patients were randomized as above.

If anti-tumor response is noted or if there is no tumor growth after two courses of therapy, administration of the drugs will be continued. If the patient demonstrates tumor growth while receiving a nonmyelosuppressive dose of drug, treatment will be continued and the dose of drugs will be increased until myelosuppression intervenes.

Table 1. Treatment Plan and Drug Doses for Patients with Disseminated Melanoma

BHD, Normal Marrow:
BCNU 150 mg/m²/day 1 of every other course, i.v.
Hydrea 1500 mg/m²/day 1-5, oral
DTIC 150 mg/m²/day 1-5, i.v.
}Every 28 days

BHD + Levamisole, Normal Marrow:
BHD as above
Levamisole 2.5 mg/kg/day 6-7, 13-14, 20-21 each course

Actinomycin-D + High Dose DTIC, Normal Marrow:
DTIC 750 mg/m²/day 1, i.v. Push
Actino-D 1.25 mg/m²/day 1, i.v. Push
}Every 21 days

If patients on BHD+levamisole or actinomycin−D+DTIC have no response after two courses and as above, they will be crossed over.

All tumor measurements were recorded in centimeters and consisted of the longest diameter and the perpendicular diameter at the widest portion of the lesion. Liver size was recorded at xyphoid line and 8 cm lateral to xyphoid line on both sides.

Objective tumor responses were defined as follows: complete remission (CR) is defined as disappearance of all clinical evidence of active tumor for a minimum of four weeks; partial remission (PR) is defined as 50 percent or greater decrease in the sum of the products of all diameters of measured lesions; patients with liver metastases 30 percent reduction in the sum of measurements below the costal margin; and no simultaneous increase in the size of any new lesion(s) may occur.

Stable disease (SD) is defined as steady state or response less than partial remission or progressive disease. There may be no appearance of new lesion(s) and no worsening of the symptoms.

Progression is defined as unequivocal increase of at least 50 percent in the size of any measurable lesion, appearance of new lesions, uncontrolled hypercalcemia and all clearly progressive skeletal involvement manifested by increasing number of lytic lesions.

Relapse is defined as the appearance of new lesion(s), the reappearance of old lesion(s) in patients who have complete remission or increase of 50 percent or more in the sum of the products of the diameter of all measured tumors over that which was obtained at the time of partial remission.

Results

Since this study opened for patients' entry on October 21, 1977, 125 were entered. A total of 22 patients are too early for evaluation at the present time. Of the remaining cases, 98 patients were fully evaluated and five patients are partially evaluable for response or drug toxicity. For the present analysis, these 103 patients from the current study have been supplemented by 95 patients randomized to the BHD arm of the previous Phase III trial for patients with disseminated malignant melanoma.

The overall response rate (CR+PR) of the 198 patients was 31 percent. In the BHD arm 38/117 (32 percent) had responded as compared with 12/39 (31 percent) BHD+levamisole and 12/42 (29 percent) with DTIC+actinomycin−D therapy. These responses were not statistically different (p = 0.893).

The response rate comparisons appear to be reasonably consistent over subgroups determined by patient pre-treatment characteristics. However, with respect to age, the chemoimmunotherapy group does better among patients younger than 40 (7/10 CR+PR), and worse among patients older than 60 (0/13 CR+PR). This contrasts with the experience in the previous Southwest Oncology Group Study trial in disseminated melanoma patients in which the immunotherapy patients did better among older patients.

Length of response for complete or partial responders and survival durations in weeks are shown in Table 2 and Figure 1. No difference of the length of remission was found among the three groups.

The median survival of DTIC+actinomycin−D arm is 35 weeks as compared with 26 weeks for the BHD group and 23 weeks for the chemoimmunotherapy group. The advantage for the DTIC+actinomycin−D group is significant with p = 0.03 relative to the BHD group and p = 0.02 relative to the BHD+levamisole group.

Survival experience is relatively better for patients with no major organ involvement (brain, liver, bone or lung) at the time of starting treatment, with medians beyond 10 months for the BHD and BHD+levamisole treated patients, and the median was not yet reached in the DTIC+actinomycin−D group. While survival is somewhat worse for

Table 2. Median Duration of Response and Survival of the Three Groups and According to Sites of Metastases and Performance Status

	No. Response	No. Relapse	Median Duration of Response (wk)	No. Patients	No. Deaths	Median Survival (wk)
All Patients:	62	42	26	198	136	29
BHD	38	31	24	117	101	26
BHD + Levamisole	12	7	17	39	21	23
DTIC + Actinomycin-D	12	4	16+	42	14	35
No Major Organ Involvement:						
BHD	16	14	29	32	28	46
BHD + Levamisole	6	2	23	9	3	44
DTIC + Actinomycin-D	3	1	12+	14	2	33+
Major Organ Involvement:						
BHD	22	17	16	80	69	21
BHD + Levamisole	6	5	11	27	16	16
DTIC + Actinomycin-D	9	3	16+	28	12	30
Good Performance Status:						
BHD	19	14	27	41	30	49
BHD + Levamisole	9	5	22	18	6	57
DTIC + Actinomycin-D	10	3	16+	24	6	36
Poor Performance Status:						
BHD	19	17	19	75	71	18
BHD + Levamisole	3	2	14	21	15	11
DTIC + Actinomycin-D	2	1	9+	18	8	20

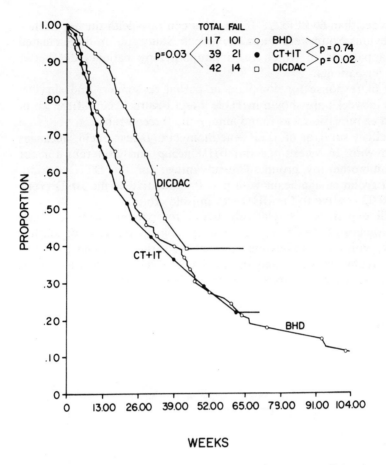

Figure 1. The overall survival from the start of treatment of the three groups.

patients presenting with major organ involvement, and also for those patients treated with DTIC+actinomycin–D although it seems to give a definite advantage, this is statististically significant (Table 2 and Figure 2).

For patients with good performance status, the overall survival did not differ significantly among the three groups (Table 2). Patients with relatively poor performance status had median survival of 20 weeks on DTIC+actinomycin–D as compared with 11 weeks for those patients treated with BHD+levamisole (p = 0.05). The survival of the BHD group does not differ significantly from either of the other two groups.

Table 3 shows type and degree of drug-induced toxicity for each of the treatment groups. As expected, nausea and vomiting has been the

predominant type of toxicity. There has been one death in the BHD+
levamisole group attributed to pulmonary fibrosis.

Discussion

Tetramisole is a synthetic antihelmintic described by Thienpont et al. in
1966.[11] Renoux and Renoux[12] were first to report that tetramisole
augmented the protective effect of a Brucella abortus vaccine in mice.
Since then more than 400 papers have appeared in the literature about
the effect of levamisole on the immune system.[13]

The accumulated evidence from studies on isolated cells, on experi-

Figure 2. Survival from the start of treatment in patients with major organ—
brain, liver, bone or lung—involvement.

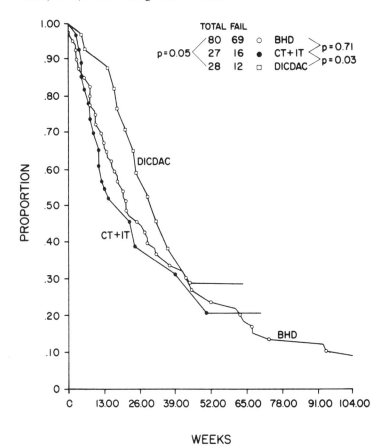

WEEKS

Table 3. Drug Toxicity Encountered in Patients Treated in the Three Therapy Group

	BHD					BHD + Levamisole					DTIC+Actinomycin			
	None	Mild	Mod[a]	Sev[b]	L.T.[c]	None	Mild	M	S	L.	None	Mild	M	S
Leukopenia	19	4	3			32	1	5	3	1	37	1	4	3
Thrombocytopenia	22	1	2		1	38		1	3		43		1	1
N and V	12		9	5		25		9	8		16	2	17	10
Diarrhea	26					42					43		2	
Mucositis	23					34					34			
Chills/Fever	23					32		1	1		34	1		

[a] Mod: Moderate.

[b] Sev: Severe.

[c] L.T.: Life Threatening.

mental animals and on patients and healthy volunteers, suggests that levamisole restores to normal the functions of phagocytes and lymphocytes from compromised hosts. Therapeutic doses of levamisole do not seem to increase the immune response above normal level. B cells do not seem to be directly influenced by this agent.[13]

In experimental animals, levamisole does not consistently repress a primary invasion by virulent bacteria, viruses or tumor cells. It may, however, increase the protective effect of certain vaccines and stabilize tumor remission.[13]

Chirigos et al.[14,15] have shown that levamisole prevented tumor relapse in animals when given during the critical period after cytoreductive therapy. They reported that stabilization of tumor remission is closely related to a faster recovery of the immune system after cytotoxic therapy.

In experimental animals or in patients with advanced cancer, levamisole increased or restored the delayed hypersensitivity reaction to various antigens even when they were suppressed by chemotherapy or radiotherapy.[9,10,16-18]

In animals the effect of levamisole on primary growth and dissemination of malignant melanoma varied. Ibrahim et al.[19] reported no effect of levamisole on Fortner melanotic melanoma transplanted in hamsters. The same results were attained for melanoma B16 transplanted (subcutaneous or intraperitoneal) in mice which has been reported by other investigators.[20,21] While Proctor et al.[22] found increase and decrease in the primary growth of melanoma B16 transplanted sub-cutaneously in mice, Fidler and Spitler[20] reported an increase and decrease of melanoma B16 transplanted intravenously in mice.

Levamisole was reported to be effective in reducing the secondary growth and dissemination of melanoma B16 in mice after surgical cytoreduction therapy.[22]

Available clinical data tend to show the usefulness of levamisole in prolonging the remission of lung cancer after surgical resection[23,24] and in breast cancer after irradiation therapy.[25] There were no significant differences with the use of levamisole as adjuvant in patients with transitional cell cancer of the urinary bladder,[26] malignant melanoma[27] or as adjuvant immunochemotherapy in breast cancer patients.[28]

Hortobagyi et al.[29] reported that the addition of levamisole, or the combination of BCG and levamisole prolonged the duration of remission and survival of responding patients with advanced breast cancer treated with chemotherapy. The overall remission rates were the same in the three groups.

In this preliminary analysis of the Southwest Oncology Group study the overall remission rates in patients with disseminated malignant melanoma treated with levamisole plus chemotherapy or chemotherapy alone were identical.

There are no differences in the duration of response among the three treatment modalities at present time. While patients who received DTIC+ACTINO−D had significantly longer survival as compared with those who received BHD (p = 0.03) or to patients who received BHD+levamisole (p = 0.02), there was no difference in survival between patients who received levamisole and/or BHD therapy (p = 0.74).

Also survival was improved significantly for patients with poor prognostic characteristics (poor performance status, or major visceral organ involvement) on DTIC+ACTINO−D as compared with the other two groups.

We concluded that the addition of levamisole to combination chemotherapy in patients with metastatic melanoma does not decrease or increase response rate, duration of remission or survival.

References

1. Nathanson, L, Wolter, J, Horton, J et al.: Characteristics of prognosis and response to an imidazole carboxamide in malignant melanoma. *Clin. Pharmacol. Ther.* 12:966–972, 1971.

2. Luce, JK, Thurman, WG, Isaacs, BL et al.: Clinical trials with anti-tumor agent 5-(3,3-dimethyl-l-triazino) imidazole-4-carboxamide (NSC-45388). *Cancer Chemo. Rep.* 54:119–124, 1970.

3. Cowan, DH, Bergsagel, DE: Intermittent treatment of metastatic malignant melanoma

with high dose 5-(3,3-dimethyl-l-triazino) imidazole-4-carboxamide (NSC-45388). *Cancer Chem. Rep.* 55:175–181, 1971.

4. Comis RL: DTIC (NSD-45388) in malignant melanoma: a perspective. *Cancer Treat. Rep.* 60:165–176, 1976.

5. Costanzi, JJ, Al-Sarraf, M, Dixon, DO: Chemoimmunotherapy for disseminated melanoma (DM). A Southwest Oncology Group Study. *Proc. ASCO* 20:362, 1979.

6. Golomb, FM et al.: Induced remission of maligant melanoma with actinomycin–D. *Cancer* 20:656–662, 1967.

7. Benjamin, RS et al.: A pharmacokinetically based phase I-II study of single dose actinomycin–D (NSC-3053). *Cancer Treat. Rep.* 60:289–291, 1976.

8. Samson, MK, Baker, LH, Talley, RW et al.: Phase I-II study of intermittent bolus administration of DTIC and actinomycin–D in metastatic malignant melanoma. *Cancer Treat. Rep.* 62:1223–1225, 1978.

9. Shibata, HR, Jerry, LM, Lewis, MG et al.: Immunotherapy of human maligant melanoma with irradiated tumor cells, oral BCG and levamisole. *Ann. N.Y. Acad. Sci.* 277:355–366, 1976.

10. Wilkins, SA, Olkowski ZG: Immunocompetence of cancer patients treated with levamisole. *Cancer* 39:487–493, 1977.

11. Thienpont, D, Vanparijs, OFJ, Raeymaekers, AHM et al.: Tetramisole (R8299), a new potent broad spectrum anthelmintic. *Nature* 209:1084–1086, 1966.

12. Renoux, G, Renoux, M: Effect immunostimulant d'un imidothiazole dans l'immunisation des souris contre l'infection par brucella abortus. *C.R. Acad. Sci.* 272D:349–350, 1971.

13. Symoens, J, Rosenthal, M: Levamisole in the modulation of the immune response: the current experimental and clinical state. *J. Reticulo-endoth. Loc.* 21:175–221, 1977.

14. Chirigos, MA, Pearson, JW, Fuhrman, FS: Effect of tumor load reduction on successful immunostimulation. *Proc. Ann. Acad. Can. Res.,* 15:116, 1974.

15. Chirigos, MA, Fuhrman, F, Pryor, J: Prolongation of chemotherapeutically induced remission of a synomeic murine leukemia by L-2,3,5,6 tetrahydro-6-phenylimidazo (2,1-b) thiazole hydrochloride. *Cancer Res.* 35:927–931, 1975.

16. Levo, Y, Rotter, V, Ramot, B: Restoration of cellular immune response by levamisole in patients with Hodgkin's disease. *Biomedicine* 23:198–200, 1975.

17. Lods, JC, Dujardin, P, Halpern, GM: Levamisole and bone-marrow restoration after chemotherapy. *Lancet* 1:548, 1976.

18. Woods, WA, Fliegehmen, MJ, Chirigos, MA: Effect of levamisole (NSC-177023) on DNA synthesis by lymphocytes from immunosuppressed C57BL mice. *Cancer Chemother. Rep.* 59:531–536, 1975.

19. Ibrahim, AB, Triglia, R, Dau, PC, Spitler, LE: Anti-tumor effects of levamisole on allogeneic hamster melanoma and syngeneic rat hepatoma. In: Chirijos, MA, ed. *Control of Neoplasia by Modulation to the Immune System,* p. 31, Raven Press, New York, 1977.

20. Fidler, IJ, Spitler, LE: Effects of levamisole on *in vivo* and *in vitro* murine last response to syngeneic transplantable tumor. *J. Natl. Cancer Inst.* 55:1107–1112, 1975.

21. Johnson, RK, Houchens, DP, Gaston, MR, Goldin, A: Effects of levamisole (NSC-177023) and tetramisole (NSC-1020631) in experimented tumor systems. *Cancer Chemother. Rep.* Part I 59:697–705, 1975.

22. Proctor, JW, Auclair, BG, Stokowski, G et al.: Comparison on effect of BCG, glucon and levamisole on B16 melanoma metastatic. *Eur. J. Cancer* 13:115–122, 1977.

23. Study-group for bronchogenic carcinoma. Immunopotentiation with levamisole in resectable bronchogenic carcinoma: a double-blind controlled trial. *Brit. Med. J.* 3:461–464, 1975.

24. Amery, WK: Final results of a multicenter placebo-controlled levamisole study of respectable lung cancer. *Cancer Treat. Rep.* 62:1677–1683, 1978.

25. Rojas, AF, Feierstein, JN, Milkiewicz, L et al.: Levamisole in advanced human breast cancer. *Lancet* 2:211–215, 1976.

26. Smith, RG, deKernian, J, Lincoln, B et al.: Preliminary report of the use of levamisole in the treatment of bladder cancer. *Cancer Treat. Rep.* 62:1709–1714, 1978.

27. Gonzalez, RL, Spitler, LE, Sagebiel, RW: Effect of levamisole as a surgical adjuvant therapy for malignant melanoma. *Cancer Treat. Rep.* 62:1703–1707, 1978.

28. Hirshaut, Y, Kesselheim, H, Pinskey, CM et al.: Levamisole as an immunoadjuvant: phase I study and application in breast cancer. *Cancer Treat. Rep.* 62:1693–1701, 1978.

29. Hortobagyi, GN, Yap, HY, Blumenschein, GR et al.: Response of disseminated breast cancer to combined modality treatment with chemotherapy and levamisole with or without Bacillus Calmette-Guérin. *Cancer Treat. Rep.* 62:1685–1692, 1978.

Characterization and Analysis of Complete Responders to Chemotherapy in Metastatic Breast Cancer[a]

D.A. Decker, D.L. Ahmann, H.F. Bisel, J.H. Edmonson, R.G. Hahn, J.R. O'Fallon

Division of Medical Oncology, Mayo Clinic, Rochester, Minnesota

Summary

Four hundred and thirty-eight patients with metastatic breast cancer treated on nine prospective randomized trials were reviewed to analyze, characterize and compare the complete regression (CR), 49/438 (11%) with the noncomplete regressions (NON-CR), 389/438 (89%). Site of dominant disease was identical in the CR and NON-CR patients. However, CR was statistically more likely when the disease-free interval and the postmenopausal status was equal to or less than five years. Survival and time to progression were statistically similar for osseous, visceral, and soft tissue dominant disease. Relapses generally occurred at sites of prior dominant disease, except that CNS relapsed in 14 percent. Six CR received prolonged chemotherapy and were believed to be "cured" when treatment was discontinued; however, all but one patient have relapsed. The definition of complete regression with abnormal bone radiographs is addressed.

Introduction

Complete responses are no longer unusual in metastatic breast cancer. With present combination chemotherapy programs and more effective single agents, such as Adriamycin, complete responses have been reported in four to 28 percent of treated patients.[1-9] These reports indicate

[a]Supported in part by Contract #NO1-CM-12185.

that complete responses are more likely to occur in patients with soft tissue or visceral dominant disease,[2,4,8] complete response in osseous disease being less common. Furthermore, complete responders are reported to survive and remain in remission longer than partial responders.[2,4] Unfortunately, these reports do not characterize their complete responders further, thus leaving many questions unanswered.

The definition of complete response is sometimes ambiguous. Usually, complete responses have been defined as the disappearance of all clinically evident cancer with return of bone radiographs and serum chemistry tests to normal. However, some responses are complete in that all palpable or visible disease disappears, yet there may be a persisting abnormality of the serum chemistry or bone radiograph (i.e., recalcification occurs, but the radiographic remains abnormal). It remains unclear whether these patients should be included in the complete response category.

In an attempt to assess the nature of complete responses as they occur utilizing chemotherapy in metastatic breast cancer, we reviewed our experience of 438 patients comparing the 49 complete remissions with 389 patients who did not achieve a complete remission with the intent of defining the incidence of complete response, the chemotherapy programs producing complete response (i.e., agents and toxicity), the characteristics of patients experiencing complete responses (i.e., age, performance score, menopausal status, disease-free interval, site of dominant disease, and site of relapse), the duration of response and survival, and attempted to clarify the definition of complete response.

Materials and Methods

In nine prospective randomized chemotherapy trials at the Mayo Clinic, complete regression of breast cancer was observed. Four hundred and thirty-eight patients were treated with 11 different chemotherapy programs in these nine studies. Forty-nine patients improved clinically to be included in three categories we chose to define as "complete responses" (Table 1). These studies are either in progress, in press or reported elsewhere.[10-16] Complete responders had not been separated from responders in our earlier reports.[10-13]

The groups of "complete responses" are defined as follows: Group I includes those patients with complete disappearance of all clinical disease, return of abnormal blood chemistry tests to normal and return to normal of all abnormal bone radiographs; Group II includes those patients with complete disappearance of all clinical disease, return of abnormal blood chemistry tests to normal and bone radiographs with abnormalities which had improved (i.e., decreased size or number of lytic lesions and/ or ossification of lytic lesions), but did not return to radiographic

Table 1. Chemotherapy Programs with Number of Complete Responses for Each Treatment

Chemotherapy[a]	Number of Complete Responders (Percent)	Total Study
CTX/5-FU/PRED	14 (9.6%)	146
CTX/5-FU/PRED/VCR	7 (17%)	41
CTX/5-FU/PRED/CAL	4 (18%)	22
ADR	4 (20%)	20
ADR/CTX	4 (17%)	24
ADR/CTX/5-FU	3 (13%)	23
ADR/L-PAM	4 (10.5%)	38
ADR/VP-16	1 (3.2%)	31
ADR/L-PAM cross CTX/5-FU/PRED[b]	4 (8.0%)	50
ADR/MTX/VCR	3 (13%)	23
Ifosp.	1 (5.0%)	20
TOTAL	49 (11%)	438

[a] Abbreviations: Ifosp. = Ifosfamide; MTX = Methotrexate; CAL = Calusterone; CTX = Cytoxan; 5-FU = 5-Fluorouracil; PRED = Prednisone; VCR = Vincristine; ADR = Adriamycin; L-PAM = L-phenylalanine mustard; Cross= fixed cross between ADR/L-PAM and CTX/5-FU/PRED.

[b] Two of 27 patients initially treated with ADR/L-PAM and two of 23 initially treated with CFP/5-FU/PRED were complete responders.

normalcy; Group III includes those patients with complete disappearance of all clinical disease, return of bone radiographs to normal and persisting elevation in blood chemistry tests (elevation in alkaline phosphatase in all cases). Bone radiographs were reviewed blindly by Ahmann. Patients not achieving complete remissions were those with progression, stability, improvement or partial response.

Of the 49 complete responders, 34 (69%) were in Group I, 13 (27% were in Group II and two (4.1%) were in Group III. Two patients in Group I and one patient in Group III had osseous disease with abnormal bone radiographs which reverted to normal after chemotherapy. Thirty-two patients in Group I had no radiographic evidence of osseous disease.

Results

Of the 166 patients initially treated with Adriamycin containing combinations, 17 (10%) achieved a complete response (Table 1). Of the 232 patients initially treated with CTX/5-FU/PRED containing combinations, 27 (12%) achieved a complete response. Single agent chemotherapy resulted in five complete responses, 5/40 (12.5%), with ifosfamide in one and Adriamycin in four. It should be noted that 46 of 49 complete responders (94%) had not received prior chemotherapy, but achieved a complete regression with their first chemotherapy exposure.

Of the 49 complete responders, 28 (57%) were five years or less postmenopausal and 21 were more than five years postmenopausal. Of the 389 patients not achieving a complete response, 162 (42%) were five years or less postmenopausal and 227 were more than five years postmenopausal. When compared by the chi-square method, complete responses are more likely if the patient were within five years of menopause (p = 0.039), indicating disease which is more chemotherapy-sensitive in this group of patients.

Of the 49 complete responders, 47 (96%) had disease-free intervals of five years or less and two had more than five years. Of the 389 other patients in the study, 323 (83%) had disease-free intervals of five years or less and 66 had more than five years. When analyzed by the chi-square method there are significantly more complete responders in the group with disease-free intervals of five years or less (p = 0.0325).

When the 49 complete responders were analyzed by the site of dominant disease, there were 10 (20%) with osseous disease, 13 (27%) with soft tissue disease, and 26 (53%) with visceral dominant disease. Of the 389 patients in the study who did not achieve a complete response, 80 (21%) had osseous disease, 114 (29%) had soft tissue disease, and 195 (50%) had visceral disease. Thus, the distribution of dominant disease in complete responders is strikingly similar to that of the other patients in the study with no statistical difference, which indicates chemotherapy sensitivity regardless of dominant disease site.

Several other characteristics of the complete responders were examined including age, performance score, prior radiation therapy treatment, prior hormonal treatment, tumor grade (Broder's grade), and cell type. There were no obvious differences between these characteristics of the complete responders and those not achieving a complete response.

The duration of response (progression-free interval) for Groups I and II are displayed in Figure 1. Because of the small number of patients in Group III, meaningful comparative analysis was not possible. Therefore, these patients are not included in this analysis. The median duration of response in Group I was 13.5 months and for Group II, 19.0 months. Comparing these two groups by the Gehan-Wilcoxon test of equality indicates no significant difference (p = 0.20).

The survival curves for Groups I and II are shown in Figure 2. Again, meaningful comparative analysis of Group III is not possible. The median survival for Group I was 21 months and for Group II, 28 months. As with duration of response, there is no statistical difference in survival between Groups I and II (Gehan-Wilcoxon test p = 0.75).

In a similar manner, duration of response curves and survival curves according to the site of dominant disease were compared. The median duration of response was 19 months for osseous disease, 14 months for soft tissue and 13 months for visceral dominant disease. The median

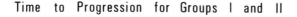

Time to Progression for Groups I and II

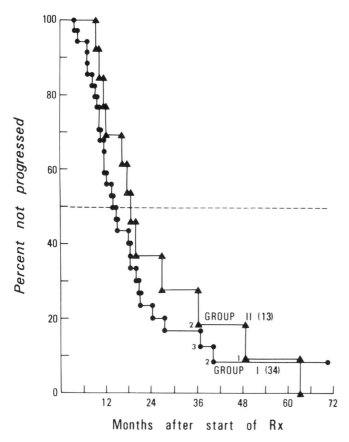

Figure 1.

survival for osseous disease was 31 months, soft tissue disease 21 months and visceral dominant disease 18 months. Even though the median duration of response and survival appear to favor those with osseous dominant disease, when the respective duration of response and survival curves are compared by the Gehan-Wilcoxon test of equality there is no significant difference statistically.

The sites of relapse in the complete responders are shown in Table 2. Forty-two have relapsed and seven responders are either disease-free or died while still in complete remission. Relapses tended to occur in sites of prior bulk disease, visceral disease relapsed at visceral sites and soft tissue at soft tissue sites. However, osseous disease did not necessarily relapse at osseous sites. Central nervous system (CNS) relapse occurred

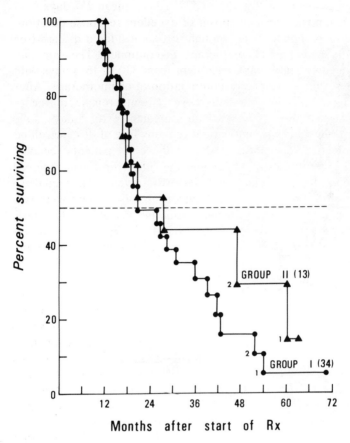

Figure 2.

in six, 6/42 (14%). None of these had CNS disease when treatment began. These relapses occurred throughout the CNS, including spinal cord, cauda equina and cerebral cortex. Furthermore, two patients of these six had other evidence of progression almost simultaneous with central nervous sytem relapse. Three patients died while free of disease from causes other than cancer. One died in an automobile accident while still in complete remission and two patients died with Adriamycin cardiotoxicity while still in complete remission. One of these was found at autopsy to have no evidence of cancer.

Twenty-five of these 49 patients have subsequently received chemotherapy after relapse. Ten of 25 (40%) have responded, seven had partial responses with a duration of 98 to 368 days, mean 225 days, and three achieved complete responses for 135 to 427+ days, mean 257 days.

Six patients compose a special subset of excellent response duration. These six patients responded well enough to be considered disease-free and subsequently had their chemotherapy discontinued. The same six received prolonged chemotherapy treatment from 830 to 1655 days with a median of 1099.5 days prior to discontinuation of chemotherapy. After the chemotherapy was discontinued, these patients remained free of relapse for a range of 68 to 727 days with a median of 265.5 days. Five of the six have relapsed; only one patient remains free of disease, on no active treatment after 455+ days. Three of these six patients received CTX/5-FU/PRED as initial treatment and the other three had received combination chemotherapy which included Adriamycin. Three of these six had osseous and three soft tissue-dominant disease. There were two additional patients who refused further chemotherapy after achieving a complete response. These two received 154 and 272 days of chemotherapy and relapsed 169 and 79 days, respectively, after their chemotherapy was discontinued.

The major toxic side effect of chemotherapy in these complete responders was Adriamycin-induced cardiomyopathy, 6/21 (29%), with two deaths secondary to cardiomyopathy. Severe myelosuppression was not encountered. White blood cell nadirs less than $1500/mm^2$ occurred in nine, 9/49 (18%), and platelet nadirs less than $100,000/mm^2$ in seven, 7/49 (14%). Thirty-four patients (69%) had white blood cell nadirs between 1,499 and $3,000/mm^3$ and 28 (57%) had platelet nadirs greater than $150,000/mm^3$. Alopecia occurred in 36, most of these from Adriamycin. Mild nausea and vomiting occurred in 37. Seven had mild stomatitis and/or diarrhea. Severe neuropathy secondary to vincristine occurred in one patient and mild to moderate neuropathy in seven. Mild virilization caused by calusterone and severe cystitis from cytoxan occurred in three patients and one patient, respectively.

Table 2. Dominant Disease Versus Site of Relapse

Dominant Disease Site	Site of Relapse					
	Visceral	Osseous	Soft Tissue	CNS	Non[a]	Total
Visceral	13	1	3	4	5	26
Osseous	3	2	3	1	1	10
Soft tissue		2	9	1	1	13
TOTAL	16	5	15	6	7	49

[a] Seven patients without relapse.

Discussion

Complete responses were acheived in 49 patients (11%) of 438 treated with chemotherapy for metastatic breast cancer. Our most effective combination chemotherapy programs have included CTX/5-FU/PRED while our most effective single agent has been Adriamycin. Adriamycin containing combinations accounted for 39 percent of the complete responses and CTX/5-FU/PRED combinations 51 percent. However, when all patients treated with either combination are considered, both combinations resulted in a complete response rate of approximately 11 percent.

When the complete responders were compared with the patients who did not achieve a complete response, it became apparent that there were significantly more complete responders within five years of the menopause. Prior experience with polychemotherapy has suggested a negative influence on response rate associated with increasing postmenopausal status.[10] The reason for this higher response rate in perimenopausal women remains speculative.

As with menopausal status, when the disease-free interval of the complete responders was compared to that of the other study patients, there were significantly more complete responses in those patients with a disease-free interval of five years or less. If a short disease-free interval implies a high growth fraction and rapid doubling time and if malignancies with high growth fractions and rapid doubling times responded well to chemotherapy (i.e., oat-cell carcinoma of the lung), then we should expect more complete responses in breast cancer patients with short disease-free intervals. Our results support this concept in metastatic breast cancer.

The distribution of dominant disease site was similar in the complete responders and those not achieving a complete response. Others have reported complete responses predominantly in visceral and soft tissue dominant disease[2,4,8] with few complete responses in osseous dominant disease. Undoubtedly, our inclusion of patients with bone radiographs who improved, but did not return to normal, accounts for the larger number of complete responders with osseous dominant disease. Indeed, there are only two patients in Group I whose bone radiographs returned to normal. However, inclusion of these patients with improved bone radiographs in the complete responses category seems reasonable (*vida infra*).

The duration of response and survival between the 34 patients with complete disappearance of all disease and the 13 "complete responders" with persisting abnormality of bone radiographs was identical. These data suggest a biologic similarity between these groups of patients. We cannot account for this similarity by the site of dominant disease (i.e., osseous-dominant disease carries a better prognosis than visceral-dominant or soft tissue-dominant disease), since the duration of response and survival by site of dominant disease shows no advantage for any one site of dominant disease. Whether or not the persisting abnormality on the bone radiograph represented residual cancer or healed bony disease is unknown. However, the data suggest that patients with complete disappearance of all disease and bony disease which on bone radiograph improves (but does not return to normal), could be included in the complete response category. Also, persisting bony abnormalities in the presence of an otherwise complete response does not indicate a poor prognosis.

We have shown previously that patients who respond to polychemotherapy survive longer than nonresponders.[10] However, we do not know from this study if the complete responders survive longer than the partial responders since the survival curves for these two groups were not compared. The median survival for all patients responding to polychemotherapy, CTX/5-FU/PRED $\pm$ VCR in our previous report was 17.5 months. These responders included those with both partial and complete responses. The median survival for complete responders in Groups I and II was 21 and 28 months, respectively. In a similar manner, the median time to progression for complete responders in Group I was 13.5 months and in Group II, 19.0 months. The median time to progression for patients responding to CFP/5-FU/PRED $\pm$ VCR was eight months. Therefore, complete responders have a longer median duration of response and survival than those treated with a standard polychemotherapy program. Unfortunately, we do not know if this difference is statistically significant.

Complete responses generally occurred without severe myelosuppression. Most patients, 69 percent, had mild leukopenia (nadir $\geq$ 1,500 to 3,000 $\leq$ leukocytes/mm^3) with only 18 percent of patients developing white blood cell nadirs less than 1,500/mm^2. Our experience with CFP/5-FU/PRED $\pm$ VCR has been similar with severe myelosuppression being accompanied by lower rather than higher response rates.[10] In that series,[10] a response rate of 33 percent was achieved with leukocyte nadirs less than 1,500/mm^3, 66 percent response rate with leukocyte nadirs between 1,500 and 2,999/mm^3, and 46 percent response rate with leukocyte nadirs greater than 3,000/mm^3.

Unfortunately, Adriamycin-induced cardiotoxicity developed in six patients (29%) with two deaths. Our prior reports have indicated approximately a ten percent incidence of Adriamycin cardiotoxicity.[12] The majority of the complete responders, because of the prolonged and favorable nature of their response, received large cumulative doses of Adriamycin. These large cumulative doses resulted in more cardiotoxicity.

Finally, progression has occurred in the majority of the complete

242

responders. Only one patient remains disease-free and off chemotherapy. Once a complete response has been achieved, and then maintained with chemotherapy, discontinuation of treatment can be considered. Our practice has been to continue treatment once a complete response has been achieved for at least two years. Unfortunately, relapse is to be expected even after two years of maintained complete response. This implies that cure with present chemotherapy remains elusive. It is to be hoped that with the development of new treatment modalities even better palliation and possible cure will be realized in the future.

References

1. Baker, LH, Vaughn, CB, All-Sarraf, M et al.: Evaluations of combination vs sequential cytotoxic chemotherapy in the treatment of advanced breast cancer. *Cancer* 33:513–518, 1974.

2. Creech, RH, Catalano, RB, Mastrangelo, MJ et al.: An effective low-dose intermittent cyclophosphamide, methotrexate, and 5-fluorouracil treatment regimen for metastatic breast cancer. *Cancer* 35:1101–1107, 1975.

3. Brunner, KW, Sonntag, RW, Martz, G et al.: A controlled study in the use of combination drug therapy for metastatic breast cancer. *Cancer* 36:1208–1219, 1975.

4. Camellos, GP, Devita, VT, Gold, LG et al.: Cyclical combination chemotherapy for advanced breast carcinoma. *Brit. Med. J.* 1:218–220, 1974.

5. DeLema, M, Brambilla, C, Morabito, A et al.: Adriamycin plus vincristine compared to and compared with cyclophosphamide, methotrexate, and 5-fluorouracil for advanced breast cancer. *Cancer* 35:1108–1115, 1975.

6. Brambilla, C, DeLema, M, Bonadonna, G: Combination chemotherapy with Adriamycin (MSC-123127) in metastatic mammary carcinoma. *Cancer Chemotherapy Reports*, Part 1, Vol. 58, No. 2, 251–253, 1974.

7. Waterfield, WC, Tashima, CK, Hortobagyi, GN et al.: Adriamycin and l-(2-chlorethyl)-3-cyclohexy-l-nitrosourea (CCNU) in the treatment of metastatic breast cancer. *Cancer* 41:1235–1239, 1978.

8. Russell, JA, Baker, JW, Dady, PJ et al.: Combination chemotherapy of metastatic breast cancer with vincristine, Adriamycin and prednisone. *Cancer* 41:396–399, 1978.

9. Brambilla, C, DeLema, M, Tossi, A et al.: Response and survival in advanced breast cancer after two noncross resistant combinations. *Brit. Med. J.* 1:801–804, 1976.

10. Ahmann, DL, Bisel, HF, Hahn, RG et al.: An analysis of a multiple-drug program in the treatment of patients with advanced breast cancer utilizing 5-fluorouracil, cyclophosphamide, and prednisone with or without vincristine. *Cancer* 36:1925–1935, 1975.

11. Ahmann, DL, Bisel, HF, Hahn, RG et al.: Phase II clinical trial of isophosphamide (NSC-109724) in patients with advanced breast cancer. *Cancer Chemotherapy Report* 58 (Part I):861–865, 1974.

12. Ahmann, DL, Bisel, HF, Eagan, RT et al.: Controlled evaluation of Adriamycin (NSC-123127) in patients with disseminated breast cancer. *Cancer Chemotherapy Reports* 58:877–882, 1974.

13. Ahmann, DL, O'Connell, MJ, Bisel, HF: An evaluation of cytoxan/Adriamycin (CA) versus cytoxan/Adriamycin/5-fluorouracil (CAF) versus cytoxan/5-fluorouracil/prednisone (CF) in advanced breast cancer. Abstract, 278, *Proceedings Twelfth Annual Meeting of the American Society of Clinical Oncology,* Toronto, Vol. 17, March 1976.

14. Ahmann, DL, O'Fallon, J, O'Connell, MJ et al.: Evaluation of a fixed alternating treatment in patients with advanced breast cancer. *Cancer Clinical Trials,* Vol. 1, No. 3, 219–226, 1978.

15. Rubin, J, Decker, DA, Ahmann, DL et al.: An evaluation of two schedules of UP-16 and Adriamycin in patients with advanced breast cancer (unpublished).

16. Britell, JC, Bisel, H, Ahmann, DL et al.: Cytoxan, 5-fluorouracil and prednisone (CFP) and immunotherapy in advanced breast cancer. ASCO-AACR Abstract, 1979.

Limits of Chemotherapy in Management of the Multiple Stages of Advanced Breast Cancer

George R. Blumenschein

Department of Medicine, The University of Texas System Cancer Center, M.D. Anderson Hospital and Tumor Institute, Houston, Texas

Summary

Analyses of disease-free survival curves for Stage II, III, IV NED and IV in complete remission breast cancer treated with 5-fluorouracil, Adriamycin, cyclophosphamide drug combination and, in most cases, nonspecific immunotherapy demonstrate a repetitive break in disease-free survival curves at 27 and 32 months. Assuming the observed mean doubling time for early breast cancer to be between 25 and 30 days and multiplying this time by the 30 doublings required for one cell to increase to a measurable 10^9 results in a calculated time for the disease-free survival curve to be 25 to 30 months. This calculated time closely approximates the observed time to break in widely different tumor burdens of metastatic breast cancer. An extrapolation by stage for an assumed distribution of microscopic metastatic tumor by stage provides the estimate that Adriamycin combination therapy may kill a breast cancer burden of slightly less than 10^6 cells. Thus, in considering chemotherapy for cure of metastatic breast cancer at whatever stage, more effective regional therapeutic measures must be considered whenever appropriate in their sequential application and in their tumor-destructive capability.

Discussion

Effective combination drug programs developed for the treatment of clinically evident metastatic breast cancer have improved remission rates and length of remissions and of survival for these patients.[1-4] 5-fluorouracil, Adriamycin, cyclophosphamide (FAC) combination chemother-apy consistently has shown response rates in the range of 70 to 80 percent.[2,3,5] Unfortunately, complete remissions rarely have exceeded 20 percent with the use of this combination program and modifications and alterations in dose and schedule of these active chemotherapeutic agents have not resulted in a cure for the metastatic stage of the disease. In an effort to decrease the mortality rate of breast cancer, this effective drug combination has been used for treatment of stages of breast cancer which have a high probability of harboring systemic microscopic meta-static breast cancer (stages II, III, and IV NED). The disease-free survival curves for these multiple stages of breast cancer (Figure 1)

Figure 1.

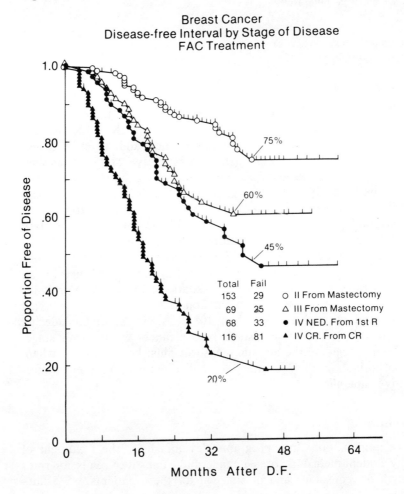

Breast Cancer
Disease-free Interval by Stage of Disease
FAC Treatment

treated with Adriamycin combination programs may provide an estimate as to the absolute number of tumor cells eliminated by FAC treatment.

One hundred and fifty-three patients with stage II breast cancer were treated following mastectomy and irradiation with FAC plus Bacillus Calmette-Guérin (BCG) to a total dose of 300 mg/m^2 of Adriamycin. Cyclophosphamide, methotrexate, and 5-fluorouracil (CMF) plus BCG were then continued for a total of 24 months of treatment. The disease-free survival for this group of patients with a median followup of 37 months appears to plateau at 40 months for approximately 75 percent of the patients (Figure 2).[6] The great majority of relapses in this clinical trial occurred prior to 28 months from beginning FAC chemotherapy. When compared to a similar staged group of patients treated only with surgery and irradiation at M. D. Anderson Hospital, this combination chemotherapy appears to provide significant disease-free survival advantage for stage II patients. The stage II patients not receiving FAC chemotherapy following mastectomy and irradiation do not show a plateau in their disease-free survival. After 40 months of followup, 55 percent remain free of clinical metastases while less than 45 percent are free of disease at 60 months (Figure 2).

Sixty-nine patients with stage III breast cancer treated in a similar fashion to stage II patients, with a median followup time of 37 months, show a plateau in their disease-free survival curve for 60 percent of the patients at 40 months (Figure 2).[6] A stage matched control population of breast cancer patients treated by surgery and irradiation alone show a continually declining disease-free survival with 45 percent of the patients remaining free of the disease at 40 months and less than 37 percent at 60 months (Figure 2).

A population of stage IV breast cancer patients who presented with a single solitary site of first metastasis was treated with surgery and/or radiation therapy for regional cure, making them clinically free of disease (IV NED). FAC plus BCG combination chemotherapy was then given to a total dose of 450 mg/m^2 of Adriamycin and CMF plus BCG chemotherapy was continued for a total treatment period of two years.[7] With a median followup for this group of patients of 44 months, the disease-free survival curve appears to plateau for 45 percent of the patients at 40 months (Figure 3). This disease-free survival for a group of patients with a very high probability of significant microscopic tumor burden compares favorably with the disease-free survival of stage IV NED patients treated by regional cure of a solitary metastasis with surgery and/or irradiation alone (Figure 3). Diagramed in the same figure is the disease-free remission curve for 116 metastatic breast cancer patients who entered complete remission (IV CR) after treatment with one of several FAC combination chemotherapy programs with and without immunotherapy.[8] This curve, as with other disease-free survival curves for lesser stages of

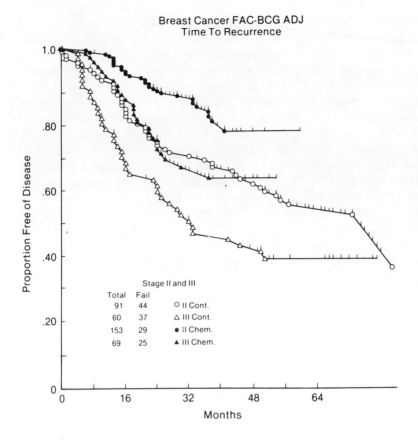

Figure 2.

metastatic breast cancer in complete remission, appears to plateau for about 20 percent of patients at 36 to 40 months.

While the relatively short median followup periods of 37 to 44 months for these groups of clinically disease-free breast cancer patients (with varying probabilities of occult and microscopic metastases) cast some doubt on the permanence of the demonstrated plateaus at around 40 months, the consistency of the plateauing or breaks in the disease-free survival curves for each group suggests that we may be observing a biological effect, which may be a function of tumor cell numbers killed in each stage of disease by FAC therapy. Plateauing of disease-free survival curves has been used to predict the therapeutic efficacy of chemotherapy with reasonable accuracy in animal tumor models and in human cancer.[9,10]

In the animal tumor models and human malignancies so studied, either a close approximation of the number of residual metastatic tumor cells was known or the distribution of microscopic tumor burden among the populations of patients was reasonably predictable. Breast cancer is recognized to be a disease with a broad spectrum of biological behavior. Doubling times of tumors range widely[11] and the natural history of each stage of disease shows great variability. By observing the disease-free survival curves for each of several stages of breast cancer, we have made semiquantitative predictions about the distribution of microscopic metastases by stage following curative regional and systemic therapy.

Figure 4 is an estimate of the distribution of tumor burden remaining in populations of patients in the four stages under discussion, e.g., stages II, III, IV NED and IV CR. In this model, a stage II population of breast cancer patients following regional cure of their clinically evident disease

Figure 3.

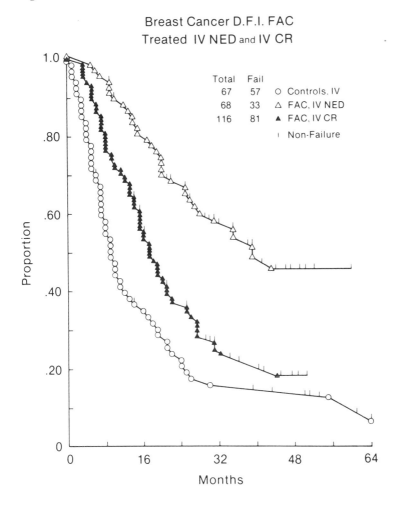

Breast Cancer D.F.I. FAC
Treated IV NED and IV CR

Total	Fail	
67	57	O Controls. IV
68	33	△ FAC, IV NED
116	81	▲ FAC, IV CR
		ı Non-Failure

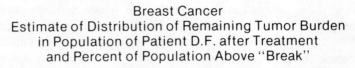

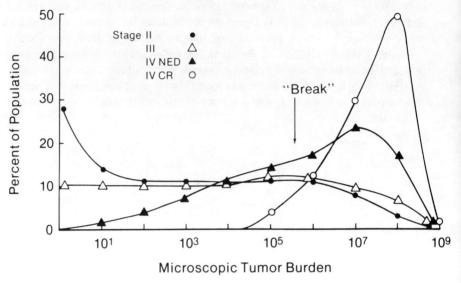

Figure 4.

would be assumed to have at least 30 percent of the patients with no remaining tumor cells and another 15 percent of the patients with 10 or less remaining cancer cells. A very small percentage of the stage II patients would probably have greater than 10^7 cancer cells remaining. For stage III patients, the prediction is that there would be a more even distribution of microscopic tumor burden among the population of patients following mastectomy and irradiation, and that these patients would be evenly distributed between zero and 10^8 microscopic tumor burden. The remaining microscopic disease in stage IV NED patients following regional cure would undoubtedly be skewed toward the 10^7 and 10^8 tumor burden, while the stage IV CR patients would have microscopic tumor burden highly skewed toward 10^8 remaining cancer cells.[12]

In order to use the disease-free survival curves for the various stages of metastatic breast cancer to predict the number of metastatic breast cancer cells that a type of chemotherapy can completely eliminate, the assumption has to be made that the disease-free survival curves will plateau at a point where one or less tumor cell remains in the patient. Thus the time from the plateau to the ordinate is a reflection of the time required for one cancer cell to multiply to a measurable 1,000,000,000 tumor cells. From the data shown, we would estimate that the time required for the 30 doublings between one and 10^9 tumor cells would require approximately 40 months. If we consider the percent of patients at the break in the curve for each stage of disease, 75 percent of stage II, 60 percent of stage III, 45 percent of stage IV NED and 20 percent of stage IV CR patients appear to be on the plateau or to have achieved a reduction in their microscopic tumor burden to one or less tumor cell. Thus, the percent of patients noted at the break on each of the disease-free survival curves could be assumed to be free of or cured of cancer.

If the percentage of patients presumed cured for each stage of disease by systemic therapy is located on each of the respective theoretical curves depicting the distribution of microscopic tumor burden among each population after regional cure, we see that 75 percent of stage II patients, 60 percent of stage III patients, 45 percent of stage IV NED patients and 20 percent of stage IV CR patients would be predicted to have a microscopic tumor burden remaining after entering complete remission of between 10^5 and 10^6 tumor cells. From these speculations, the assumption follows that FAC chemotherapy may be curative for a tumor burden of only 100,000 to 1,000,000 cancer cells. While it is understood that the cytotoxic effect of chemotherapy is dependent upon multiple factors, such as doubling time of cancer cell population, phenotypic expression of cancer cell clones, tumor blood supply and host defense mechanisms, these crude estimates of the microscopic tumor burden killed by a specific chemotherapy program provides us with some estimate of how we should weigh the effectiveness of one regime when we are considering its use for cure. With this apparent limited effectiveness cure of metastatic breast cancer by a combination drug program which provides the highest remission rate for metastatic breast cancer, one is encouraged to reconsider the timing and sequence of chemotherapy in the treatment of specific stages of the disease. Renewed consideration has to be given to the more aggressive use of other therapeutic modalities such as surgery, irradiation and immunotherapy in an effort to achieve cure of metastatic breast cancer, and the sequencing of these multiple modalities of treatment should become a major effort in the research of improved therapy for each stage of disease.

References

1. Cannellos, GP et al.: Combination chemotherapy for advanced breast cancer: response and effect on survival. *Ann. Int. Med.* 84:389–392, 1976.
2. Blumenschein, GR et al.: FAC chemotherapy for breast cancer. *Proc. Am. Assoc. Clin. Oncol.* 15:193, 1974.
3. Jones, SE, Durie, BGM, and Salmon, SE: Combination chemotherapy with Adriamycin and cyclophosphamide for advanced breast cancer. *Cancer* 36:90–97, 1975.

252

4. Carbone, PP, Davis, TE: Medical treatment for advanced breast cancer. *Semin. Oncol.* 5(4):417–427, 1978.

5. Bull, JM et al.: A randomized comparative trial of Adriamycin vs methotrexate in combination drug therapy. *Cancer* 41:1649–1657, 1978.

6. Buzdar, AU et al.: Postoperative adjuvant chemotherapy with 5-fluorouracil Adriamycin, cyclophosphamide and BCG: a followup report. *JAMA* (in press), 1979.

7. Blumenschein, GR et al.: Adjuvant chemoimmunotherapy following regional therapy of initial solitary metastases of breast cancer (stage IV NED). In: Jones, SE, Salmon, SE, eds. *Adjuvant Therapy of Cancer II,* pp. 303–310, Grune & Stratton, New York, 1979.

8. Legha, SS et al.: Complete remissions in metastatic breast cancer treated with combination drug therapy, *Annal. of Int. Med.* (in press), 1979.

9. Schabel, FM: Surgical adjuvant chemotherapy of metastatic murine tumors. *Cancer* 40:558–568, 1977.

10. Frei, E et al.: Adjuvant chemotherapy of osteogenic sarcoma: progress and perspectives. In: Jones, SE, and Salmon, SE, eds. *Adjuvant Therapy of Cancer,* p. 49, Elsevier/North-Holland Biomedical Press, Amsterdam, 1977.

11. Schackney: Growth rate of cancers. *Annal. of Int. Med.* 89:107–121, 1978.

12. Blumenschein, GR: Tumor burden killed by Adriamycin-combination therapy in metastatic breast cancer, In: *Proceedings of 2nd International Conference on the Adjuvant Therapy of Cancer,* March 28–31, 1979.

Treatment of Disseminated Sarcomas[a]

Frederick R. Eilber, James Huth,
E. Carmack Holmes, Donald L. Morton

*Division of Oncology, Department of Surgery, UCLA School of Medicine,
University of California, Los Angeles, California and Surgical Service,
Sepulveda Veterans Hospital, Sepulveda, California*

Summary

The treatment of patients with metastatic sarcoma is a controversial and extremely difficult clinical problem. Our group has achieved objective responses of 40-50 percent with Adriamycin whereas results with combination chemotherapy (CyVADTIC) have been disappointing. Pilot studies indicate that multidisciplinary treatment with preoperative Adriamycin and radiation therapy may allow selection of those patients who would benefit from surgical resection of their metastatic disease and also might reduce subsequent disease recurrence in the chest. Until additional chemotherapeutic agents are available for the treatment of metastatic soft tissue sarcomas, the multidisciplinary approach, chemoradiation therapy and surgical resection, is the most effective way to treat metastatic sarcomas.

Discussion

Natural History

Soft tissue sarcomas often resist therapy and, consequently, relatively few patients survive this malignancy. Russell and associates found an overall 10-year survival rate of only 30 percent in 1215 patients with various histologic types of soft tissue sarcomas.[1] Only 5 percent of the

[a]These investigations were supported by Grants CA 12582, CB 53941 from the National Cancer Institute (DHEW) and Medical Research Service of the Veterans Administration.

patients with histologically aggressive tumors (clinicopathologic Stage III or IV) were alive 10 years after diagnosis.

Despite advances in radiation therapy and chemotherapy, complete surgical excision of the primary tumor is still the treatment of choice. Local control can be achieved in nearly 80 percent of the patients by operation and radiation therapy.[2,3] However, 50 percent of these patients who are free of recurrent local disease will develop distant metastases to the lung within six to 12 months and will die.[2] Obviously, undetectable, microscopic metastasis is present at the time of surgical resection of the primary tumor and accounts for the recurrent systemic illness. Thus, the treatment of disseminated sarcoma becomes the primary concern regardless of the clinical stage of the disease at presentation.

Single Agent Chemotherapy

Of the multiple single agent chemotherapeutic drugs used against metastatic sarcoma, Adriamycin appears to be the most effective. Objective responses to Adriamycin range from 30-45 percent whereas responses to other agents such as actinomycin-D and cytoxan are from five to 15 percent.[4]

Combination Chemotherapy

The VAC (vincristine, actinomycin-D and cytoxan) combination which has been the most successful treatment for childhood sarcomas (rhabdomyosarcoma) has less than a 10 percent response for adult disease.[5] The combination of CyVADTIC (cytoxan, vincristine, Adriamycin and DTIC) has been reported to induce a 40-65 percent objective response by M.D. Anderson and the Southwest Oncology Group,[6,7] although other investigators have reported much lower response rates.[8]

Twenty patients with recurrent or metastatic soft tissue sarcomas were treated by the UCLA Division of Oncology.[9] The chemotherapy regimen consisted of CyVADTIC (cytoxan 500 mg/m^2, vincristine 1 mg/m^2, Adriamycin 50 mg/m^2, and DTIC 250 mg/m^2) on Day one through five. This drug combination was repeated every 22 to 28 days; treatment was withheld if the white blood cell count fell below 4000. All patients had histologically-proved soft tissue sarcomas and clinically evident metastatic disease in the chest which could be evaluated by chest X-ray. Nine patients already had received some chemotherapy—three with Adriamycin, three with actinomycin-D, vincristine and cytoxan and three with postoperative Adriamycin plus high dose methotrexate. All patients were ambulatory with no significant weight loss and received treatment as outpatients.

Of the 20 patients who received the CyVADTIC, two experienced a complete response and one patient had a partial response. However, the remaining 17 patients had no measurable response to the CyVADTIC chemotherapy; the objective response rate was 3/20 (15 percent). The mean duration of treatment for all patients was 4.2 months and the mean number of completed courses was 4.1.

Reports of responses up to 60 percent in patients treated with Cy-VADTIC are in marked contrast to only 15 percent that we observed. Since nearly half of these patients had failed to respond to previous chemotherapy, it is conceivable that their sarcomas represented a particularly aggressive type of tumor. Furthermore, only 30 percent of our patients developed total white cell counts less than 3000, whereas 56 percent of the Southwest Oncology Group patients had a median white count less than 1000. Increasing the toxicity could, perhaps, account for an increased partial response rate; however, increased toxicity often requires a life island support system to prevent infection.

Surgical Resection

Holmes and Morton[10,11] recently reviewed experiences with surgical resection of sarcomas metastatic to lungs. In this series, 38 patients with soft tissue (20 percent) or osteosarcoma (18 percent) metastastic to lung were subjected to thoracotomy. All patients in this series had tumor doubling times greater than 60 days. Of this group of patients, 12/38 (32 percent) remain disease-free with a median followup of 29.0 months. Of the patients whose disease recurred, 34 percent of the recurrences were found to be in the ipsilateral chest and 33 percent in the contralateral chest, indicating that 66 percent of recurrent disease was limited to the lungs. The number of metastases, or the bilaterality of metastases did not correlate with disease recurrence.

Present Trials

Since it was apparent that the CyVADTIC regimen (at least in our hands) had a very low objective response rate, the reasons for this dramatic difference were examined. The Adriamycin dosage in the CyVADTIC regimen is approximately one half the dose prescribed when Adriamycin is used as a single agent, i.e., a total dose of 90 mg/m^2, whereas in the CyVADTIC regimen the total dose of Adriamycin is 50 mg/m^2/course. The myelosuppressive characteristics of the cytoxan and DTIC limit the amount of Adriamycin.

Radiation therapy has been used extensively in the treatment of metastatic sarcomas to the chest with a documented 30 percent response rate. The radiation has been limited to approximately 2000-3000 rads because of radiation pneumonitis. A recent report by the E.O.R.T.C. Cooperative Group has indicated the rationale for the use of whole-lung irradiation in inpatients with metastatic sarcomas.[12] In a randomized prospective trial, 86 Stage I patients with osteosarcoma received either amputation alone (42) or amputation and whole-lung irradiation (44) at a dose of 2000 rads delivered over two weeks to the entire lung parenchyma. The patients who received the whole-lung irradiation had a 15 percent increase in survival rate compared to patients treated by amputation alone. Therefore, it appears that under selected circumstances, whole-lung irradiation may be beneficial for destruction of microscopic disease in the chest.

Using this information, a recent pilot trial was started at UCLA for patients with metastatic sarcomas. To date, 15 patients have been treated with systemic Adriamycin (45 mg/m^2), divided over two consecutive days followed by 2000 rads of whole-lung irradiation. Tumor doubling times are calculated before treatment starts and again after the course of combined chemo-radiation therapy. To date, 2/4 postthoracotomy patients remain free of disease 12-18 months following therapy. Of 10 patients treated preoperatively, five had an objective response and one had complete disappearance of all metastatic disease. Of the patients treated thus far, the five who had no objective response were not subjected to pulmonary resection and have expired of their disseminated sarcomas. Of the five who had the objective responses, one was not subjected to thoracotomy because all gross disease and visible disease had disappeared whereas the remaining four patients had surgical resection. All patients remain free of recurrence with a median followup of 10 months.

Conclusion

In conclusion, the treatment of patients with metastatic sarcoma is a controversial and extremely difficult clinical problem. Adriamycin appears to be the most successful single agent for chemotherapy and our group has achieved objective responses of 40-50 percent with this agent. The results obtained with combination chemotherapy have been disappointing in our experience—a 15 percent objective response rate. It appears that in order to achieve a more significant response rate (50-60 percent), escalating dosages of these combination chemotherapeutic agents must be given, an increase that can lead to fatal leukopenia.

Our pilot studies indicate that the multidisciplinary treatment with preoperative Adriamycin and radiation therapy may allow selection of those patients who would benefit from surgical resection of their metastatic disease and also might reduce subsequent disease recurrence in the chest. However, only time and additional patients will allow us to determine whether this preoperative chemo-radiation therapy and surgical resection will, in fact, improve the overall survival for patients with metastatic sarcoma. Until other therapeutic agents are available or are developed, it is our opinion that the multidisciplinary approach, the combination of surgery, radiation and chemotherapy, is the most effective way to treat these patients.

References

1. Russell, WO, Cohen, J, Enzinger, F et al.: A clinical and pathological staging system for soft tissue sarcoma. *Cancer* 40:1562-1570, 1977.

2. Suit, HD, Russell, WO, Martin, RG: Management of patients with sarcoma of soft tissue in an extremity. *Cancer* 31:1247-1255, 1973.

3. Eilber, FR, Townsend, CM, Weisenburger, TH et al.: Preoperative intra-arterial Adriamycin and radiation therapy for extremity soft tissue sarcomas: a clinicopathologic study. In: *Management of Primary Bone and Soft Tissue Tumors*, pp. 411-422, Year Book Medical Publ., Chicago, 1977.

4. Tan, C, Etcubanas, E, Wollner, N et al.: Adriamycin—an anti-tumor antibiotic in the treatment of neoplastic disease. *Cancer* 32:9-17, 1973.

5. Gottlieb, JA, Baker, LH, Burgess, MA et al.: Sarcoma chemotherapy. In: *Cancer Chemotherapy: Fundamental Concepts and Recent Advances*, pp. 445-454, Year Book Medical Publ., Chicago, 1974.

6. Gottlieb, JA, Bodey, GP, Sinkovics, JG et al.: An effective new 4-drug combination regimen (CyVADIC) for metastatic sarcomas. *Proc. Amer. Soc. Clin. Oncol.* 15:162, 1974.

7. Gottlieb, JA, Baker, LH, O'Bryan, RM et al.: Adriamycin (NSC-123127) used alone and in combination for soft tissue and bony sarcomas. *Cancer Chemother. Rep.* 6:271-282, 1975.

8. Creagan, ET, Hahn, RG, Alman, DL et al.: A comparative clinical trial evaluating the combination of Adriamycin, DTIC, and vincristine, combination of actinomycin-D, cyclosphosphamide, and vincristine and single agent methyl-CCNU, in advanced sarcomas. *Cancer Treat. Rep.* 60:1385-1387, 1976.

9. Giuliano, AE, Larkin, K, Eilber, FR, Morton, DL.: Failure of combination chemotherapy (CyVADTIC) in metastatic soft tissue sarcomas: implications for adjuvant studies. *Proc. Amer. Soc. Clin. Oncol.* 19:359, 1978.

10. Morton, DL, Joseph, WL, Ketcham, AS et al.: Surgical resection and adjunctive immunotherapy for selected patients with multiple pulmonary metastases. *Ann. Surg.* 178:360-366, 1973.

11. Holmes, EC, Ramming, KP, Eilber, FR, Morton, DL: The surgical management of pulmonary metastasis. *Semin. Oncol.* 4:165-169, 1977.

12. Breur, K, Cohen, P, Schweisguth, O, Hart, AMM: Irradiation of the lungs as an adjuvant therapy in the treatment of osteosarcoma of the limbs. An E.O.R.T.C. randomized study. *Europ. J. Cancer* 14:461-471, 1978.

Panel Discussion

UNKNOWN: I would like to pose a question to Dr. Decker and Dr. Blumenschein. How would you treat a post-menopausal female with four positive nodes, laterally located lesion?

GEORGE BLUMENSCHEIN: We consider the risk of recurrence in a post-menopausal woman with four positive nodes significant. I think the estrogen receptor status of her tumor would be important. If her estrogen receptor status is negative, we would recommend that she receive radiation therapy to the peripheral lymphatics. If less than 20% of the lymph nodes contain metastatic disease we would probably limit the radiation therapy to the regional lymphatics. If there was an adequate axillary dissection, we would not irradiate the axilla. If greater than 20% of the nodes were involved, we would use electron beam therapy to the chest wall. The reason I am emphasizing radiation is that it has come under a lot of disservice, I believe, because of the way it has been done in our country and not because radiation therapy is an ineffective modality. Following the radiation therapy, we would give FAC-BCG chemoimmunotherapy as an adjuvant treatment. The reason we choose an Adriamycin combination is because in our study post-menopausal women with four or more nodes benefitted more than pre-menopausal women in that category. In our post-menopausal women with four or more axillary nodes with a median followup in excess of 40 months, 82% of the women remained free of disease with no relapses after 28 months. Adriamycin is a less cycle-dependent agent than methotrexate, 5-fluorouracil and to some degree cyclophosphamide. We believe that Adriamycin is more effective in the post-menopausal woman because of a higher incidence of estrogen receptive positivity and presumably slower growing tumors with lower doubling times.

UNKNOWN: What is the incidence of local recurrence at M.D. Anderson?

BLUMENSCHEIN: The incidence of local recurrence in patients who have received radiation is under 4%.

UNKNOWN: What was the incidence of local recurrence before radiation therapy was initiated?

BLUMENSCHEIN: I don't know what it was at M.D. Anderson; but comparative studies show the local recurrence rate to vary between 12 and 40% in most studies depending upon the tumor burden. The CMF study from Bonadonna which did not use radiation has a disastrously high local recurrence rate.

UNKNOWN: Do you feel that radiation defers your chemotherapy or your effective adjuvant chemoimmunotherapy?

BLUMENSCHEIN: Yes it does.

UNKNOWN: Doesn't that have some bearing on your proposed increasing tumor burden?

BLUMENSCHEIN: Yes. The logical way to treat breast cancer, if we assume that chemotherapy is effective from microscopic tumor burden and we have an effective combination chemotherapy program, is to start with chemotherapy and then do the regional treatment after you have given some adequate therapeutic dose of drugs. The beauty of surgery is that it can be intermingled with chemotherapy. You do not have to break the sequence or the cycle of the chemotherapy in order to do surgery. Radiation therapy has the burden of not being able to be given in conjunction with chemotherapy. If I had the best of all situations, I would use the radiotherapy following the initial 300 mg/m^2 of Adriamycin. However, it's important to add, despite this important kinetic delay with our adjuvant program in patients with a significant tumor burden, we still have results that are superior to those from studies in which chemotherapy was started within two weeks of surgery indicating the therapeutic efficacy of Adriamycin combinations in the treatment of breast cancer.

UNKNOWN: If you look at the NASBP studies, they no longer are radiating the axilla either in patients with one to three positive nodes or in patients with more than four positive nodes. They are treating all those patients, depending upon the protocol, with L-Pam 5FU, L-Pam 5FU plus tamoxiffen. I'm not clear what role radiation therapy would have in the patient presented with four positive nodes. Continuing on in that vein, I wanted to ask you to further explain your concluding statement because I'm not sure what you mean by "thus in considering chemotherapy for cure of metastatic breast cancer of whatever stage, you need more effective regional therapeutic measures." I don't know what role that plays in advanced disease.

BLUMENSCHEIN: I'll be happy to explain both questions. We'll start with the last question first, since it is really the sum and substance of the discussion. We have effective regional therapies; but we do not have effective strategies to use the regional therapies and the word strategy should be substituted in an abstract for therapy. Let's assume we have a patient with multiple sizes of metastases that we can measure. When a patient goes into a partial remission, with chemotherapy or hormonal therapy or whatever therapy you think is applicable, and that partial remission is then maintained in a stable situation in which about 37% of the tumor volume still remains, it does not seem sensible to continue the chemotherapy to maintain the stable partial remission status. A more logical approach to us would be to try and cure those sites regionally that are clinically evident with surgery and/or radiation therapy, local application of heat, regional immunotherapy or other treatments such as that, and then go on to effective second-line programs with chemotherapy. Now the question about radiation therapy, I think is very important. With radiation therapy we can probably cure a larger microscopic tumor burden than we can with chemotherapy. I think there is reasonable evidence that radiation therapy is very effective against microscopic disease in breast cancer. All of the studies that have been done between surgery versus surgery plus radiation have shown no benefit to those who had surgery plus radiation in terms of over-all survival. However, it has been beneficial in decreasing the incidence of local recurrence. Now, when we look at all radiation therapy, what we are looking at is a potpourri of things that have been called radiation therapy. I'm not a radiation therapist; but, I have been around enough to know that if there is any variability in the quality of therapy in our society it's in radiation therapy. We are many times comparing apples to oranges when we compare one person's radiation therapy to another. In the incidence of breast cancer, for instance, Toronto has just reviewed their cases in terms of radiating the internal mammary nodes and they have shown that in around 40% of the cases, when they attempted to do radio isotope investigation of the location of the internal mammary nodes, they were missing the nodes. A large group of radiation therapists in this country have been trained to use a tangential port with cobalt to treat the internal mammary nodes in the chest wall. When they do that, the internal mammary nodes which lie right on the margin of the radiation beam are under-dosed. So, a good deal of radiation therapy is not really accomplishing what it is supposed to accomplish. There are studies, however, in which good radiation therapy has been done and compared to equal series in which it hasn't been done. In these studies done in Sweden, radiation therapy has not only shown a decrease in regional recurrence but also a significant prolongation in survival. I choose to believe these studies that are well done rather than take a common denominator of a larger group of studies which aren't well done.

FRED EILBER: Dr. Decker, in your presentation you found a longer tumor-free interval, longer than five years, to be a less favorable sign. Certainly in our studies at UCLA and other studies where surgery is used for metastasis, one of the single most determinants of favorable prognosis is a long tumor-free interval.

DAVID DECKER: These are patients who had metastatic disease. If the theory of short doubing time is correct, i.e., oat-cell carcinoma of the lung, you would have a disease that would have a short disease-free interval and respond better to chemotherapy. From a surgical standpoint, I understand what you are saying; but, we have evidence of oat-cell carcinoma of the lung where rapid doubling time, short disease-free interval might indicate that it would respond better to chemotherapy.

EILBER: That was in terms of weeks, six to eight weeks. We are talking about years. I don't know the answer.

DECKER: I don't either and the only explanation I can give is the analogy of the rapid growing tumor that might respond better to chemotherapy.

EILBER: Dr. Al-Sarraf, did you in your analysis look at the weight of the patient? The reason I ask is because of a European study in which it was found that patients under 70 kilograms did better than those over 70 kilograms for a standard dose of levamisole.

MUHYI AL-SARRAF: We did not look at weight.

LAWRENCE ALLEN: I would like to address a question to Dr. Decker and then maybe Dr. Blumenschein and to anyone else who cares to comment on long term remitters or complete remitters. Your conclusion, Dr. Decker, was to stop chemotherapy in your patients even though there was no long term cure of their breast cancer. Is it possible that had the chemotherapy been continued the remissions would have lasted longer? Perhaps we should not stop chemotherapy on patients after long term complete remissions?

DECKER: I can not answer that directly; but I can tell you the results of the study and let you draw your own inferences. There were two patients who had about six months of chemotherapy and they elected to stop because of toxicity. These patients interestingly enough relapsed at approximately the same time as those who received very prolonged chemotherapy or those who received the 36 months or 24 months of chemotherapy. I think this raises the question do we, indeed, have to treat them for approximately two years which is the common treatment for these patients? Of our eight patients, six stopped treatment because they were disease-free at approximately two years and two patients quit treatment; one subsequently had a CR. All the other patients had minor responses with partial remissions but rapidly failed and died within a short period of time.

UNKNOWN: In the patients who were retreated, were they treated with the same chemotherapy or with a different chemotherapy?

DECKER: They were almost all treated with a different chemotherapy.

EILBER: Isn't that almost an inescapable conclusion from your study that chemotherapy should not be terminated?

DECKER: I think the morbidity of the treatment, the problems with the patients losing their veins from administration of long term chemotherapy and the fact that they all relapse anyway and that few of them can be rescued are reasonable considerations for stopping treatment. I think the only way this question is going to be answered is to have a group of patients and stop their treatment at varying times and see what happens to them in terms of relapse.

BLUMENSCHEIN: We have a slightly different experience in our long term complete remission patients. Those, who have visceral and soft tissue disease and have remained in complete remission beyond the traditional two years of chemotherapy, have tended to do very well. The late relapsers have been those few patients who have gone into complete remission in bone and have had normal remodeling of the bone. There is another group of patients who have not gone into complete remission in bone. They are in partial remission and their bones never completely heal. In these patients we have been afraid to stop chemotherapy. This is a very interesting subset of patients and they fall into two groups. We usually tire of giving them chemotherapy after three years for the reasons that were mentioned. They become fatigued, they run out of veins and we begin to wonder what sensible good we are doing. At that point, usually at two years and again at three years, we do a bone biopsy. If we find the biopsy to be normal, we get up our courage to stop the chemotherapy. Of course, the problem is, a normal biopsy means nothing; it is only a positive biopsy in that situation that means something. In the group of patients in whom we stopped chemotherapy with this type of bone situation about half of them have relapsed in bone in the time period described by Dr. Decker. There's another subset, however, who have clinical evidence of bone metastases and have not relapsed. Now, about three of these patients have for one reason or another broken or fractured a bone and they have had to have open reduction. The biopsy specimens of the lytic areas with recalcified borders have not shown metastatic cancer but fibrous tissue; so, in bone disease we are confronted with the dilemma of how to interpret radiographs. I believe there is a subset of patients with metastatic disease to the bone who, in fact, do go into complete remission even though their boning metastases on X-ray doesn't improve completely. To date, we have not had any late relapses in our patients who have a 60-month survival. This is not to say that these patients are cured because the natural history of breast cancer is such that we will have to wait 15 or 20 years before we can begin to make that assumption. I am certain, as in your study, we will begin to see patients drop out between the five-year and ten-year period. But, I am encouraged to think that we are beginning to see for the first time a plateau in the treatment of breast cancer. It's beginning to indicate that maybe systemic treatment does have a role to play. I am encouraged to think that possibly by combining hormonal therapy, in those patients where it is indicated, with chemotherapy in a sensible kinetic fashion and by possibly consolidating our remission gains with chemotherapy and regional therapy we may be able to see true cures in metastatic breast cancer.

UNKNOWN: Dr. Blumenschein, they are using the more potent drug Adriamycin in FAC BCG radiation combination and getting good results. But, when a relapse comes there isn't a good backup program. CMF in my view is not a good backup program for a FAC failure. Whereas, if you go the other way, using FAC and regional therapy and the patient relapses, you still have the best drug left, Adriamycin. Has anyone done a study similar to your group and Hersh's group at M.D. Anderson with CMF-BCG radiation rather than Adriamycin in that combination?

BLUMENSCHEIN: No, we haven't. I think there are some interesting studies that are being done in the post-menopausal patient with tamoxiffen plus CMF which may be just as positive as the FAC study. There are some CMFEP studies that are positive. The Southwest Oncology Group's CMFEP study is very positive and the trial that was conducted by Dr. Cooper over 10 years ago is very interesting where he used an intensive CMFEP beginning immediately post-operative. I'm not saying that FAC is the standard for all adjuvant therapy; at the moment we happen to have very good results. The results are such that we're not too concerned about what to do with those who relapse because we are not interested in seeing relapses. We're not planning for relapses. We do see relapse; but, we'd just as soon devise a treatment and ask a question which would try to eliminate that chance of relapse. So far the figures speak for themselves.

UNKNOWN: You suggested the use of regional therapy for consolidation but then suggested giving it early in breast cancer. It seems to me that the local failure rate in Bonadonna's studies was about 20% as opposed to the 70 to 80% failure for both local plus distant metastases or just distant metastases alone. In other recent studies, it has been suggested that patients who had CMF plus radical mastectomy had equivalent or greater pre-survival relapse than patients who had radio therapy plus CMF plus modified radical mastectomy.

BLUMENSCHEIN: I think those observations are all valid. The question is the effectiveness of CMF when you begin it eight to 12 weeks after the mastectomy. My bias is that CMF has the ability to cure a smaller tumor burden than I am estimating FAC has the ability to cure. So, if you want to use CMF it seems to me that it would be necessary to use it earlier than you would use Adriamycin. In fact, in Cooper's study, which is a selected patient study that was retrospective, the relapse rate in patients who had surgery, radiation, than CMFEP was 50 to 65%. The relapse rate in patients who had radical mastectomy and CMFEP within the two weeks of mastectomy and many times within a week, had a 10 to 15% relapse rate with a median followup in excess of five years. It is a very impressive study and it suggests that the timing of CMF is very important. I think the timing of FAC is also important and this is the question we have to address. It may be that radiation therapy is not necessary; but, for the moment I'm in the position that radiation therapy is effective against regional recurrence. It is effective in reducing significant microscopic tumor burden. I find it very difficult to discard a proven treatment for which there is evidence that it can actually improve survival in a few studies for a treatment for which there is no evidence it can cure you, so that is why I am including both.

UNKNOWN: I would like to ask Dr. Sweet a question. In your patients with histiocytic lymphoma, who did not have a complete remission because of a particular area of bulky tumor that doesn't respond totally, do you treat any of them with radiation in order to produce a complete remission? If so, how do these patients survive as compared to those who had a complete remission with chemotherapy alone?

DONALD SWEET: The patients in the slide that I showed achieved a complete remission without the benefit of chemotherapy, radiation therapy or debulking procedures. There's no doubt that a number of the patients, who were not responders or partial responders, have persistent disease usually in the abdomen. We have recently modified our protocol. Now if these patients have a good response to their initial partial cycle of COMLA and if there is still persistent palpable disease, we debulk that tumor either by surgery and/or radiation therapy, then continue with chemotherapy. I don't have any numbers to show you. The most difficult patient management problem in histiocytic lymphoma is the huge abdominal mass.

UNKNOWN: We have a patient who nearly had complete remission except for a sonogram positive area after chemotherapy was completed. We did treat further and at six months the patient had a relapse in the sono positive area which is now strongly clinically positive. We are going to attempt to reinduce remission with chemotherapy and radiation. Do you feel this will lead to a better clinical response?

SWEET: Well, I hope so. At the end of chemotherapy, for example, we are restaging the patient. If there was equivocal data on either ultrasound or CAT scan, we would explore the patient to confirm the absence or presence of disease. If there is disease, our surgeon would try to resect or debulk the area and then we would give radiation therapy followup. The definition of complete remission has to be stringently controlled and there is no doubt that at the site of bulk disease there is likely to be recurrence.

EILBER: Certainly in an area where we have such effective chemotherapy, it would seem logical to have a combined approach.

Immunochemotherapy of Clinical
Metastasis

Specific Immunotherapy with Autologous Tumor Cells and C. Parvum for Advanced Renal Cell Carcinomas[a]

Craig S. McCune, David V. Schapira,
Edgar C. Henshaw

*The University of Rochester Cancer Center and Department of Medicine,
University of Rochester School of Medicine and Dentistry, Rochester, New
York*

Summary

A successful application of specific immunotherapy has been demonstrated experimentally in several animal tumor systems. The procedure requires autologous tumor cells prepared as a cell suspension and bathed in a media containing an adjuvant. We have employed this concept in a clinical trial of the treatment of renal cell cancer using the patients' cryopreserved autologous tumor tissue and employing *C. parvum* as the adjuvant. Twelve patients have completed treatment and of these, four have demonstrated a clinical effect with some metastases regressing completely. The observations made in this study give additional support to the hypothesis that specific immunotherapy approaches may have a useful role in advanced neoplasia.

Introduction

The hypothesis that human malignancy might be treated by immunization using a tumor cell vaccine was probably first investigated in a human trial by von Leyden and Blumenthal.[13] They reported in 1902 that no effect was seen. There has been renewed interest in this concept in the past 15 years. In the laboratory, there has been remarkable success at immunizing mice against tumors using their syngeneic tumor cells. This

[a]Supported by the Marie C. and Joseph C. Wilson Foundation and by Grant CA 11198 from the National Cancer Institute, DHEW.

led to several clinical trials in which patients were immunized with their own autologous irradiated tumor cells. Bloom et al.[4] treated glioblastoma multiforme in a prospective randomized trial. Ikonopisov[9] and Currie[5] in separate trials treated melanoma patients with autologous tumor cells. All of these attempts to immunize using an autologous tumor cell vaccine were negative. Retrospectively, Alexander,[1] Baldwin[2] and others have pointed out that the early animal models were misleading. The animal tumors were highly immunogenic and unrepresentative of the human problem. This led to the gradual discarding of unrealistic animal models and their clinical trial counterparts.

A later development in the concept of specific immunotherapy by tumor cell vaccines was the use of adjuvants. One of the classic immunologic techniques for sensitizing the immune system is to inject intradermally the foreign target antigen bathed in an adjuvant such as Freund's adjuvant. This is particularly useful when the target antigen itself is poorly immunogenic. In 1972, Bartlett and Zbar[3] demonstrated that BCG could be used effectively as the adjuvant in their model of guinea pig hepatoma. Later Scott[12] demonstrated that *C. parvum* could be used effectively as the adjuvant in a mouse mastocytoma system. Scott's mouse model is a parallel with the clinical study which we are reporting.

During the 1970s, a few clinical trials using autologous tumor cells with an adjuvant were conducted.[6–8,10] However, in the translation to human trials, the successful animal models were modified in two major ways. First, allogeneic tumor cells often were used rather than autologous. Second, frozen rather than fresh tumor cells were used. The substitution of frozen cells for fresh was later evaluated by Bartlett in a guinea pig model and found to have a very detrimental effect on the immunogenicity of the tumor cell preparation.

In spite of the liberties taken in the transition from laboratory to clinic, Laucius et al.[10] obtained four objective regressions in 18 melanoma patients treated with autologous tumor cells administered in a medium containing BCG as the adjuvant. Although the remissions were brief, the actuality of objective responses which included two complete regressions that had been produced solely by an immunologic means is noteworthy.

We undertook a Phase I clinical trial[11] with autologous tumor cells and incorporated the formalin-killed bacterium *C. parvum* as the adjuvant. During the Phase I study, one patient with metastatic renal carcinoma had a remarkable remission and this prompted us to investigate this therapy in others with the same diagnosis. A series of 12 patients having metastatic renal carcinoma have now completed treatment and are the subject of this report. No chemotherapy or radiation was given concurrent with the immunotherapy, but may have been employed later in those who developed progressive disease. Measurable or evaluable disease was present for assessment from the start of treatment in 10 of the 12 patients. The other two had intra-abdominal disease and postoperatively had developed intra-abdominal abscesses. Both of these patient expired within three months, and no followup by CT scan was performed.

Materials and Methods

At the time of surgical excision, the tumor tissue was minced and placed in freezer vials containing tissue culture medium with 7.5 percent DMSO. These were stored in a liquid nitrogen freezer and several vials removed each day that a patient was to be treated. The thawed mince was disaggregated enzymatically using hyaluronidase, collagenase and pronase sequentially. The tumor cells obtained from the supernatant of the last incubation were collected and irradiated with 10,000 rads. *C. parvum* was then added at a ratio of 37.5 mcg/10^7 tumor cells. The cells were resuspended in serum-free medium and injected intradermally in the shoulders. The volumes injected ranged from 0.5 to 2.0 ml. Patients consistently developed a small wheal at the site of injection which was tender to touch. It resolved in one to four days. Slight induration and discoloration sometimes was permanent. The local reactions did not become more severe with repeated weekly injections. There were no ulcerations or skin breakdown. No other side effects were attributable to the treatment.

Results

The clinical data pertaining to the patients are shown in Table 1. Their performance was graded by the scale developed by the Eastern Cooperative Oncology Group. The source of tumor tissue was from the primary hypernephroma lesion in seven of the 12 patients. Of those five patients where metastatic lesions were used, the tissue was obtained from the skin or from intra-abdominal masses that were removed surgically. The number of weekly injections and the total number of tumor cells administered was dependent largely on the quantity of tumor tissue that had been obtained at surgery. From four to 14 weekly injections were given and the total tumor cells ranged from 3.4×10^7 to 71.3×10^7. Two patients, Cases one and five, had objective regressions of a portion of their metastatic lesions. Two others had stabilization of disease as indicated by prolonged stabilization of lesions and dramatic relief of symptoms. Eight patients had progressive disease.

Two patients who underwent objective regressions provided some particularly pertinent information which bears on the concept of specific immunotherapy. Case One was a 67-year old woman who had multiple pulmonary nodules identified prior to her nephrectomy. In a five-week

Table 1. Clinical Data of Patients Treated with Specific Immunotherapy

Patient Number	Perf.[a] Status	Tissue[b] Source	Number of Weekly Injections	Total Tumor Cells (x10[7])	Response[c]	Response[d] Duration (mo)	Survival (mo)
1	1	Pri	4	3.4	R	11	29
2	0	Met	7	8.4	P		22+
3	0	Pri	4	6.6	P		21+
4	1	Met	5	27.0	S	20+	20+
5	0	Pri	11	35.0	R	7	18+
6	0	Pri	14	71.3	S	6	16+
7	3	Met	4	5.6	P		3
8	3	Met	7	26.7	P		4
9	4	Met	4	5.2	P		6
10	3	Pri	6	24.3	P		2
11	0	Pri	8	13.3	P		3+
12	2	Pri	4	13.1	P		2+

[a] 0 = asymptomatic; 1 = ambulatory but symptomatic; 2 = in bed < 50 percent of time; 3 = in bed > 50 percent of time; 4 = in bed 100 percent of time.

[b] Primary or metastatic lesions.

[c] R = regression; S = stabilization; P = progression.

[d] Described in case reports.

postoperative period, these lesions grew rapidly and she was symptomatic with fatigue. A bleeding biopsy-proven vaginal wall metastasis also developed. Weekly injections of her irradiated autologous cells with *C. parvum* as adjuvant was begun. At four weeks the beginning of regression was observed and at three months, 18 out of the 22 pulmonary nodules had undergone complete regression and the vaginal bleeding had ceased. The four remaining pulmonary nodules were stable for 11 months until slight enlargement was noted. At 20 months, definite relapse occurred with growth of the pulmonary nodules, brain lesions and bone metastases.

One observation is of particular interest. Of the 18 pulmonary nodules that had undergone complete regression only two reappeared at the time of relapse. The predominant growth in the lungs was of those nodules which had not regressed on initial treatment. The mixed response observed in this patient gave clinical evidence to the concept that metastases may be polyclonal in nature. Hence, in this patient, we had successfully immunized against the antigens expressed on certain metastatic clones and may well have eliminated completely those particular metastatic lesions. Others were unaffected by the immunotherapy and eventually these metastatic deposits grew and produced lethal disease.

Evidence of a polyclonal antigenic makeup of metastases is also seen in Case Five. This was a 36-year old woman who had pulmonary metastases at the time of nephrectomy and also was noted to have liver metastases during the surgical procedure. She received weekly immunotherapy injections for three months, during which time the pulmonary metastases increased in size and number. However, the chest X-ray at three and one half months which followed the start of treatment showed a definite decrease in the size of some nodules. In the next few months three of nine pulmonary nodules underwent complete regression. The largest was initially 5 cm in diameter. The nonregressing nodules continued to enlarge. Those in the mediastinum became symptomatic and were radiated and chemotherapy was started. The striking mixed response in this case illustrated that the tumor-specific antigens against which we were directing our therapy were not a single entity but were heterogeneous. This polyclonal character of metastases represents an important challenge which any specific immunotherapy approach will probably have to surmount.

Two other patients have had a stabilization of their disease course that is suggestive of a clinical effect from this specific immunotherapy program. Case Four is a 49-year old man who presented with back pain and hematuria. He was found to have a large hypernephroma in one kidney, and either a second primary or a metastasis in the opposite kidney, and a massive involvement of retroperitoneal lymph nodes. He was explored and a sizable portion of the retroperitoneal tissue removed and this was used for the immunotherapy. Following five weeks of the immunotherapy injections, his back pain had improved. There was no further hematuria; he felt well enough to return to a very active job and he continued completely stable for 20 months. Serial CAT scans of the abdomen showed the lesions in both kidneys and retroperitoneal areas had not changed in size over this period. Case Six is a 51-year old man whose primary renal tumor was obtained at the time of surgery. He developed lesions at three sites, which gave evidence of rapid growth. A cutaneous lesion was observed over two months to be rapidly enlarging and concurrently, two pulmonary nodules were observed to be enlarging rapidly. At the same time, a large painful lesion developed in the bone of the pelvis which gave him pain when walking and caused him to use a cane. Following treatment there was a six-month period with no growth of the pulmonary nodules, a slight regression of the skin lesion, but insufficient to call a partial response and his painful bony lesion became totally asymptomatic.

Patients who develop a stable disease pattern can never be called a response to treatment with 100 percent certainty since it is hard to distinguish it from the natural history. However, because these two cases had accompanying striking symptomatic changes, their overall course was suggestive of a clinical effect from the immunotherapy. Using a definition of a response to include these two stable disease patients, the following analyses may be made with relation to other parameters.

In Table 2 we compare the outcome for the patients with their

Table 2. Ambulatory Status Compared With Clinical Effects

Ambulatory Status	No. Having Clinical Effect/Total Patients
0	2/5
1	2/2
2	0/1
3	0/3
4	0/1

Table 3. Total Tumor Cells Given Compared With Clinical Effects

Total Tumor Cells	No. Having Clinical Effect/Total Patients
$> 20 \times 10^7$	3/5
$< 20 \times 10^7$	1/7

ambulatory status at the start of treatment and see that we have only had an effect on those patients who were of a high level of ambulatory status either asymptomatic or fully ambulatory with minimal symptoms. In Table 3 we have analyzed patients who have had an affect according to how successful we were at giving them a large quantity of immunizing tumor cells. Three of the five clinical effects have occurred in patients who received greater than 20×10^7 tumor cells. One of the seven patients who received less than 20×10^7 tumor cells has also had evidence of an effect.

Conclusion

In summary, we believe this specific immunotherapy program using a patient's autologous tumor cells and using *C. parvum* as a bacterial adjuvant is indicative of the potential of the immune system for producing regressions of cancer. In renal carcinoma where regressions by chemotherapy are uncommon and of short duration, we believe this approach may represent a worthwhile alternative. In interpreting our experience, we realize that one must always take into consideration spontaneous regressions with renal carcinoma. It is reported that a spontaneous regression may occur once in every 200 patients. We realize that in the two patients who have had clearcut objective regressions, spontaneous regressions would be an alternate explanation. However, the fact that both patients underwent their regressions at the end of a course of immunotherapy makes it highly likely that the treatment and regressions were cause and effect.

References

1. Alexander, P: Back to the drawing board—the need for more realistic model systems for immunotherapy. *Cancer* 40:467, 1977.

2. Baldwin, RW: Relevant animal models for tumor immunotherapy. *Cancer Immunol. Immunother.* 1:197, 1976.

3. Bartlett, GL, Zbar, B: Tumor-specific vaccine containing *Mycobacterium Bovis* and tumor cells: safety and efficacy. *J. Natl. Cancer Inst.* 48:170, 1972.

4. Bloom, HJG, Peckham, MJ, Richardson, AE et al.: Glioblastoma multiforme: A controlled trial to assess the value of specific active immunotherapy in patients treated by radical surgery and radiotherapy. *Br. J. Cancer* 27:253, 1973.

5. Currie, GA, Lejeune, F, Hamilton Fairley, G: Immunization with irradiated tumor cells and specific lymphocyte cytotoxicity in malignant melanoma. *Brit. Med. J.* 2:305, 1971.

6. Currie, GA, McElwain, TJ: Active immunotherapy as an adjunct to chemotherapy in the treatment of disseminated malignant melanoma: a pilot study. *Br. J. Cancer* 31:143, 1975.

7. Gerner, RE, Moore, GE: Feasibility study of active immunotherapy in patients with solid tumors. *Cancer* 38:131, 1976.

8. Hudson, CH, McHardy et al.: Active specific immunotherapy for ovarian cancer. *Lancet* 2:877, 1976.

9. Ikonopisov, RL, Lewis, MG, Hunter-Craig, ID et al.: Autoimmunization with irradiated tumor cells in human malignant melanoma. *Brit. Med. J.* 2:752, 1970.

10. Laucius, JM, Bodurtha, AJ, Mastrangelo, MJ, Bellett, RE: A Phase II study of autologous irradiated tumor cells plus BCG in patients with metastatic malignant melanoma. *Cancer* 40:2091, 1977.

11. McCune, CS, Patterson, WB, Henshaw, EC: Active specific immunotherapy with tumor cells and *Corynebacterium parvum:* a phase I study. *Cancer* 43:1619, 1979.

12. Scott, MT: Potentiation of the tumor-specific immune response by *Corynebacterium parvum. J. Natl. Cancer Inst.* 55:65, 1975.

13. Von Leyden, VE, Blumenthal, F: *D. Med. Wschr.* 28:637, 1902.

Specific Active Immunotherapy with Vaccinia Oncolysates

Marc K. Wallack

Department of Surgery, Washington University School of Medicine, St. Louis, Missouri

Summary

A live vaccinia vaccine virus-augmented tumor cell vaccine (vaccinia oncolysate) is used as a specific active immune mechanism stimulator against certain advanced human cancers. The Phase I trials in 29 patients have shown the vaccine to be safe, nontoxic and potentially effective. The heterogeneity of this early tumor group only reflects the type of patient available to the study during the early phase of vaccine testing. Randomized, prospective trials have begun in a more homogeneous tumor group so as to make analysis easier.

Introduction

Cancer immunotherapy continues to excite the imagination of investigators with its promise of cure. Although immunotherapy is in its earliest developmental phases, it already has demonstrated activity in terms of increasing the remission and survival durations in acute and chronic leukemia, soft tissue sarcoma, malignant melanoma, carcinoma of the colon and carcinoma of the lung.[1] However, the message coming from most trials that the tumor burden capable of destruction by the immune system cannot be large carries the implication that immunotherapy will find its place as an adjunct to other therapeutic modalities.

The scientific basis of the clinical rationale for immunotherapy for human cancer rests on several important demonstrations: antigens are seen in tumors which are not present in adult tissue; the host is capable of an immune response against its cancer; immune competence of the host is related to prognosis, and immunologic resistance to tumor growth can be produced.[2]

The various approaches to immunotherapy can be divided into three categories: nonspecific active immunotherapy, which involves the stimulation of the immune system with adjuvants that nonspecifically enhance the patient's capacity to respond to his own neoplasm such as BCG; specific active immunotherapy, which involves the active stimulation of the immune system with tumor vaccines to induce specific autoimmunity; and adoptive immunotherapy, which involves administration of antisera, immune lymphoid cells, or subcellular fractions from another host that has been specifically immunized against cancer-specific antigens in an attempt to increase the cancer patient's level of immunity.

Specific active immunotherapy is conceptually the most attractive of all the immunotherapeutic methods because it offers the following unique advantages over other treatment modalities: selective destruction of residual tumor cells bearing the specific distinctive tumor antigen; protection against neoplastic recurrence, and specific destruction of tumor cells while sparing normal counterparts.

Specific active immunotherapy vaccines consisting of either killed autologous or allogeneic tumor cells have been used to treat certain cancer patients since the turn of the century.[3] The majority of these studies was performed out of desperation in patients with advanced disease and were very poorly controlled. Moreover, since malignant cells are only weakly immunogenic in their host, one could hardly expect to generate a strong immune response with the injection of vaccines consisting of these cells alone. However, there are now several approaches specifically developed to strengthen the tumor cell immunogenicity. One of the most promising of these methods is through antigenic cooperation which presents weak tumor antigens to the host defense mechanism against a background of stronger antigens or haptens. This approach is typified by the work of Czajkowski[4] and his group, who complexed tumor cells with xerogenic globulins by using diazotized benzidene as a coupling agent. Another rather interesting means of providing antigenic cooperation is to use virus-augmented tumor cell preparations in which the tumor cell surface may be modified by infecting them with virus that either bud from the surface and leave the cell intact or cause lysis of the cell, the so-called viral oncolysis approach.

Awareness of the potential value of viral oncolysates dates back to observations by Koprowski[5] who noted the strong antigenic effect of virus-destroyed ascites tumor cells in mice. Lindenmann[6] performed similar experiments and presented a detailed immunologic study which established the value of viral oncolysates in contrast to lysates prepared by other means. The viruses employed in the preceding studies were neuropathic and there were many reservations as to their employment in human studies. This difficulty was circumvented by Wallack[7] who produced immunizing oncolysates with live vaccinia vaccine. Humans evidenced no ill effects from this virus since this was the same strain used to immunize them against smallpox. Furthermore, live vaccinia vaccine virus has the additional advantage of being able to cause a lytic infection in a wide variety of human tumor cells cultivated *in vitro*.[7] With the completion of successful murine tumor trials,[8] a Phase I human trial was instituted to determine the safety and potential efficacy of the vaccinia oncolysates. The following report is a summary of the Phase I study.

Materials and Methods

Preparation of Vaccinia Oncolysates

Tumor tissue removed from the patient in the operating room was processed as follows:

1. Those portions of the tumor which were not necrotic, fatty or hemorrhagic were finely minced by scalpels and placed in Eagle's MEM with 20 percent FBS plus penicillin and gentamicin.
2. The minced tissue was placed in an Erhlenmeyer flask with 30 ml of 0.25 percent trypsin, one percent versene solution and stirred with a magnetic bar to effect a suspension of single cells.
3. Approximately 1×10^7 $TCID_{50}$/ml of vaccinia virus was used to infect 1×10^6 ml of tumor cells in suspension.
4. The virus-tumor cell suspension was incubated for 72 hr at 37°C in Spinner's media with five percent human serum while both tumor cell lysis and virus titer were monitored.
5. The live vaccinia vaccine virus-augmented tumor cell suspension was spun at 20,000 rpm for 60 min at 0°, the supernatant was removed, and the pellet homogenized and suspended in enough Eagle's MEM to effect a concentration of 1×10^6 live vaccinia vaccine virus-augmented tumor cells/ml. These 1 ml aliquots were frozen at $-70°$ for use later.

Virus

The Wistar Institute's vaccinia virus is harvested from Wi 38 cells. Vaccine titers were determined on monolayers of Wi 38 cells in Eagle's MEM, containing three percent human serum. The vaccinia titer was approximately 1×10^7 $TCID_{50}$/ml.

Vaccine Administration

The vaccinia oncolysates were injected in 1 ml doses intradermally into the anterior thigh, upper arm and anterior thorax to stimulate regional lymph node groups. Oncolysate injections were given every two weeks for three months. Thereafter, I ml doses were given every month until recurrence.

Skin Tests for Delayed Hypersensitivity

The following skin tests were performed: dermatophytin, candida, mumps and tuberculin-PPD. All skin tests were injected intracutaneously and readings were made daily for three days. Also, testing was done with 1-chloro, 2, 4-dinitrobenzene (DNCB) which followed closely the method of Blewmink.[8]

Selection of Patients

The following cancer patients were selected for treatment with the vaccinia oncolysate in the Phase I study:

1. Cancer patients who had tumor resection and showed overwhelming metastasis to regional lymph nodes.
2. Patients with disseminated disease who were treated previously by chemotherapy or immunotherapy but were considered to have progressive disease.
3. Patients with disease so far advanced that they were declared untreatable by surgery, radiotherapy or chemotherapy.

All patients involved in these trials gave informed consent and showed a delayed hypersensitivity response to one or more common recall antigen skin tests used to gauge immunocompetence. All patients were prevaccinated with vaccinia vaccine one week prior to receiving the immunotherapy. Lastly, an essential requirement was that cells from the tumor could be surgically obtained and grown in suspension tissue cultures so that autochthonous vaccines can be prepared.

Results

A total of 29 patients received the vaccinia oncolysate immunotherapy in the Phase I trial. These patients represent 10 cases of melanoma, nine cases of colon carcinoma, two cases of gastric carcinoma, one case of cervical carcinoma, one case of lung carcinoma, one case of hepatoma, one case of fibrosarcoma, one case of ovarian carcinoma, one case of renal carcinoma, one case of breast carcinoma and one case of thyroid carcinoma.

Side effects of the immunotherapy were minimal except for pain and inflammation at the injection sites which seemed to correlate well with the host's response to the tumor burden (Table 1).

Patient response to the vaccinia oncolysate immunotherapy was as follows:

1. 0/29 patients with generalized vaccinia, allergy, anaphylaxis, tumor growth at injection site.
2. 20/29 patients have died.
3. 9/29 patients died in early part of study.
4. 15/29 patients had delayed hypersensitivity reactions at the vaccine injection sites.
5. 9/15 patients who had delayed hypersensitivity reactions at the vaccine injection sites remain alive with marked control of tumor growth.
6. 9/9 patients with control of tumor growth had elevated vaccinia antibody titers.

The nine patients who seem to have responded to the vaccine are summarized in Table 2. The majority of the patients in this Phase I study had either malignant melanoma or colon carcinoma. Tables 3 and 4 summarize the results from these two groups of patients and show three responders in the melanoma group and three responders in the colon group.

Discussion

The first hints that viral invasion of a tumor might lead to the development of anti-tumor immunity were provided by the work of Sharpless et al.[9] on a transplantable lymphoid tumor of chickens, and more clearly by

Table 1. Side Effects of Vaccinia Oncolysates

Side Effects	Percent of Patients Intradermal
Fever	20
Chills	7
Shaking	2
Malaise	7
Headache	5
Nausea	7
Vomiting	0
Increased blood pressure	0
Decreased blood pressure	0
Diarrhea	0
Pain at site of injection	45
Inflammation at site of injection	65

Table 2. Nine Responders to Vaccinia Oncolysate Immunotherapy

Name	Age/Sex	Tumor	Clinical Condition	Previous Therapy	No. of Injections	Results	Survival in Months from Time of First Injection
RS	46/M	Thyroid (Undiff.)	Liver and neck mets	R[a]	16	Regression	28
VV	47/M	Renal Carcinoma	Plus nodes plus lumbar spine mets	S	24	Stable	24
EO	51/M	Melanoma	Recurrent Stage II	S	12	Stable	20
JN	53/M	Colon	Dukes' C plus Liver mets	S	16	Stable	20
EK	61/F	Melanoma	Recurrent Stage II	S	20	Stable	20
EN	68/F	Colon	Dukes' C, plus nodes plus vessels	S	12	Stable	17
VS	59/F	Breast	Plus nodes plus Liver mets	S	14	Stable	18
WM	71/M	Colon	Dukes' C, plus Liver mets	S	16	Stable	17
MM	53/M	Melanoma	Recurrent Stage II	S and C	14	Stable	12

[a] S = surgery; C = chemotherapy; R = radiation; Mets = metastasis.

Table 3. Treatment of Ten Advanced Melanoma Patients with Vaccinia Oncolysates (U.S. Trials)

Name	Age/Sex	Tumor	Stage	Previous Therapy	No. of Injections	Results	Survival in Months from Time of First Injection
EK	61/F	Melanoma	Recurrent Stage II	S[a]	20	Stable	18
EO	51/M	Melanoma	Recurrent Stage II	S and C	18	Stable	18
MM	53/M	Melanoma	Recurrent Stage II	S	12	Stable	10
Nonresponders:							
RC	55/F	Melanoma	Stage III	S and C	10	Progress	11
GJ	49/M	Melanoma	Recurrent Stage II	S and C	8	Progress	6
EH	56/M	Melanoma	Stage III	C and I	5	Progress	3
PS	62/M	Melanoma	Recurrent Stage II	S and C	7	Progress	6
MS	55/M	Melanoma	Recurrent Stage II	S and C	3	Progress	3
FA	52/M	Melanoma	Recurrent Stage II	S	5	Progress	3
MG	56/F	Melanoma	Stage III	S and R	3	Progress	3

[a] S = surgery; C = chemotherapy; R = radiation; I = immunotherapy.

Table 4. Treatment of Nine Advanced Colon Cancer Patients with Vaccinia Oncolysates

Name	Age/Sex	Disease/Stage	Previous Therapy	No. of Injections	Results	Survival in Months from Time of First Injection
WM	71/M	Colon C plus Liver	S[a]	18	Stable	17
EN	68/F	Colon C plus Peritoneum	S	19	Stable	17
JN	53/M	Colon C plus Liver	S	15	Stable	19
Nonresponders:						
DJ	46/F	Colon C plus Liver, Lung	S	6	Progression	4
FM	56/F	Colon C plus Lung	S	3	Progression	1
JM	39/F	Colon C plus Abdominal Wall	S	3	Progression	10
MP	51/F	Colon C plus Liver	S and C	1	Progression	1
MS	52/F	Colon C plus Peritoneum	S	5	Progression	1
MT	73/F	Colon C plus Lung, Liver	S	6	Progression	1

[a] S = surgery; C = chemotherapy.

that of Koprowski et al.[5] on oncolysis of tumors in mice genetically resistant to the lethal action of the oncolytic virus used. These researchers demonstrated that animals which recovered from a tumor after West Nile viral infection were able to resist subsequent challenges with same tumor. Utilization of murine strains genetically resistant to a particular virus provided an opportunity to study viral oncolysis without killing the host and was subsequently employed by Lindenmann[10] who used a mouse-adapted strain of neurotropic influenza-A virus against Ehrlich ascites tumor growing in A_2G mice. In his early experiments Lindenmann used virus fully adapted to the Ehrlich ascites tumor; the influenza was inoculated into a 7–8 day ascites and within 48–72 hours oncolysis occurred; animals that showed definite tumor collapse were sacrificed, their solidified tumor masses removed, homogenized, frozen and thawed. This viral oncolysate which was initiated *in vivo* was used to immunize intraperitoneally A_2G mice; these animals were subsequently able to resist a challenge with 100 LD50 of Ehrlich ascites seven days later, while control animals immunized with uninfected mechanical lysate of Ehrlich ascites cells were unable to survive.[11] From these experiments, post viral oncolytic immunity was explained as a viral adjuvant effect induced by the interaction of virus-specific and host cell-specific determinants, a situation analogous to a carrier-hapten system.[12]

The viruses employed in the preceding studies were considered to be pathogenic and reservations were in order regarding their employment in human studies. As a result, we tested *in vitro* six live viral vaccines (measles, mumps, smallpox, rubella, yellow fever, rabies) against four human tumor lines (ovary, lung, melanoma, colon); only the smallpox (vaccinia) vaccine duplicated the lytic action of the influenza virus on the Ehrlich ascites cells.[7] Moreover, and even more important, this virus (a viral vaccine) would be safe to use in humans.

The vaccinia oncolysate was first tested in an SV40 transformed BALB/c male mouse peritoneal macrophage tumor system. These immunoprophylaxis experiments confirmed both the safety and potential efficacy of the vaccine in the animal model. There was no vaccine-associated mouse deaths; furthermore, tumors failed to grow in animals pretreated with the vaccinia oncolysate.[13]

Because of the encouraging results in the murine tumor system, the vaccine was evaluated as an immunotherapeutic in Phase I trials in human cancer. All patients involved in this study had advanced disease, but showed delayed hypersensitivity reactions to one or more common recall antigen skin tests and had tumors that could be safely incised in the operating room. The Phase I trials have been concluded. These trials have shown the vaccine to be safe, nontoxic and potentially effective in stimulating the patient's tumor immune response. The heterogeneity of this early tumor group only reflects the type of patient available during the early phase of testing vaccine safety. Obviously, positive responses to the vaccine in certain of these patients were interesting but difficult to evaluate. With completion of the Phase I trials, randomized prospective trials have begun in a more homogeneous tumor group so as to make analysis easier.

Lastly, one may conclude that a budding virus such as influenza or Newcastle Disease Virus would be more promising for generating cell-mediated tumor immunity (CTL) than a nonbudding virus such as vaccinia. However, experimental evidence that bears directly on the use of vaccinia virus for the generation of cytotoxic T lymphocytes has been forthcoming; Zinkernagel et al.[14] demonstrated in 1977 that CTLs with dual specificity for vaccinia and H-2 were generated after vaccinia infection. More recently, Hapel et al.[15] have presented evidence that vaccinia virus generates potent CTL responses in mice, even when UV irradiated, noninfectious virus was used. It is unclear from their data whether the virus is adsorbed to the cells or whether it enters the cells and initiates an abortive cycle of replication. The point is that the choice of vaccinia virus for the generation of viral oncolysis may be in fact very promising even if we don't understand at present the mechanism of action. Finally, Chang and Metz[16] have reported that vaccinia virus entered HeLa cells by a process of direct fusion between the virus envelope and the plasma membrane of the cell. After fusion, components of the virus envelope become rapidly dispersed in the plasma membrane producing the juxtaposition of a strong viral antigen with a weak tumor antigen, which could produce an increase in the immunogenicity of the tumor antigen.

Conclusion

A live vaccinia vaccine virus-augmented tumor cell vaccine (vaccinia oncolysate) is used as a specific active immune mechanism stimulator against certain advanced human cancers. The Phase I trials in 29 patients have shown the vaccine to be safe, nontoxic and potentially effective. The heterogeneity of this early tumor group only reflects the type of patient available to the study during the early phase of vaccine testing. Randomized, prospective trials have begun in a more homogeneous tumor group so as to make analysis easier.

References

1. Hersh, EM, Gutterman, JV, Mavligit, GM: Immunotherapy of human cancer. *Adv. Int. Med.* 22:145–185, 1976.
2. Prager, MD: Specific cancer immunotherapy. *Cancer Immunol. Immunother.* 3:157–161, 1978.
3. Currie, G: Cancer and the immune response. In: Turk, J, ed. Yearbook Medical Publishers Inc., Chicago, p. 75, 1975.

4. Czajkowski, NP, Rosenblatt, M, Wolf, PL, Vasquez, J: A new method of active immunization to autologous human tumor tissues. *Lancet* ii: 905, 1967.

5. Koprowski, H, Love, R, Koprowska, I: Enhancement of susceptibility to viruses in neoplastic tissues. *Tex. Rep. Biol. Med.* 15:559–576, 1957.

6. Lindenmann, J, Klein, PA: Immunological aspects of viral oncolysis. *Rec. Res. Cancer Res.* 9:1–84, 1967.

7. Wallack MK, Steplewski, Z, Koprowski, H et al.: A new approach in specific, active immunotherapy. *Cancer* 39:560–564, 1977.

8. Blewmink, E, Nater, JP, Koops, HS, The, TH: A standard method for DNCB sensitization testing in patients with neoplasms. *Cancer* 33:911–915, 1974.

9. Sharpless, GR, Davies, MC, Cox, HR: Antagonistic action of certain neurotropic viruses toward a lymphoid tumor in chickens with resulting immunity. *Proc. Soc. Exp. Biol. Med.* 73:270, 1950.

10. Lindenmann, J: Resistance of mice to mouse adapted influenza-A virus. *Virology* 16:203, 1962.

11. Lindenmann, J, Klein, P: Viral oncolysis: increased immunogenicity of host cell antigen associated with influenza virus. *J. Exp. Med.* 126:93, 1967.

12. Lindenmann, J: Viruses as immunological adjuvants in cancer. *Biochemica et Biophysica Acta.* 355:79, 1974.

13. Wallack, M: Vaccinia virus-augmented tumor vaccines as a new form of immunotherapy. *Gann. Mono. on Ca. Res.* 23:273, 1979.

14. Zinkernagel, RM, Athage, A: Antiviral protection by virus-immune cytotoxic T cells: infected target cells are lysed before infectious progeny is assembled. *J. Exp. Med.* 145:644, 1977.

15. Hapel, AJ, Bablanian, R, Cole, GA: Inductive requirements for the generation of virus-specific T lymphocytes. I. The nature of the host cell-virus interaction that triggers secondary pox virus-specific cytotoxic T lymphocyte induction. *J. Immunol.* 121:736, 1978.

16. Chang, A, Metz, DH: Further investigations on the mode of entry of vaccinia virus into cells. *J. Gen. Virol.* 32:275, 1976.

Immunotherapy of Advanced Disease

A. Hollinshead, T. Stewart, R. Yonemoto, M. Arlen, H. Takita

Department of Medicine, Division of Hematology and Oncology, The George Washington University Medical Center, Washington, D.C.; Department of Medicine, Ottawa General Hospital, The Ottawa University Medical Center, Ottawa, Canada; Department of Surgery, City of Hope National Medical Center, Duarte, California; Department of Surgical Oncology, Brookdale Hospital Medical Center, New York; Department of Surgery, Roswell Park Memorial Institute Medical Center, Buffalo, New York

Summary

The selection of the most effective cancer therapeutic modalities for patients with advanced disease includes considerations as to whether or not surgery might be considered useful for reducing or debulking the amount of tumor present, and whether it might be helpful to use chemotherapy before surgery. These considerations are based upon whether or not such procedures might make it possible to have more effective treatment using selected combinations which may or may not include radiotherapy, chemotherapy or immunotherapy in combined modality post-surgical treatment.

Immunopharmacologic studies of the interreactions between chemical drugs and biological drugs permit additional information which may be useful in the rational selections of multimodality therapy. Three examples of the way in which chemical drugs interreact with suppressor substances, lymphokines, tumor associated antigens and other biological agents will be described.

Cooperative pilot studies of the effects of various combinations of immunotherapy, chemotherapy and surgical debulking in 39 patients with recurrent melanoma and 20 lung cancer patients will be discussed.

Discussion

The first therapeutic human trial which uses separated human tumor antigens has entered its sixth year. This trial involves the use of human lung cancer cell antigens selected for their association with the different histologic forms of lung cancer and used for specific active therapeutic studies of patients with early stage cancer.[1] As shown in Figure 1, the usefulness of these biological drugs was suggested, and in Figure 2 the analyses now possible up through five years, indicate that this form of therapy will be a useful addition to multi modality treatment. Theoretically, TAA would be best used for immunoprophylaxis in individuals at high risk for a particular form of cancer,[2] or, as shown in the aforementioned trial, in the treatment of patients with a minimal tumor burden. The experience with these biologic drugs in a single center is being repeated (Table 1) by another group[3] with the addition of an adjuvant arm. This permitted two single institution studies prior to a multicenter trial with larger numbers of patients. Although it is too early to assess the second trial, it may be seen (Table 1) that the results at 20 months parallel the experience in the earlier trial. The multicenter trial was undertaken starting in June 1978, with 80 patients accrued, in which 300 lung cancer patients will be tested in a three-arm, randomized trial by many cancer centers in order to see whether or not the multicenter study will repeat the experience of the two centers conducting specific active immunotherapy trials.

No one considered the use of such biologic drugs in patients with

Figure 1. (Courtesy of Springer-Verlag)

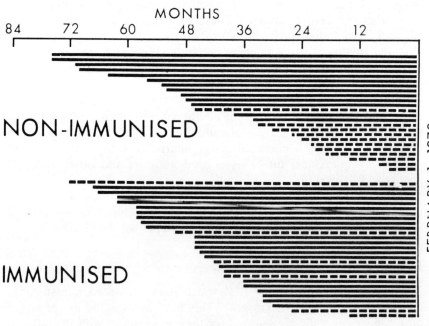

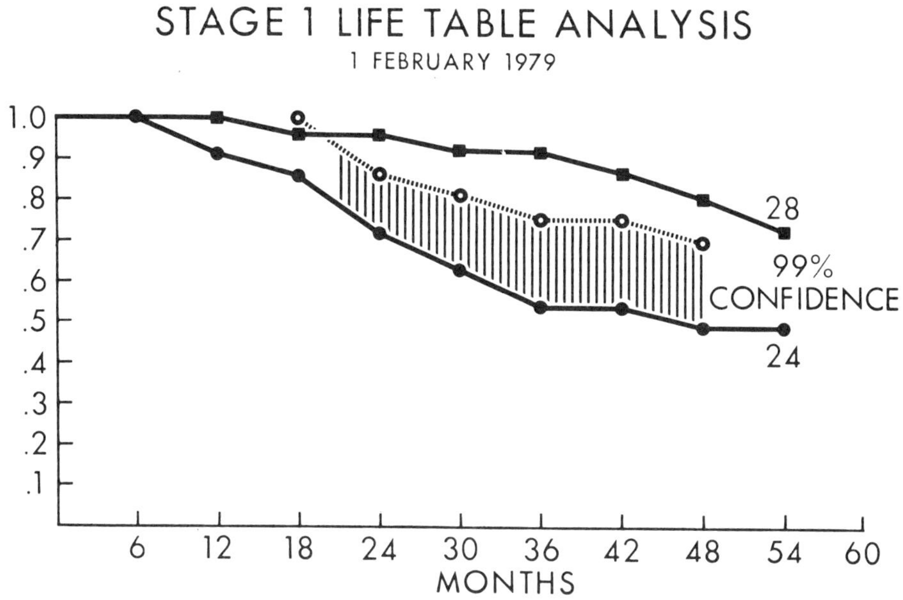

STAGE 1 LIFE TABLE ANALYSIS
1 FEBRUARY 1979

Figure 2. Stage 1 life table analysis. (Courtesy of Springer-Verlag)

metastatic disease, and our experience has been that, for the most part, in the presence of disseminated or bulk tumor, this form of treatment would be highly inadequate. Indeed, our experience in the treatment of a small number of later-stage lung cancer patients was negative.[4] For the past three years we have worked with three surgeons, conducting pilot studies, in order to determine whether or not different combinations of chemotherapy, surgery and chemoimmunotherapy might be useful in the treatment of patients with late stage malignant melanoma and with late stage lung cancer. These two forms of cancer are totally different and diverse and demand very different approaches.

The course of melanoma is highly unpredictable and it is difficult to appoint the time of recurrence after resection of Stage I lesions. Unfortunately, when recurrence is seen, the clinical course of these patients is usually short-lived and this permits a fairly rapid assessment. We therefore chose to work with Stage III recurrent, metastatic malignant melanoma patients in order to compare the effects of chemotherapy alone, immunotherapy alone and immunochemotherapy. These procedures followed aggressive surgical/debulking. The experience of Robert Yonemoto[5] at the one-year level for 13 patients with recurrent melanoma shows that there was no benefit for two of four patients on immunotherapy, four of five patients on chemoimmunotherapy and three of four patients on chemotherapy. However, only three of the 13 patients had

Table 1. Roswell Park Memorial Institute Study

Squamous Cell Carcinoma:

Phase II specific active immunotherapy trial, ongoing:

> Control arm: 21 patients: 4 dead, 1 recurr. (5,7,8,19 and 20 mo)
> TAA + FcA arm: 17 patients: 1 recurr. (13 mo responded to chemo.)
> FcA arm: 20 patients: 1 dead (15 mo)

Adenocarcinoma:

Phase II specific active immunotherapy trial, ongoing:

> Control arm: 6 patients: 1 dead
> TAA + FcA arm: 7 patients: 1 dead
> FcA arm: 4 patients: 1 dead

Comparison of Ottawa and RPMI Data at Twenty Months:

> RPMI: Adenocarcinoma + squamous cell carcinoma: 75 patients[a] stages
> 1 and 2: Control: 5 dead 1 recurrence
>   Immuno. 1 dead 1 recurrence
>
> Ottawa: real data at 20 months of 6 year trial: 52 patients[a] stage
>   1: Control: 5 dead 2 recurrences
>   Immuno.: 1 dead 2 recurrences

[a] RPMI trial: patients' skin tested with 100 μg TAA eleven times and Ottawa trial: patients' skin tested with 100 μg TAA three times before and during therapy. Different lots of TAA used both for skin testing and therapy in the two institutes.

debulking: two are alive, free of disease at 12 and 13 months. During the pilot studies with Myron Arlen, we found the use of DTIC in combination with TAA gave the best results. DTIC has a special biologic effect which has been described elsewhere.[6,7] This drug induces a reduction of the amount of inhibitory nonspecific antigen antibody complexes in the blood stream for a period of up to three days after chemotherapy. Therefore, if one combines the use of melanoma TAA introduced during this three-day period, the effectiveness of the biological drug and access to the tumor is greater since these complexes may be prevented from blocking the distribution of TAA.

When Arlen started treating patients with melanoma, he chose those with terminal disease. At that time we were using fairly crude extracts. Some of these patients exhibited regression of nodal disease; however, within a short period of time disease returned. TAA were used alone and we did not have enough antigen for repeated injection to maintain humoral levels.

Since then 26 patients have been placed on a protocol combining antigen (TAA) and chemotherapy (DTIC) for the aforementioned reasons. Three patients were treated initially with TAA alone, but were reimmunized after one week of IV DTIC (200 mg/day) followed by 500 μg TAA homogenized with 0.25 ml complete Freund's adjuvant. This regimen was repeated monthly over a three-month period. Six of the 26 patients so treated displayed total regression of clinical disease over a period of one to three years. Six additional patients showed greater than a 50 percent regression in tumor size for a six-month to a two-year period. Their course was characterized by a sense of well-being not present prior to the initiation of therapy. These responses were felt to be consistent with an enhancement in immune reactivity which resulted from the specificity of this form of immunotherapy.

The first patient treated using the above protocol was a 33-year old female presenting with bulky visceral disease secondary to metastatic melanoma arising from the back. She was given TAA without adjuvant or chemotherapy. This failed to alter her clinical condition so she was explored in an attempt to debulk tumor. Large areas of tumor were resected, with diffuse areas of involvement being left. She was given three monthly courses of TAA and FcA and DTIC starting one-week post surgery. Her postoperative course was characterized by a feeling of well-being and during the next three months she gained 30 pounds. Within six months she had increased her weight by 60 pounds above her presurgical weight. Shortly thereafter she became septic. Work-up revealed an abscess in the region of the splenic flexure. Reexploration showed the peritoneal cavity virtually free of disease. A necrotic tumor mass near the splenic flexure had caused perforation of bowel. Despite resection of the area of involvement, her clinical course deteriorated and resulted in expiration from uncontrolled sepsis.

A long-standing survivor in the present series was seen in June 1975 for bulky paraspinal metastasis from melanoma of the shoulder treated one year previously. The tumor was debulked without free margins of resection. TAA was given alone (800 μg) monthly for four doses. One year following surgery, a coin lesion was noted in the right lower lung field consistent with metastatic melanoma (Figure 3). This failed to respond to TAA or DTIC alone. The combination of agents with FcA homogenized with TAA produced prompt, complete regression (Figure 4). One year later, there was suspicion of reappearance of the lung lesion. Repeat immunization resulted in clearing the lung field. In February 1979 reappearance of tumor was again noted in the same region of the right lung (Figure 5). This region was resected to obtain histologic evaluation. The tumor proved to be metastatic melanoma. No other foci of disease have appeared and the patient remains free of disease.

Twelve of the 26 patients were initially placed on DTIC or a combination of chemotherapy with BCG. No tumor regression was seen among any patient so treated. These 12 patients were then crossed over to the protocol of immunochemotherapy in spite of the failure to respond

294

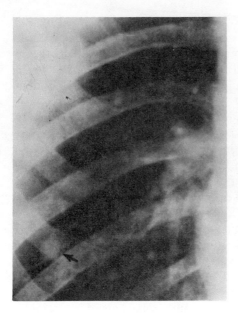

Figure 3. R.L. 6/76—One yr after resection of back primary melanoma; arrow indicates coin lesion.

Figure 4. R.L. 8/76—Repeat film one mo after immunochemotherapy shows complete regression of coin lesion.

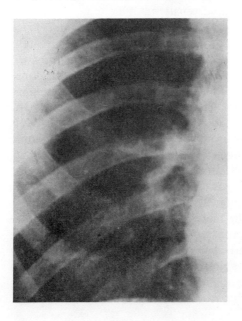

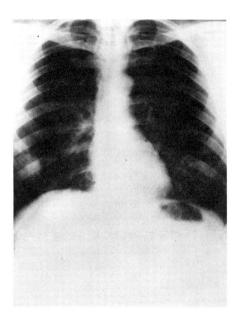

Figure 5. R.L. 2/79—Repeat chest film nearly 3 yr following regression of nodule shows tumor at site of original metastasis. Resection proved it to be metastatic melanoma.

initially to DTIC. Four of these patients were among the six who showed complete tumor regression. Two of these patients remain alive, but with disease. Six expired within two to four months of TAA therapy from tumor involving liver or the CNS.

The information obtained to date suggests that: disseminated metastasis involving liver, bone marrow (diffuse) and CNS precludes response probably caused part by overwhelming immune suppression; debulking tumor enhances immune reactivity; the immune response can destroy tumor burden in excess of 10^9 cells; combination therapy including chemotherapy and immunotherapy is more effective than immunotherapy alone; reimmunization at yearly intervals may be necessary; and escaping populations of tumor cells may be unresponsive to immunotherapy because of varying antigenic composition necessitating polyvalent TAA in Stage III disease.

The concept that therapy with biologic drugs will be useful in the treatment of patients with disseminated melanoma must be studied in great detail. We do not know optimal doses and whether pretreatment of the surgical patient with earlier stages of disease will be of benefit. In short, further studies must be engineered and designed for future clinical trials.

Hiroshi Takita has used the combined modality approach in order to see whether or not the treatment of patients with inoperable lung carcinomas might result in longer survival.[8,9] He selected 20 patients with inoperable lung carcinoma who responded to combination chemotherapy which included the use of cis-diamminedichloroplatinum, for a series of from two to 12 courses in a period of two to 16 months, with a mean of three courses of chemotherapy for a mean of 3.9 months. Two of the patients received localized radiation therapy for bone metastases and one patient had radiation therapy for brain metastasis and subsequent craniotomy to remove a solitary brain metastasis.

The study[8,9] consisted of 17 males and three females, from 43 years of age to 61 years of age. Eight patients had squamous cell carcinoma, seven had adenocarcinoma, two bronchioalveolar, two large-cell and one mixed adeno-squamous cell cancer. Eleven of these patients had disease limited to the hemithorax and nine patients had distant metastases. Six patients had previous thoracotomy in attempt for lung resection but were proven to be inoperable.

All of these patients underwent lung resection to remove all visible evidence of tumor (in two cases gross tumor was left behind). Nine of the patients had pneumonectomies, 10 patients lobectomies and one had local excision of bilateral lung lesions by median sternotomy.

Postoperatively, the patients received three more doses of chemotherapy, alternating appropriately with lung TAA therapy. It was necessary to allow the appropriate intervals, since the combination chemotherapy caused immunosuppression, and appropriate timing for the use of the biologic drugs allowed a better effect.

The result of this study[8,9] is of interest. There were two postoperative deaths. Two additional patients died six and eight months, respectively, postoperatively because of cardiac disease. In all four patients, autopsy failed to show evidence of carcinoma. The remaining 16 patients are alive from four to 28 months from onset of chemotherapy and one to 22 months postoperatively (one with recurrent disease). Survival distributions from onset of chemotherapy and from surgery were calculated using actuarial life table analysis, and median survival from chemotherapy was estimated to be 35 months and postoperatively 21.7 months.

Two of these cases may be of interest. A 52-year old man had a left thoracotomy in April 1977. The operative report described a "tumor 6 cm in diameter invading the wall of the descending thoracic aorta over a 5–6 cm length. The mass was invading the pericardium and the left atrium. In addition, it was extensively adherent to the esophageal muscle." He was referred to Takita in May 1977 and received two courses of chemotherapy which consisted of a combination of cis platinum, Adriamycin and vincristine; the lesion was no longer visible in the chest X-ray (Figure 6). On July 13, 1977, a repeat left thoracotomy

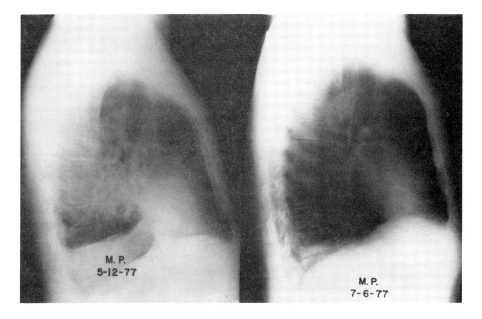

Figure 6. M.P. 52-yr lung cancer, advanced disease. **Left:** Lateral roentgenogram showing large lesion, lower lobe. **Right:** After two courses chemotherapy, lesion not visible. (Courtesy of *Ann. Thoracic Surgery.*)

and pneumonectomy was performed (Figure 7). The tumor then measured 2 cm in diameter adherent to the pericardium, but was free from the aorta, esophagus and atrium. Postoperatively, this patient received three courses of appropriately timed chemoimmunotherapy. The biologic drug used was lung TAA. This patient is doing well without recurrence.

A second case was a 53-year old man found to have bilateral lung lesions following hemoptysis. Bronchoscopy revealed a lesion of the superior segment, right lower lobe and blood at the orifice of the left upper lobe. Cytology was positive for squamous cell carcinoma from right bronchial washings. After three courses of chemotherapy with a combination of five drugs, including DDP, a repeat bronchoscopy, chest X-ray and tomogram showed a complete disappearance of the right lung lesion (Figure 8). He underwent a left upper lobectomy for squamous cell carcinoma. Postoperatively, the patient received three more doses of chemotherapy alternated with lung TAA. The patient is doing well without recurrence at present. Takita concludes that combination chemotherapy alone is probably not effective against a neoplasm which consists of heterogeneous cell populations and that combination chemotherapy would not be effective enough to destroy all of the neoplastic cells. However combination chemotherapy used in conjunction with

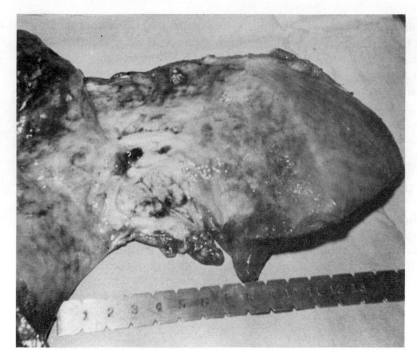

Figure 7. M.P. (see Figure 6) resected left lung with residual tumor measuring approximately 2 cm diameter. (Courtesy of *Ann. Thoracic Surgery.*)

appropriate lung resection and followed by the use of chemical drugs and biologic drugs in appropriate combination may be helpful in many cases.

In conclusion, these anecdotal cases do not in any way suggest that the use of combined modality pre- and post-surgical treatment is effective in the treatment of advanced disease. We would suggest, however, that these studies do indicate that a negative conclusion would be premature. We suggest that these studies have made it possible to conclude that use of biologic drugs in future multimodality treatment of advanced cancers is *an open question.*

In our early studies of the treatment of patients with Stage 1 lung cancer, we noted that the use of methotrexate in 1 arm of the study was ineffective. However, the biologic responses to this drug were of interest. Methotrexate induced a rebound overshoot phenomenon, which peaked at approximately seven days after initiation of drug treatment.[1,4] If, at this point, the biologic drug, lung TAA, were introduced, we noted a striking increase over the months that followed, in the parameters which measure cell-mediated immune response. Although at this time, patients on immunotherapy are doing as well as patients on immunochemotherapy, these parameters indicate that the patients may possibly live longer. We have mentioned also that the use of DTIC in the treatment of patients with advanced melanoma produced a three-day period when the blood stream was much more free of nonspecific, immunosuppressive immune complexes.[6,7] Thus, DTIC might well be effective as a biologic response modifier for use in combination with melanoma TAA therapy. The two drugs act in ways totally different upon the immune system. We recently have described the chemical nature of certain suppressor materials which exist on the surface of tumor cells. These suppressors are DNA nucleoproteins which exist in patches or lines along the surface of the tumor cell.[2] *In vitro,* we have shown that ovarian cancer cells grown in tissue culture can be treated with cis platinum, which strips away these DNA nucleoprotein patches. However, after washing and regrowing the cells, the suppressors reappear after a period of time. We have described the existence of these suppressor substances on several types of tumor cells, including lung cancer cells. It is possible that the cis platinum base treatment used by Takita is useful in stripping away these suppressor or inhibitory DNA nucleoprotein patches off the tumor cells which permits

Figure 8. J.S. 53-yr lung cancer, advanced disease. **Left:** Chest roentgenogram of left upper and right lower chest lesions. **Right:** After three courses of chemotherapy, the right lower lobe lesion is not visible. (Courtesy of *Ann. Thoracic Surgery.*)

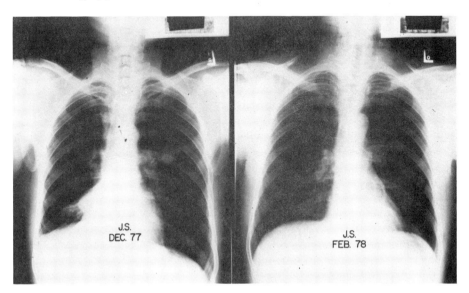

greater accessibility to the effects of the biologic drugs. The immuno-pharmacology of several other drugs are now under study, with a view to providing further insight as to the interreactions between chemical drugs and biologic drugs.

References

1. Stewart, THM, Hollinshead, AC, Harris, JE et al.: Specific active immunochemotherapy in lung cancer: a survival study. In: *Proceedings EORTIC Plenary Session on Adjuvant Therapies and Markers of Post-surgical, Minimal Disease*, Springer Verlag, Paris, *(in press).*

2. Hollinshead, A, Stewart, THM: Specific active immunotherapy and specific active immunoprophylaxis in lung cancer. In: *Symposia, XII International Cancer Congress,* Pergamon Press, Ltd., Buenos Aires, 1978.

3. Hollinshead, A, Stewart, THM, Takita, H: Phase II trials of specific active immuno-therapy for lung cancer patients. *Proceedings of American Society of Clinical Oncology* C-76:325, 1978.

4. Stewart THM, Hollinshead, AC, Harris, JE et al.: A survival study of specific active immunochemotherapy in lung cancer. In Crispen, RG, ed. *Neoplasm Immunity: Solid Tumor Therapy,* pp. 37–48, Franklin Institute Press, Philadelphia, 1977.

5. Yonemoto, R et al.: Personal communication, 1979.

6. Arlen, M, Hollinshead, A: Tumor specific immune stimulation in patients with recurrent malignant melanoma. 30th annual meeting of the Society of Surgical Oncology, Inc., 1977.

7. Hollinshead, AC: Active specific immunotherapy. In: *Immunotherapy of Human Cancer,* pp. 213–233, Raven Press, New York, 1978.

8. Takita, H, Hollinshead, AC, Bjornsson, S: Chemotherapy, surgery and immunotherapy of inoperable lung cancer. In: Weinhouse, S, ed. *Proceedings of the American Society of Clinical Oncology,* Vol. 19, Abstract C-50, p. 319, Waverly Press, Inc., Maryland.

9. Takita, H, Hollinshead, A, Rizzo, D et al.: Treatment of inoperable lung carcinoma: a combined modality approach. *Ann. Thoracic Surgery* (in press).

Immunotherapy of Human Malignancies with Immune RNA

Kenneth P. Ramming, Jean B. deKernion

Department of Surgery, Division of Oncology, UCLA School of Medicine, Los Angeles, California; Tulane University School of Medicine, New Orleans, Louisiana

Summary

RNA preparations extracted from lymphoid organs of animals immunized with specific antigens can mediate immune responses in lymphoid cells not exposed to that antigen but incubated with immune RNA. Transfer of immunity to tumor specific antigens has been demonstrated in animals by autologous and xenogeneic RNA (RNA derived by immunization of a species different from that of the tumor origin) both by sensitization of autologous lymphocytes and by direct injection of immune RNA. In humans, more than 100 patients with advanced malignant melanoma, colon carcinoma and hypernephroma have been treated with immune RNA. There is some evidence of increased cellular immune responses in patients receiving immune RNA injections, but little impact on survival with the exception of hypernephroma. Survival was significantly greater in RNA treated hypernephroma patients who had multiple metastases limited to the lungs when compared with matched untreated controls. RNA therapy did not influence survival of hypernephroma patients with metastases to other sites. A randomized, prospective, postsurgical, adjuvant therapy trial of immune RNA in patients at high risk to develop recurrent hypernephroma is current.

Introduction

The mediation of immune reactions by lymphoid ribonucleic acid has been accomplished in a variety of animal systems since first described as an *in vitro* experiment by Fishman and Adler in 1961.[1] Common to most of these experimental models has been an extraction of RNA from the lymphoid tissues of specifically immunized donors, an intimate association of nonimmune lymphoid cells with the immune RNA, usually by incubation, and the subsequent demonstration of immune response in the RNA-treated cells identical to that which had been induced in the RNA donor.

The term "immune RNA" (I-RNA) refers to RNA-rich extracts of immune lymphoid cells. The initial interest in immune RNA was stimulated by the observation that RNA extracted from lymphoid cells which had been exposed to specific antigens *in vitro,* or extracted from lymphoid tissues of animals immunized *in vivo,* could convert normal, nonimmune lymphoid cells to specific immunologic activity.[2] As demonstrated in various systems, accelerated rejection of skin allografts *in vivo*[3] and specific immune cytolysis of target cells *in vitro*[4] mediated by RNA from specifically sensitized donors confirm the mediation of immune responses to histocompatability antigens by tbe immune RNA.

Alexander et al.[5] reported the induction of anti-tumor immunity with RNA. They administered I-RNA extracted from lymphoid cells of sheep which had been immunized against primary benzpyrene-induced rat sarcomas to sarcoma-bearing rats. This treatment often inhibited the growth of the specific sarcoma used to immunize the RNA donor and occasionally resulted in regression of growing tumors.[6] Other observations confirmed that this xenogeneic immune RNA was capable of mediating immune responses against other chemically-induced tumors. Ramming and Pilch[7] immunized guinea pigs with a benzpyrene-induced sarcoma grown in C3H mice, after which RNA was extracted from the guinea pig lymphoid tissues. Spleen cells from normal, nonimmune C3H mice were incubated with the guinea pig I-RNA *in vitro* and then injected intraperitoneally into normal, syngeneic C3H mice. These immunized animals rejected transplants of the same tumor which had been used to immunize the guinea pigs. The reaction seemed to be specific, since RNA preparations extracted from lymphoid organs of guinea pigs immunized with normal mouse tissues or with Freund's adjuvant or with other benzpyrene-induced sarcomas did not affect growth of the tumor transplants. The activity of the I-RNA was abolished by pretreatment with ribonuclease, which indicated that the active moeity was one or more species of RNA. Numerous other studies with a number of different tumors in several rodent species have confirmed the induction of specific tumor immunity *in vivo* by syngeneic, allogeneic, or xenogeneic immune RNA preparations, either by the administration of syngeneic lymphocytes incubated with I-RNA *in vitro,* of by the direct systemic administration of I-RNA.[8]

Immune cytolysis of tumor cells *in vitro* mediated by immune RNA was then demonstrated by Ramming and Pilch in a totally syngeneic animal system.[9] Normal syngeneic spleen cells preincubated with syngeneic I-RNA extracted from spleens of inbred Strain 2 guinea pigs, which had been immunized by excision of growing tumor transplants, produced areas of cytolysis in a monolayer of the same tumor cells. This suggested that the immune response was directed against tumor-associated antigens. In another syngeneic system, Kern et al., using a quantitative microcytotoxicity assay, reported the mediation of immune cytolysis of cells from a methylcholanthrene-induced sarcoma of Fischer 344/N rats by syngeneic lymphocytes preincubated with syngeneic I-RNA extracted from spleens of Fischer rats bearing growing transplants of the same tumor.[10] Kern et al. later described the *in vitro* lysis of human tumor cells by normal human autologous and/or allogeneic lymphoid cells incubated with RNA extracted from xenogeneic donors.[11]

The mediation of cellular immune responses to human tumor-associated antigens *in vitro* by immune RNA extracted from the lymphoid organs of immunized animals provided a logical basis for the immunotherapy of cancer with xenogeneic immune RNA. Xenogeneic immune RNA offers several theoretical advantages over other methods of immunotherapy. First, large quantities of immune RNA can be produced for relatively inexpensive and plentiful animals, without dependence on human donors. Secondly, since histological similar human tumors may share common, group-specific tumor-associated antigens, many patients with the same tumor type could be treated with immune RNA from an animal immunized with a single patient's tumor. Finally, RNA appeared to cause insignificant local or systemic toxic reactions in treated animals.

Materials and Methods

Preparation and Purification of RNA

Xenogeneic RNA was prepared from spleen and lymphoid tissues excised from sheep which had been immunized with human tumors. Sheep were chosen since they are a convenient size and since they harbor no known oncogenic viruses. When possible, tumor from the patient to be treated was used to immunize the animal. After four weekly injections of a fixed suspension of human renal carcinoma cells with an equal volume of complete Freund's adjuvant, the animals were sacrificed and lymph nodes were removed and quick-frozen in dry ice. After extraction of RNA by a hot phenol method,[13] the RNA was purified by precipitation with potassium acetate and treated with pronase to remove protein contaminants. It was then dialyzed against sterile distilled water and sterilized by passage through 0.22 mc filters.

Sterility was determined by fungal and bacterial cultures. No preparations were found to be contaminated. Integrity of the RNA was determined by disc gel electrophoresis which had been previously described. Degraded preparations were discarded. The method for measuring the concentrations of RNA and protein has been previously reported.[14] RNA was lyophilized and stored at −40° C.

Patient Population—Renal Cell Carcinoma

In the past, patients with metastatic renal cell cancer have exhibited rare, but documented spontaneous regressions of lesions. Occasionally, erratic growth patterns of metastatic foci are observed, and not uncommonly, a very long interval between primary treatment and development of metastasis has been noted. These observations have caused speculation that this disease may be responsive to immunologic tumor host factors and immunotherapeutic manipulation may be feasible. In addition, no proven effective systemic therapy has been devised in this disease. For these reasons, a trial of immunotherapy in renal cell carcinoma using xenogeneic immune RNA was instituted.

Since this was considered to be a Phase I study, 25 patients with advanced metastatic renal carcinoma comprised the majority of the study population. Patients had objective evidence or biopsy evidence of metastases to skin, bone and viscera. The only criteria for exclusion were patients who had a life expectancy of less than three months or those who refused therapy.

After initiating the study, 10 other patients received immune RNA after undergoing surgical excision of either primary tumor or solitary metastases. These patients were all believed to have a high probability of developing recurrence or of having micrometastatic disease, and were designated as having minimal residual disease (MRD). Included were patients who had excision of tumor from the diaphragm, excision of tumor metastatic to lymph nodes, patients with extension through the renal capsule and patients who had undergone resection of locally recurrent tumor or metastatic foci.

Patients initially received 2 mgs of immune RNA which had been resuspended in sterile saline and injected intracutaneously in multiple wheals in lymph node-bearing areas of the groins or axillae. The dose was subsequently increased to 4 mgs, although single doses as high as 64 mgs per week have been administered.

Historical Control Group

Since the study was a Phase I study mainly to define feasibility and toxicity, patients were not randomized and a simultaneous control group was not included. However, it appeared that survival of treated patients was greater than that reported in most series of patients with metastatic carcinoma.[15] It therefore seemed appropriate to construct an institutional control group of patients with metastatic renal carcinoma from the same institution as those who received the immunotherapy. Sufficient data for 86 patients were retrieved retrospectively and survival, location and type of metastases, and methods of therapy were entered into a data bank for computer analysis. The frequency distributions of age, site and number of metastases, sex, and disease-free interval following nephrectomy were similar in the RNA treated and nontreated groups. Specific subpopulations were compared with the study group by means of Life-Table Analysis (cumulative survival) and the significance between survival of the two populations was determined by Students' t-test.

Immunologic Testing

Delayed cutaneous hypersensitivity was assayed by skin test response to dinitrochlorobenzene (DNCB) and common skin test antigens. The method has been described previously.[16]

Serial absolute lymphocyte counts were also determined using the conventional microscopic evaluation of the Wright's stain of the peripheral blood smear.

Peripheral blood lymphocytes were assayed for cytotoxicity by a modification of the assay described by Cohen et al.[17] Lymphocytes were stored at two-month intervals by gradual freezing in a Linde biologic step down freezer and stored in the vapor phase of a liquid nitrogen freezer. The lymphocytes were separated by layering on ficol-hypaque gradients. Viability of the lymphocytes was determined by trypan blue exclusion.

Serum was obtained at eight-week intervals and tested for complement-fixing antibody levels by a method previously described.[18]

Results

Toxicity

Total dosage in a single patient has exceeded 700 mgs over a 40-month period and single dosage as high as 60 mgs (including several intravenous injections) have resulted in few side effects. Three patients experienced erythema and discomfort at the site of injection and six patients reported a mild flu-like syndrome with low grade fever 24 months after injection. No allergic or anaphylactic reactions have occurred and no patient required dose modification or discontinuation of therapy because of toxicity.

Clinical Response

Of the patients with metastatic disease, no complete responses were noted. Eight patients exhibited partial regression (50 percent or less) of measurable lesions or had stability of documented previously growing lesions for at least three months. Two patients received an insufficient trial of therapy (less than one month). Fifteen patients had no measurable response of the metastatic lesions.

Of the ten patients classified as having MRD, two have developed recurrence, 16 and 36 months after initiation of treatment. The remaining seven are free of tumor after 34–58 months.

Patients appeared to have longer survival than that reported in the literature. Comparison of the RNA treated patients with the computer-matched controls showed that the patients were similar with respect to previously identified poor prognostic indicators[19] as well as with respect to site of metastases. When all RNA treated patients were compared with the retrospective control group, survival was improved in patients receiving RNA, although this was not consistently significant at all points of observation (Figure 1). However, patients with metastases limited to the lungs appeared to have the best survival. Survival of I-RNA treated patients with metastases limited to the lungs was greater than a similar

Figure 1. Life table analysis comparing survival of all patients with metastatic renal cell carcinoma who received immune RNA compared with survival in patients in a historical control group with metastatic renal cell carcinoma who did not receive immune RNA.

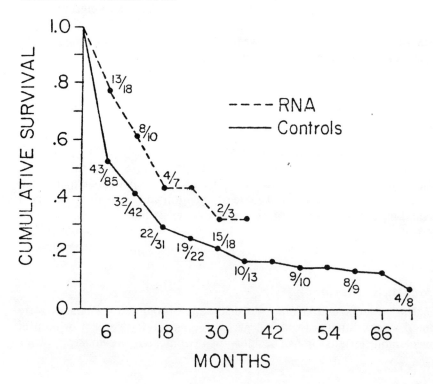

matched group of controls (Figure 2). This statistically significant difference in survival was not observed when comparing groups of patients
with metastases to other areas.

Immunologic Studies

Since no untreated prospective control group was included, the changes
in the immune assays which were noted cannot be ascribed to the RNA
therapy, but perhaps were caused by host-immune factors related to the
progressive changes in tumor burden.

Initial DNCB response was correlated with tumor burden. Patients
were arbitrarily divided into those with presumed minimum residual
disease (MRD) and those with small (three or less than 3 cms) or large
(more advanced metastases) tumor burden. Most patients, even with
small tumor, had very low DNCB response scores. In addition, little
correlation was found between patients who demonstrated a partial
response and those who had rapid progression. Responses to common
antigens did not correlate with tumor burden and were not predictive of
clinical course.[20] Similarly, absolute lymphocyte count bore no correlation to the extent of tumor involvement or clinical course.

Although patients who were stable or who had evidence of a partial
response maintained a higher mean cytotoxicity index compared with
patients who were failures at therapy, these changes were more likely
attributable to the tumor burden than to interposition of immunotherapy.
The changes noted in the level of complement-fixing antibody titers
reflected those observed in other patients with renal cell carcinoma.[21]
Antibody titers fell to zero within 12–14 months following complete
removal of tumor in the MRD group. The patients with small tumor
burden had a higher mean antibody titer than those with far-advanced
tumor. The antibody titers fell in patients with tumor progression once
the tumor became far-advanced.

It is of interest that in the group with minimum residual disease, there
have been only two recurrences in 10 patients followed for a period of 34
to 58 months. Five of these patients had RNA immune therapy discontinued, and after six to nine months, treatment was then reinitiated. In
every instance, antibody titer fell when RNA was discontinued and then
rose at least two dilutions or more when the RNA treatment was
reinstituted. In three of these five patients, RNA was begun,
discontinued, begun again and then discontinued again. In every instance,
antibody titer was increased when RNA therapy was reinstituted.

Prospective Randomized Trial of Postoperative Adjuvant
Immune RNA Therapy in Renal Cell Cancer Patients

A prospective randomized trial of adjuvant immune RNA therapy has
been instituted at UCLA. Candidates are those patients who are found
at nephrectomy to have pathologic findings which suggest a high likeli-

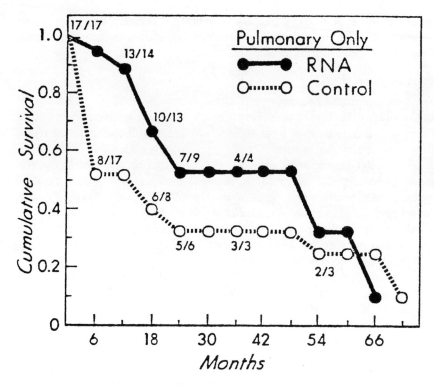

Figure 2. Life table analysis comparing survival of renal cell carcinoma patients with metastases confined to the lung who received immune RNA therapy compared with patients whose metastases were confined to the lungs who did not receive immune RNA therapy.

hood of recurrence, as invasion of the capsule by tumor and/or metastases in the regional lymph nodes. Those who are randomized to receive immune RNA get weekly injections of four milligrams intradermally as described for one year. Controls receive no therapy. Thirteen patients are currently in this study, with a median followup of less than six months, so obviously, no conclusions can yet be made. It is hoped, however, that this simple two-arm study will yield a definitive result on therapeutic efficacy of immune RNA.

Immune RNA Therapy of Other Tumors

Early in our experience with immune RNA, other cases of advanced malignancies were given trials of direct injection of immune RNA as described in the patients with renal cell carcinoma. Five patients with malignant melanoma, two patients with lung cancer, three patients with sarcomas, two patients with gastric cancer and two patients with advanced colon cancer were treated. The RNA treatment was well tolerated, but in this Phase I trial, therapeutic efficacy could not be determined.

Discussion

Immunotherapy does not appear to be ideally suited for patients with extensive metastatic disease. Yet, as described, patients with large tumor burden were entered on protocol. This was believed to be appropriate since the goal was not primarily to measure response, but to determine such factors as toxicity and dose-response relationships. Many patients were significantly immunosuppressed, as determined by delayed cutaneous hypersensitivity and lymphocyte cytotoxicity prior to therapy, and this correlated most closely with large tumor burden. It would be unlikely for regression to occur in such patients following adoptive immunotherapy, although the temporary stabilization of growth in metastases and partial regressions which were documented seemed to be secondary to RNA therapy. The ideal patient for immunotherapy, i.e., the patient with minimal tumor burden, might be much more responsive to immunologic manipulation and a group of such patients are currently the subject of randomized trial of RNA immunotherapy. However, several similar Phase I studies have reported regression of metastatic disease secondary to other methods of immunotherapy, including transfer factor.[22,23]

The survival of patients with metastatic renal cell carcinoma has been reported to be extremely poor. The survival of untreated patients at UCLA appeared to be better than that reported in the literature. It was therefore necessary to construct an institutional historic control group for comparison with treated patients. When the entire RNA treated group was compared with the entire control group, some apparent improvement in survival was noted, although this was not consistent at every point of observation. Although every attempt was made to match historic controls in treated patients, it is impossible to exclude selection and other factors which could influence favorably the outcome of the treated group. It is therefore difficult to attach significance to the differences noted in Figure 1.

Although survival of patients with metastases limited to the lung has not been reported to be improved over those with other sites of metastases, pulmonary metastases from renal carcinoma behave in a singular manner. Most documented regressions of renal carcinoma have been regressions of pulmonary metastases.[12] The unusual waxing and waning of pulmonary metastases, not uncommonly noted, has been cited. Finally, most responses to immunotherapy have been in patients with pulmonary metastases.[22,25,26] Our patients with metastases confined to the lungs seemed to survive longer than expected from reported data. Indeed, when survival of this group was compared with the control, the RNA treated patients had significantly greater survival. It is important to note, however, that all of these patients had extensive bilateral metastases and all eventually succumbed to progressive tumor growth. It is possible that RNA may be a useful adjuvant following excision of limited pulmonary metastases.

An aim of the study was to determine toxicity. Clearly, the toxicity following RNA therapy is acceptable and considerably less than that reported from most methods of immunotherapy. However, the goal of establishing dose-response relationship was not accomplished completely, because of the relatively small number of responders and the varying periods of response.

Although, initially, patients with advanced malignancies of all types were treated with immune RNA, we have confined our studies currently to patients with renal cell carcinoma. The experience with the clinical application of immune RNA is not large. Pilch has treated approximately 25 patients with malignant melanoma. More than half of these were patients with presumed minimal residual disease following surgery for malignant melanoma thought to have a high likelihood of recurrence. To date, the recurrence rate in the treated group has been less than that observed in historic controls. However, this was not a randomized prospective study. Twenty-five patients were randomized to a prospective trial of immune RNA following apparently curative resections for Dukes' B² and Dukes' C colon cancer. Median followup in this group of patients is more than two years and there has been no difference in the incidence of recurrence between those patients receiving immune RNA and untreated controls.[27] Steele and his associates have, at the time of this writing, treated six patients with RNA immunotherapy. These patients were all patients with renal cell carcinoma. Autologous lymphocytes were incubated *in vitro* with RNA extracted from guinea pigs immunized with human renal cell carcinoma. These lymphocytes were then reinfused into the patient. This interesting therapeutic model, which duplicates that used in the earlier animal RNA immunotherapy experiments, may well prove to be effective in inducing an anti-tumor response in humans. No conclusions can be made at this point in the study, however, except that therapy is safe and well-tolerated.[28]

Fukushima et al. recently reported on 31 patients who received immunotherapy with xenogeneic immune RNA. As part of this study, animals were given doses of immune RNA proportionately many times higher than that given to humans. No adverse effects from this therapy could be demonstrated in animals or in humans. Again, therapeutic efficacy in this heterogeneous group of patients with various tumors at various stages in tumor development could not be established definitively.[29]

Considerable debate exists regarding certain aspects of immune RNA therapy. First, the method of action has not been ascertained and it is unknown whether the agent simply acts as a nonspecific immunostimulant, or has some specific mode of action, such as initiation of immunoglobulin production. We have reported the induction of complement-fixing antibodies to renal carcinoma by immunizing rabbits with the specific tumor.[30] The rise of antibody titer after restarting RNA therapy in the few patients on whom this could be tested suggests that immune RNA may indeed induce a specific, anti-tumor response.

Another major area of debate is the role of RNA as a true immunotherapeutic agent. Most animal experiments have demonstrated immunoprotection rather than regression of established tumors. We have reported, however, some regression of established FANFT tumors in mice as well as prolonged survival following treatment with immune RNA.[31] There are theoretical advantages to RNA-adopted immunotherapy. Since I-RNA recipients do not have contact with tumor cells, sensitization to HLA antigens is avoided. Graft-vs-host reactions have not been observed in animals. Passive transfer of blocking factor is not a problem since serum products are not administered. Finally, RNA preparations are weakly antigenic and sensitization does not seem to occur. This is in contrast with the strong reactions associated with adoptive transfer of cells or serum products of human or animal origin.

The results in the treatment of metastatic renal carcinoma, the apparent absence of significant toxicity, and the extensive experience in animal models support the application of immune RNA in the treatment of patients with microscopic disease. The prospective randomized trial, which has been initiated, will measure changes in host immune function secondary to immune RNA and may determine if RNA is effective as an adjuvant to surgical excision of renal cell cancer.

References

1. Fishman, M, Adler, FL: The role of macrophage RNA in the immune response. Cold Spring Harbor Symposium. *Quant. Biol.* 32:343, 1967.
2. Askonas, BA, Rhodes, JM: Immunogenicity of antigen containing ribonucleic acid preparations. *Nature* 205:470, 1965.
3. Mannick, JA, Egdahl, RH: Transformation of nonimmune lymph node cells to a state of transplantation immunity by RNA. *Ann. Surg.* 156:356, 1962.
4. Bondevik, H, Mannick, JA: RNA-mediated transfer of lymphocyte vs target cell activity. *Proc. Soc. Exp. Biol. N.Y.* 129:264, 1968.
5. Alexander, P, Delorme, EJ, Hamilton, LDG et al.: Effect of nucleic acids from immune lymphocytes on rat sarcomata. *Nature* 213:469, 1967.
6. Deckers, PJ, Pilch, YH: Mediation of immunity to tumor-specific transplantation antigens by RNA: inhibition of isograft growth in rats. *Cancer Res.* 32:839, 1972.

7. Ramming, KP, Pilch, YH: Transfer of tumor-specific immunity with RNA: inhibition of growth of murine tumor isografts. *J. Nat. Cancer Inst.* 46:735, 1971.

8. Pilch, YH, Fritze, D, Ramming, KP et al.: The mediation of immune responses by I-RNA to animal and human tumor antigen. In: Fink, MA, ed. *Immune RNA in Neoplasia,* p. 149, Academic Press, New York, 1976.

9. Ramming, KP, Pilch, YH: Transfer of tumor-specific immunity with RNA: demonstration by immune cytolysis of tumor cells *in vitro. J. Natl. Cancer Inst.* 45:543–553, 1971.

10. Kern, DH, Drogemuller, CR, Pilch, YH: Immune cytolysis of rat tumor cells mediated by syngeneic immune RNA. *J. Natl. Cancer Inst.* 52:299–302, 1974.

11. Kern, DH, Fritze, D, Schick, PM et al.: Mediation of cytotoxic immune responses against human tumor associated antigens by allogeneic immune RNA. *J. Natl. Cancer Inst.* 57:105–109, 1976.

12. Freed, SZ, Halperin, JP, Gordon, M: Idiopathic regression of metastases from renal cell carcinoma. *J. Urol.* 118:538, 1977.

13. Ramming, KP, deKernion, JB, Pilch, YH: Immunotherapy of cancer with immune RNA: current status. In: Waters, H, ed. *Handbook of Cancer Immunology,* pp. 285–314, Garland Publishing Inc., New York, 1978.

14. deKernion, JB, Ramming, KP, Skinner, DG, Pilch YH: Clinical experience in the treatment of renal adenocarcinoma with immune RNA. In: Fink, MA, ed. *Immune RNA in Neoplasia,* p. 259, Academic Press, New York, 1976.

15. Middleton, RG: The value of surgery in metastatic renal carcinoma. In: King, JS, ed. *Renal Neoplasia,* p. 483, Little, Brown, Boston, 1967.

16. Eilber, FR, Nizze, JA, Morton, DL: Sequential evaluation of general immunocompetence in cancer patients: correlation with clinical course. *Cancer* 35:748, 1975.

17. Cohen, AM, Burdick, JF, Ketcham, AS: Cell-mediated cytotoxicity: an assay using ^{125}I-indodeoxyuridine labeled target cells. *J. Immunol.* 107:895, 1971.

18. Gupta, RK, Morton, DL: Suggestive evidence of *in vivo* binding of specific anti-tumor antibodies of human melanomas. *Cancer Res.* 35:58, 1975.

19. deKernion, JB, Ramming, KP, Smith, RB: Natural history of metastatic renal cell carcinoma—a computer analysis. *J. Urol.* 120:148, 1978.

20. Ramming, KP, deKernion, JB: Immune RNA therapy for renal cell carcinoma: survival and immunologic monitoring. *Ann. Surg.* 186, No. 4:459, 1977.

21. deKernion, JB, Ramming, KP: The detection and clinical significance of antibodies to tumor-associated antigens in patients with renal cell carcinoma. *J. Urol.* (in press).

22. Schapira, DV, McCune, CS, Henshaw, EC: Treatment of advanced renal cell carcinoma with specific immunotherapy consisting of autologous tumor cells and *C-parvum. Proc. Am. Soc. Clin. Oncol.* 17:348, 1979.

23. Bukowski, RM, Groppe, C, Reimer, R, Weick, J et al.: Immunotherapy (IT) of metastatic renal cell carcinoma. *Proc. Am. Soc. Clin. Oncol.* 17:402, 1979.

24. Mostofi, FK: Pathology and spread of renal cell carcinoma. In: King, JS, ed. *Renal Neoplasia,* p. 41, Little, Brown, Boston, 1967.

25. Minton, JP, Pennline, K, Nowrocki, JF et al.: Immunotherapy of human kidney cancer. *Proc. Am. Soc. Clin. Oncol.* 17:301, 1976.

26. Tykka, H, Oravisto, KJ, Lehtonen, T et al.: Active specific immunotherapy of advanced renal cell carcinoma. *Eur. Urol.* 4:250, 1978.

27. Pilch, YH: Personal communication, Oct., 1979.

28. Steele, G: Personal communication, Sept., 1979.

29. Fukushima, M, Fukuda, S, Machida, S, Ishikawa, Y: Experimental and clinical studies on toxicity of xenogeneic tumor-specific immune ribonucleic acid. *Tohoku Journal of Experimental Medicine* 128:285–294, 1979.

30. Ramming, KP, Gupta, RK, deKernion, JB: Induction of antibody to human renal cell cancer *in vivo* by injections of xenogeneic immune RNA. *Proc. Am. Soc. Clin. Oncol.* 17:214, 1979.

31. deKernion, JB, Ramming, KP, Fraser, K: Immunotherapy and chemoimmunotherapy of FANFT bladder tumor. *Proc. Am. Soc. Clin. Oncol.* 17:116, 1977.

Complete Remissions Lasting Over Three Years in Adult Patients Treated for Metastatic Sarcoma

Joseph G. Sinkovics

Department of Medicine, University of Texas Cancer Center, M.D. Anderson Hospital, Houston, Texas

Summary

Patient 1 had intra-abdominal rhabdomyosarcoma metastatic to the bone marrow. He received vincristine, cyclophosphamide and actinomycin-D for three years. He remains tumor-free 10 3/4 years later. Patient 2 had a pleomorphic sarcoma of the breast metastatic to both lungs. She received chemoimmunotherapy with vincristine, doxorubicin, actinomycin-D, dacarbazine, Bacille Calmette-Guérin and sarcoma lysates. She is tumor-free at 78 months. Patient 3 had rhabdomyosarcoma metastatic from the leg to both lungs. She received vincristine, cyclophosphamide, doxorubicin, actinomycin-D and dacarbazine for two years. She is tumor-free at 42 months. Patient 4 had fibrosarcoma of the femur metastatic to both lungs after amputation. She received vincristine, cyclophosphamide, doxorubicin, actinomycin-D, dacarbazine and Bacille Calmette-Guérin for two years. She is tumor-free at 42 months.

Patient 5 had malignant fibrous histiocytoma of the buttock metastatic to the pectoralis muscle. After simple excision, he received vincristine, actinomycin-D and cyclophosphamide for three years. He remains tumor-free at 87 months. Patient 6 had osteosarcoma of an index finger treated with amputation. Axillary lumph node metastases were excised. She received 10 courses of vincristine, cyclophosphamide, doxorubicin and dacarbazine and remains tumor-free at 60 months.

Patients 7, 8 and 9 were treated for metastatic leiomyosarcoma, osteosarcoma and hemangiopericytoma, respectively. They are alive and well at 80, 70, and 60 months, respectively but may harbor stable minimal residual disease.

The vast majority of patients with metastatic sarcomas succumbed despite similar treatment. Rapid achievement of complete remission and immune reactivity to sarcoma cells are possible decisive factors in long remission maintenance.

Introduction

Complete remissions (CR) of metastatic sarcomas in adult patients are difficult to achieve, occur at low rate and seldom are sustained over two years.[1,2]

The Southwest Oncology Group (SWOG) claimed 14 percent CR rate in a large adult patient population with metastatic sarcomas.[3-5] The median duration of CR was 14 months. These patients were treated with CyVADIC (VCR, CTX, Adria/Act-D DTIC)[a] regimen. Most patients relapsed with chemotherapy-resistant tumors after one year.

At the Solid Tumor Clinics (Service) of the department of medicine, more than 200 patients with locally destructive or recurrent and inoperable sarcomas, or with metastatic sarcomas were treated in the past 10 years. The case histories of most of these patients were incorporated into previous reports of the SWOG. A number of patients with locally destructive or recurrent and inoperable, but not metastatic, sarcomas (retroperitoneal and intra-abdominal fibrosarcoma, leiomyosarcoma and mesenchymoma; nasopharyngeal and paratesticular rhabdomyosarcoma, etc.) have also achieved CR for more than three years on combination chemotherapy. The case histories of some of these patients were mentioned in various previous publications.[6-10] Thus patients who recovered from inoperable recurrent or locally destructive sarcomas will not be discussed in this publication. Patients who are now in CR after treatment for metastatic sarcomas, but observed for periods shorter than three years will also be excluded. The purpose of this communication is to review briefly long term tumor-free survivors (nine of 164 patients) who were treated for distant metastases.

Case Histories

Patients Treated with Clinically Evident Metastatic Disease and Surviving Tumor-Free

Patient 1

IR, male, born in 1922 was admitted in December, 1968 with large intra-abdominal tumor. The largest diameter of the tumor was more than 18 cm. The tumor occupied the left flank and crossed the midline of the

---

[a]VCR=vincristine; CTX=cyclophosphamide; Adria=Adriamycin; Act-D=actinomycin-D; DTIC=dacarbazine.

abdomen. A 2×2.5 cm right axillary node was palpated. A bone marrow aspirate revealed metastatic tumor cells (1 per 3–5 high power fields). At laparotomy, an unresectable tumor consisting of spindle cells with cross-striations was found (Figure 1). The pathologic diagnosis was issued by J. J. Butler and W. O. Russell as "malignant neoplasm, suggesting rhabdomyosarcoma." The patient received VCR and CTX with rapid decrease of tumor size. Palliative radiotherapy (3000r) was given to the left flank. Act-D was added. From January, 1969 to December, 1973, the patient consumed a total dose of 118 mg VCR, 87 gm CTX, and 7.5 mg Act-D. He entered CR within three months and remained tumor-free until August, 1979, 10 3/4 years after the initiation and 5 3/4 years after the discontinuation of this chemotherapy. During the first three years of his treatment, this patient was tested repeatedly for his immune reaction to sarcoma cells. He circulated lymphocytes cytotoxic to sarcoma cells and unblocking serum factors.[11,12]

Patient 2

JC, female, born in 1926, developed a poorly differentiated, highly pleomorphic tumor in her left breast in March, 1972. She was treated with radical mastectomy. By October, 1972, she developed large, bilateral pulmonary metastases. One of these metastases was biopsied. The tissue

Figure 1. Elongated sarcoma cells with cross striations characteristic of rhabdomyosarcoma in the biopsy specimen of the inoperable intra-abdominal tumor.

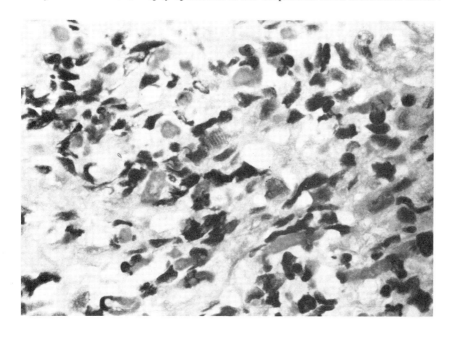

diagnosis issued by S. Gallager was poorly differentiated sarcoma (Figure 2). The patient received 10 courses at monthly intervals of VCR, Adria and DTIC (1972–1973) and 16 courses at monthly intervals of VCR, Act-D and DTIC (1973–1974). She rapidly achieved CR (Figures 3 and 4). Thereafter (1974–1975), she received two scarifications per month with Chicago strain Bacille Calmette-Guérin and two intracutaneous immunizations with viral oncolysates prepared from an established cell line of cytosarcoma phylloides. She circulated lymphocytes cytotoxic to cultured sarcoma cells and serum factors potentiating this effect (Table 1). She was clinically tumor-free in July, 1979, 78 months after the initiation and 52 months after the discontinuation of her chemotherapy.

Patient 3

MM, female, born in 1944, developed grade 3 alveolar rhabdomyosarcoma in her right calf. After excision, she received 6465r radiotherapy. By October, 1975, she developed bilateral pulmonary metastases. She received 10 courses of chemotherapy at monthly intervals with VCR 2 mg, CTX 800 mg, Adria 80 mg and DTIC 400 mg × 5. She rapidly achieved CR. She received 15 further courses of chemotherapy at monthly intervals with Act-D 0.5 mg × 5 (2.5mg) replacing Adria per course. She remains in CR in July, 1979, 42 months after the initiation and 17 months after the cessation of her chemotherapy.

Figure 2. Highly pleomorphic sarcoma cells from the biopsy of one of the pleurally based intrathoracic metastases.

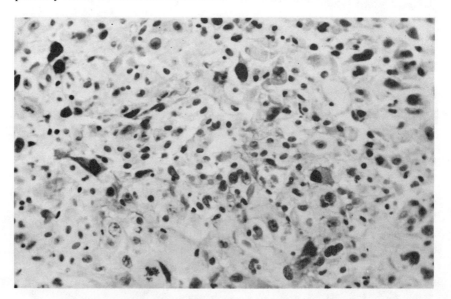

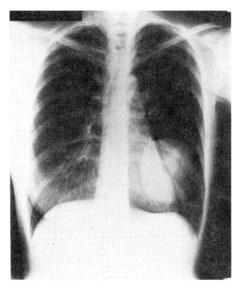

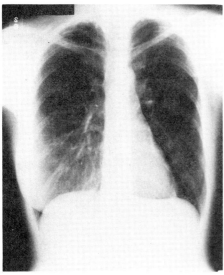

Figures 3 and 4. Large bilateral pulmonary metastases (3) completely regressed (4). Chest X-ray picture remains negative six years later.

Patient 4

AL, female, born 1928, developed a grade 3 fibrosarcoma in her right thigh and femur. She was treated with hip disarticulation. By December, 1975, bilateral pulmonary metastases became evident. She started chemotherapy in January, 1976, with VCR 2 mg, CTX 800 mg, Adria 80 mg,

Table 1. Percent Reduction of Target Tumor Cell Growth by Lymphocytes and by Serum and Lymphocytes of Three Patients

| Patient | Attacker Cells | % Target Tumor Cell Growth Reduction | | | | | | | | | | |
| | | Sarcoma Cell Lines[a] | | | | | Carcinoma Cell Lines[a] | | | | Melanoma Cell Line | Human Fetal Cells |
		2089	2322	3123	3370	3743	2043	2118	2305	3329	5145	2891
JC	Lymphocytes	63	–	–	56	61	17	32	51	31	–	–
	Serum and lymphocytes	90	–	–	67	69	46	32	61	46	–	–
QG	Lymphocytes	18	42	–	–	–	13	–	–	–	49	–
	Serum and lymphocytes	62	63	–	–	–	58	–	–	–	97	–
MM	Lymphocytes	54	25	20	–	–	40	30	–	–	–	30
	Serum and lymphocytes	78	88	60	–	–	45	48	–	–	–	48

[a] Established human tumor cell lines: 2089–rhabdomyosarcoma; 2322–chondrosarcoma; 3122–neurofibrosarcoma; 3370–synovial sarcoma; 3743–cystosarcoma phylloides; 2043–squamous carcinoma of uterine cervix; 2118–kidney carcinoma; 2305–breast carcinoma; 3329–breast carcinoma.

(*Source: Sinkovics et al.*)[8,9,12,14]

and DTIC 400 mg × 5, at monthly intervals for 24 courses; Adria was replaced by Act-D 1 mg per course after the 10th course. Two scarifications per month, on Days 17 and 24 of each course, with Chicago Bacille Calmette-Guérin were given. The patient rapidly achieved CR. She remains clinically tumor-free in July, 1979, 42 months after the initiation and 18 months after the cessation of chemotherapy.

Patients Treated After the Simple Excision of Metastatic Tumor and Surviving Tumor-Free

Patient 5

MM, male, born 1923, developed large (> 15 cm) tumor in his right buttock in February, 1972. The histologic diagnosis was pleomorphic (undifferentiated) rhabdomyosarcoma. He was treated with excision and radiotherapy (5040r). While receiving radiotherapy, metastasis in right pectoralis muscles became evident. The metastatic tumor was simply enucleated; it yielded the same tissue diagnosis, i.e., pleomorphic sarcoma. M. Luna recently suggested malignant fibrous histiocytoma (Figure 5). The patient started chemotherapy in April, 1972 and received chemotherapy until April, 1975 (three years). He consumed 31 mg VCR, 75 gm CTX, and 45 mg Act-D, total dose. In July, 1979, he was found to be

Figure 5. Highly pleomorphic metastatic sarcoma excised from the right pectoralis muscle.

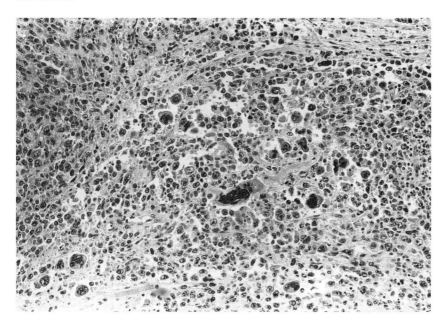

without signs of tumor recurrence. Thus, this patient remains in CR 87 months after the initiation and 51 months after the cessation of chemotherapy. Immunological testing of this patient revealed lymphocyte-mediated cytotoxicity directed toward cultured sarcoma cells and serum factors potentiating this effect (Table 1).

Patient 6

QG, female, born in 1910, developed osteogenic sarcoma in her right index finger in 1971. She was treated with amputation of the finger. In June, 1974, large tumor appeared in the right axilla. It was removed by simple excision. The tissue diagnosis was metastatic osteogenic sarcoma in lymph node. From July, 1974 to May, 1975, the patient was given 10 courses of chemotherapy at monthly intervals with VCR 2 mg, CTX 600 mg, Adria 70 mg and DTIC 375 mg × 5. In July, 1979, she was found to be tumor-free, 60 months after the initiation and 50 months after the discontinuation of chemotherapy. This patient circulated serum factors potentiating her lymphocyte-mediated cytotoxicity toward sarcoma, carcinoma and melanoma cell lines (Table 1).

Patients Treated with Clinically Evident Disease and Surviving with Residual Lesions that May Be Stable Minimal Residual Tumors

Patient 7

MH, female, born in 1937, had hysterectomy in 1963 because of uterine leiomyosarcoma. In 1966 she suffered local recurrence and developed metastases in both lungs. Recurrent tumors were repeatedly excised in 1966, 1968 and 1971. Further metastases in both lungs became evident in 1972. Chemotherapy begun in October, 1972, with VCR, Act-D and CTX. After brief tumor response, relapse occurred. Adria and DTIC were given from March to June, 1973. After brief tumor response, relapse occurred. Both lungs were irradiated with 1492r and hydroxyurea 30 mg/kg/day was given by mouth on days of radiotherapy. After brief tumor response, relapse took place. Semustine (methyl CCNU) and DTIC were given from September, 1973 to April, 1976. After stabilization of tumor size, slow and steady decrease in the size of metastatic nodules occurred. Semustine alone was given from August, 1976 to February, 1978. Further decrease of tumor nodules took place. The patient received no treatment after March, 1978. In April, 1979, she was found to have very small, ill-defined spots at sites where previously tumor nodules were identified on her previous chest film; there was no evidence of disease elsewhere. She is either tumor-free or carries stable minimal residual disease 80 months after the initiation and 16 months after the cessation of her chemotherapy.[10]

Patient 8

KC, male, born in 1957, had his right leg amputated in May, 1973 because of osteogenic sarcoma of the tibia (Figure 6). In June, 1973, bilateral pulmonary metastases and left sided pleural effusion were found. Chemotherapy calculated for body size over 2 m² began in July, 1973 with VCR 2 mg, CTX 1.5 gm, Adria 150 mg, DTIC 600 mg × 5 for 8 monthly courses. Partial remission and then progression of disease occurred. From March, 1974 to September, 1976, the patient received 20 courses of 250 mg semustine and Act-D 0.75 mg × 5 per course. He experienced reduction in the size of tumors (Figures 7 and 8). He is off treatment (at his own decision) since October, 1976. In May, 1979, he was still alive, but with small residual densities in his lungs. He is either tumor-free or has stable, minimal residual disease 70 months after the initiation and 31 months after the cessation of chemotherapy. Patient refuses thoracotomy. Contrary to expectations, this long survivor, when tested for lymphocyte-mediated cytotoxicity against a battery of established human tumor cell lines, showed poor reactivity toward cultured

Figure 6. Osteogenic sarcoma of the tibia with malignant osteoid and some cartilage.

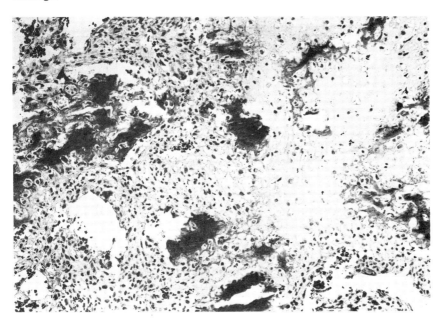

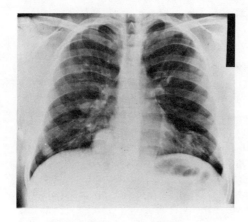

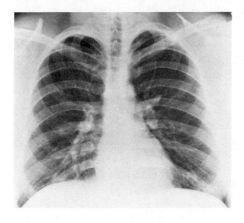

Figures 7 and 8. Bilateral pulmonary metastases of osteosarcoma regressed; stable minimal residual disease in the right hilum is possible.

human sarcoma cells and did not possess serum factors potentiating this effect.[13]

Patient 9

RW, male, born in 1914, developed large mediastinal tumor in 1964. He was treated with excision. The tissue diagnosis was hemangiopericytoma. In 1973 left supraclavicular mass appeared. It was excised; the tissue diagnosis was hemangiopericytoma. In 1974 a very large and inoperable mediastinal tumor recurred (Figure 9). From July, 1974 to February, 1975, nine courses of chemotherapy were given with VCR 2 mg, CTX 900 mg, Adria 90 mg and DTIC 450 mg × 5 per course. Partial remission with reduction of more than 50 percent of tumor size occurred. Radiotherapy with 5640r total dose (fast neutrons and 25 MEV photons) to the mediastinum was given. Patient was well with fibrotic changes in mediastinum and right upper lobe (Figure 10) in June, 1978. He is either tumor-free or may harbor stable minimal residual disease 54 months after the initiation and 40 months after the cessation of chemotherapy. At 60 months, the patient's private physician reported that the patient was free of clinically active disease.

Discussion

Cure of metastatic sarcomas in adults is achieved very seldom, especially when the only modality of treatment is chemotherapy. Well differentiated or slowly growing sarcomas may possibly be cured by surgical removal of a single or of a few metastases; well differentiated chondrosarcoma is an example. Radiotherapy of metastatic disease is palliative. Only occasionally can radiotherapy given in small doses, but with a radiosensitizing agent, achieve remission. For example, a young woman with synovial sarcoma metastatic to both lungs experienced dramatic tumor response with low dose radiotherapy and hydroxyurea.[6,8] Figures 11 and 12 show the dramatic, but temporary, regression of chemotherapy-resistant osteosarcoma metastases in the lungs of another young woman treated with low dose radiotherapy and hydroxyurea.

Among the nine patients described in this report (Table 2), there are some who were cured. It is not known why the same treatment regimen failed to cure the vast majority of patients with metastatic sarcomas. One decisive factor could be the chemotherapy-susceptibility of the tumor. Achievement of CR with dramatic rapidity apparently allows no time for the selection of chemotherapy-resistant tumor cell clones. Patients 1–4 achieved their complete remission with dramatic rapidity (within three months).

Another major factor can be sought in host resistance and tumor-specific immunity. Some of the patients described in this report displayed impressive immune faculties directed to allogeneic cultured sarcoma cells, but there is no evidence that the achievement of long, tumor-free remission depended on this particular faculty of the host. Table 1 shows growth reduction of allogeneic target tumor cells after exposure to the patients' purified lymphocytes or to the patients' heat-inactivated sera first and then to their lymphocytes. The technics and the human tumor cell lines used in these assays have been described elsewhere.[8,9,12,14] The attacker cell:target cell ratio was in the range of 100:1. The average of three to five experiments for each value shown in Table 1 was calculated; each experiment was done in duplicate or triplicate. It cannot be claimed that the lymphocytes of these patients selectively destroyed sarcoma cells or inhibited their growth. However, Table 3 shows that

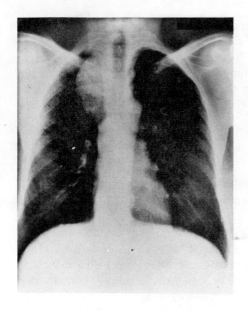

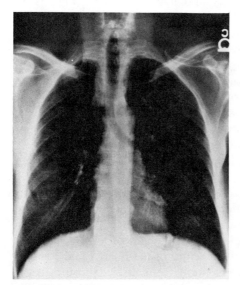

Figures 9 and 10. Large hemangiopericytoma in the mediastinum underwent partial remission on chemotherapy and regressed completely after radiotherapy. Stable minimal residual disease in the mediastinum is possible.

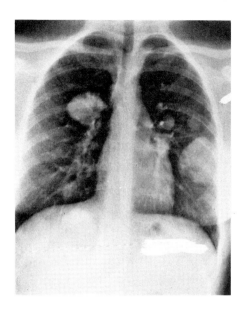

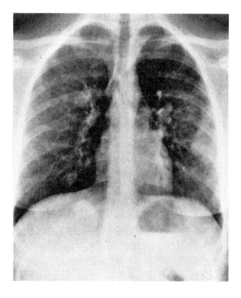

Figures 11 and 12. Large bilateral lung metastases of osteosarcoma resistant to doxorubicin and high dose methotrexate partially regress after radiotherapy (1300r to whole lung, 1000r boost to large tumor) and hydroxyurea (30 mg/kg/day on days of radiotherapy.).

Table 2. Patients Surviving over Three Years after Treatment for Metastatic Sarcomas

Number	Patient	Tumor	Treatment	Outcome	Comment
1	IR	Rhabdomyo Sc	VCR CTX Act-D	NED 129 mo	
2	JC	Pleomorph Sc	VCR CTX Adria Act-D DTIC BCG Sc lysates	NED 78 mo	Treated for clinically evident hematogenous metastases.
3	MM	Rhabdomyo Sc	VCR CTX Adria Act-D DTIC	NED 42 mo	
4	AL	Fibro Sc	VCR CTX Adria Act-D DTIC	NED 38 mo	
5	MM	Rhabdomyo Sc	VCR Act-D CTX	NED 87 mo	Treated after simple excision of metastasis.
6	QG	Osteo Sc	VCR CTX Adria DTIC	NED 60 mo	
7	MH	Leiomyo Sc	VCR Act-D CTX Adria DTIC XRt HU MeCCNU	St MRD 80 mo	Treated for clinically evident metastases; may harbor stable minimal residual disease.
8	KC	Osteo Sc	VCR CTX Adria DTIC Act-D MeCCNU	St MRD 70 mo	
9	RW	Hemangiopericytoma	VCR CTX Adria DTIC XRt	St MRD 60 mo	

VCR = vincristine; CTX = cyclophosphamide; Adria = doxorubicin; Act-D = actinomycin-D; Sc = sarcoma; BCG = Bacille Calmette-Guérin; NED = no evidence of disease; HU = hydroxyurea; XRt = radiotherapy; MeCCNU = semustine; MRD = minimal residual disease; St = stable; mo = months.

Table 3. Inhibition of Target Cell Growth in Excess of Fifty Percent

Cell Lines	Attacker Cells	> 50% Inhibition Cell Lines Tested	% of Cell Lines Inhibited >50%
Sarcoma	Lymphocytes	5/8	62
	Serum and Lymphocytes	8/8	100
Carcinoma	Lymphocytes	1/7	14
	Serum and Lymphocytes	2/7	28

inhibition of target cell growth by these lymphocytes or by these sera and lymphocytes was consistently stronger toward sarcoma than toward carcinoma cells. This finding may reflect to a greater natural susceptibility of sarcoma cells than carcinoma cells to lymphocyte-mediated cytotoxicity; or it may indicate sarcoma-specific immunity expressed by these patients. It is to be emphasized that these patients circulated lymphocytes cytotoxic to or capable of inhibiting the growth of cultured sarcoma cells and that their serum potentiated this effect. For controls, the immune reactions of 25 patients who died with metastatic sarcomas and the immune reactions of 15 healthy blood donors to sarcoma cell lines 2089 and 2322 and to carcinoma cell lines 2043 and 2118 were compared (Table 4). Healthy donors did not distinguish clearly between sarcoma and carcinoma cells, but their sera slightly potentiated lymphocyte-mediated cytotoxicity to sarcoma cells. The lymphocytes of patients who eventually died with metastatic sarcomas were only slightly more cytotoxic to sarcoma cells than to carcinoma cells; potentiating serum factors were not evident or if they occurred in an exceptional patient,[8] in the averaged results, the effect of blocking serum factors counterbalanced potentiation. In contrast, the four patients who survived long tumor-free clearly reacted better to sarcoma cells than to carcinoma cells and serum factors potentiating lymphocyte-mediated cytotoxicity were evident in their blood. This latter effect was also detectable against a carcinoma cell line. Thus, while sarcoma selectivity of the reaction pattern of surviving patients is highly suggestive, its immunologic specificity to sarcoma cells remains to be proved. The interpretation of similar results has been discussed in previous publications.[7,8,9,12]

For the cure of metastatic sarcomas, more effective chemoimmunotherapy is needed. Interferon may be utilized for long term treatment or in short, intensive courses as a cell synchronizer. If interferon acts as a tumor cell growth regulator, its cytostatic effects may be utilized for intensifying the efficacy of cell cycle-specific agents. For example, if the growth of sarcoma cells is stopped temporarily by interferon, after the withdrawal of interferon this tumor cell population may enter the S and M phases of the cell cycle in one cohort. Methotrexate given at this point may achieve a much increased cytocidal effect. Investigational protocols of this type have now been initiated.[15]

Table 4. Comparison of Immune Reactions of Surviving Tumor-free Patients, Nonresponding or Relapsing Patients and Healthy Donors

Patients	Attacker Cells	Target Tumor Cell Lines					P value
		2089	2322	2043	2118		
IR, JC, QG, MM	Ly	52	44	24	29		2089 and 2322 vs 2043 and 2118: <0.05
	Se Ly	82	80	45	37		2089 and 2322 of this group vs 2089 and 2322 of 25 patients: <0.05
25 patients with growing sarcomas	Ly	35	27	18	20		–
	Se Ly	40	20	15	29		2089 and 2322 of this group vs 2089 and 2322 of IR, JC, QG and MM: <0.05
15 healthy blood donors	Ly	32	37	33	28		–
	Se Ly	44	48	27	32		–

Figures represent averaged percent reduction of growth of target tumor cell cultures.

<0.05 = significant difference; – = difference not significant; Ly = lymphocytes; Se = serum (heat inactivated at 56°C).

2089 – rhabdomyosarcoma; 2322 – chrondrosarcoma; 2043 – squamous carcinoma of uterine cervix; 2118 – kidney carcinoma.

References

1. Sinkovics, JG: *Medical Oncology: An Advanced Course,* Marcel Dekker, Inc., New York, pp. 679, 1979.

2. Sinkovics, JG, Shirato, E, Cabiness, JR, Martin, RG: Rhabdomyosarcoma after puberty: clinical, tissue culture and immunological studies. *Journal of Medicine Clinical and Experimental,* 1:313–326, 1970.

3. Gottlieb, JA, Bodey, GP, Sinkovics, JG et al.: An effective 4-drug combination regimen (CyVADIC) for metastatic sarcomas. *Proc. Tenth Annual Meeting Am. Soc. Clin. Oncol.,* 10:162, 1974.

4. Gottlieb, JA, Baker, LH, O'Bryan, RM, Sinkovics, JG et al.: Adriamycin used alone and in combination in soft tissue and bony sarcoma. *Cancer Chemotherapy Reports, Part 3,* 6:271–282, 1975.

5. Benjamin, RS, Gottlieb, JA, Baker, LO, Sinkovics, JG: CyVADIC vs CyVADACT—a randomized trial of cyclophosphamide (CY), vincristine (V)V, and Adriamycin (A), plus dacarbazine (DIC), or actinomycin-D (DACT) in metastatic sarcomas. *Proc. 12th Annual Meeting Am. Soc. Clin. Oncol,* 17:256, 1976.

6. Sinkovics, JG: A multidisciplinary approach to the understanding and treatment of human sarcomas. In: Mackay, B, *Sarcomas.* W. B. Saunders, Philadelphia, 1980 (in press).

7. Sinkovics, JG, Campos, LT, Kay, HD et al.: Chemotherapy of metastatic sarcomas: clinical results and correlations with immune reactions to cultured sarcoma cells. *Proc. Eighth Internat. Cong. Chemotherapy,* 3:508–513, 1974.

8. Sinkovics, JG, Campos, LT, Kay, HD et al.: Immunological studies with human sarcomas: effects of immunization and therapy on cell- and antibody-mediated immune reactions. In: *Immunological Aspects of Neoplasia* pp. 367–401, Williams & Wilkins, Baltimore, 1975.

9. Sinkovics, JG, Campos, LT, Loh, KK et al.: Chemoimmunotherapy for three categories of solid tumors (sarcoma, melanoma, lymphoma): the problem of immunoresistant tumors. In: Crispen, RG, ed. *Neoplasm Immunity: Mechanisms* pp. 193–212, Chicago Symposium, Chicago, 1976.

10. Sinkovics, JG, Plager, C, von Eschenbach, A, Johnson, D: Sarcomas of the genitourinary tract: case histories. In: Johnson, DE, Samuels, ML, eds. *Cancer of the Genitourinary Tract.* pp. 281–299, Raven Press, New York, N. Y., 1979.

11. Sinkovics, JG, Williams, DE, Campos, LT et al.: Intensification of immune reactions of patients to cultured sarcoma cells: attempts at monitored immunotherapy. *Seminars in Oncology,* 1:351–365, 1974.

12. Sinkovics, JG, Plager, C, McMurtrey, M et al.: Immunotherapy of human sarcomas. In: *Current Concepts in the Management of Primary Bone and Soft Tissue Tumors,* pp. 361–410, Year Book Medical Publishers, Chicago, 1977.

13. Sinkovics, JG, Plager, C, Papadopoulos, N et al.: Immunology and immunotherapy of human sarcomas. In: *Immunotherapy of Human Cancer,* pp. 267–288, Raven Press, New York, 1978.

14. Sinkovics, JG, Gyorkey, F, Kusyk, C, Siciliano, M: Growth of human tumor cells in established cultures. In: Busch, H, ed. *Methods in Cancer Research,* 14:243–323, Academic Press, New York, 1978.

15. Sinkovics, JG, Plager, C: Project M27/gm 23: clinical trials with human interferon. *Research Report* 1978–1980, University of Texas M. D. Anderson Hospital (in preparation).

Chemoimmunotherapy for Disseminated Melanoma (DM)[a]

Muhyi Al-Sarraf, John J. Costanzi, Dennis O. Dixon

School of Medicine, Wayne State University, Detroit, Michigan; University of Texas Medical Branch, Galveston, Texas; University of Texas, M.D. Anderson Tumor Institute, Houston, Texas

Summary

A randomized study of 377 patients with DM and evaluated for response and toxicity produced response rates of 31 percent to a combination of BCNU, Hydrea and DTIC (BHD), 26 percent to BHD plus BCG and 18 percent to DTIC plus BCG ($p = 0.05$). The overall survival of patients on the three arms was not statistically different. In certain subgroups related to age, sex and sites of metastasis there were differences in survival related to the type of therapy. Total peripheral lymphocyte and delayed hypersensitivity reactions to the challenge of PPD, dermatophyton, Varidase, candida, mumps and PHA were performed before therapy. There was a statistical difference for the levels of peripheral lymphocytes and the overall response rate, but no difference in survival. Patients with no positive skin tests had a median survival of 26 weeks, those with one or two positive tests 32 weeks and 3 or more positive tests 48 weeks ($p = 0.05$). Of patients that were treated with BCG and had a pre-treatment PPD negative (47), 74 percent changed to positive on a repeat test during therapy. These 35 patients had a median survival of > 63 weeks. Those that remained negative had a median survival of 31 weeks ($p = 0.01$).

[a]This investigation was supported by Grant Nos.: CA 14028, CA 03096-22, CA 17701-05 and CA 12014 awarded by the National Cancer Institute, DHEW.

Introduction

In patients with disseminated malignant melanoma, DTIC is one of the most effective single agents.[1-3] Anti-tumor effect was noted at doses from 150–375 mg/m² daily for five days.

Utilizing BCNU alone, DeVita and Gold[4] reported objective remissions in two of three patients with advanced malignant melanoma. They reported response rate to the combination of BCNU and vincristine as 27 percent and 45 percent against disseminated melanoma.[5,6] The major dose limiting toxicity of BCNU is depression of the white blood count and platelet count.[7]

Hydroxyurea was found to have biological activity in patients with malignant melanoma.[8] Leukopenia with megaloblastosis which is not responsive to vitamin B12 or folate is the major side effect of hydroxyurea.[9]

Combination chemotherapy had been effective in the treatment of patients with disseminated melanoma.[10,11]

The combination of DTIC for five days and BCG by stratifications administered on Days seven, 12 and 17 every three weeks, has increased remission rate and prolonged survival as compared with historical control in patients with advanced malignant melanoma.[12]

This study was designed to determine the effectiveness of the combination of BCNU, hydroxyurea and DTIC (BHD) as compared with BHD plus BCG or DTIC alone plus BCG. The protocol was activated on October 8, 1974, for all SWOG institutions and was closed for patients' entry in January, 1977.

Materials and Methods

Patients with histologically proven disseminated malignant melanoma and who have not been treated with any of the protocol agents were included in this study. Patients must have adequate renal and hepatic function.

Initial prestudy evaluation included: history and physical examination, complete blood count, platelet count, urinalysis, BUN, creatinine, bilirubin, SGOT, alkaline phosphatase, bone marrow biopsy, EEG, brain scan, liver scan, chest X-rays and bone X-rays. Tumor measurement and performance status were performed and recorded. Patients were randomized to either arm of therapy (Table 1).

Patients with brain involvement were registered and randomized then placed on decadron 8–12 mg/day orally for three days then tapered off. On the third day, total brain irradiation was started to a total dose of 3,000 rads over a two-week period. Systemic therapy began during the second week of radiotherapy.

Table 1. Drug Dosage and Treatment Plan

BHD (Every 28 days):
BCNU   150 mg/m^2 day 1 every other course
Hydroxyurea   1500 mg/m^2 day 1-5, orally
DTIC   150 mg/m^2 day 1-5, i.v.

BHD+BCG:
BHD as above
BCG = lyophilized Connaught Strain, 6x10^8 (range 4-8x10^8) constituted in 1 ml of fluid, by
    scarification on days 7, 14 and 21.

DTIC+BCG (Every 28 days):
DTIC = 250 mg/m^2 day 1-5 i.v.
BCG as above

Patients with massive liver involvement were defined as a liver span of at least 16 cm at the mid-clavicular line, 12 cm at the anterior axillary line and 4 cm below the xyphoid area with diffuse involvement in both lobes by liver scan. After registration and randomization it was recommended that the patients were to receive DTIC 200 mg/m²/day over 24-hour intrahepatic artery infusion for five days. Liver measurement was recorded during this period and after five to seven days the patients were started on the randomized systemic therapy.

The sites of BCG scarification were rotated with the upper arms, upper legs or back. If, after three courses of chemoimmunotherapy, the patient was a responder, BCG maintenance was given monthly on Day 14 of the cycle, between maintenance courses of chemotherapy.

In all patients, the following skin tests were performed and recorded prior to the first two courses of therapy, then prior to every other course thereafter: PPD, Varidase, dermatophyton, candida albicans, PHA and mumps. Absolute lymphocyte counts were done prior to therapy and before each monthly course.

Objective tumor remissions were defined as follows: complete remission (CR) as complete disappearance of all clinical evidence of tumor; partial remission (PR) as decrease of 50 percent or more in the sum of the products of two diameters of all measurable tumors for a minimum of four weeks.

No change (NC) was defined as an increase or decrease of less than 50 percent of the sum of the products of the two diameters of measurable lesions.

Increasing disease (ID) was defined as an increase of 50 percent or more in the product of two diameters of any measurable tumor or appearance of new lesion(s). Relapse was defined as an increase of 50 percent or more in the product of two diameters of the tumor being measured over that which was obtained during maximum remission;

reappearance of old lesions in patients who achieved a complete remission; or appearance of new lesions.

Therapy with at least two courses was considered as an adequate trial for this study.

Results

Three hundred and ninety-seven patients were registered, 394 were eligible and 377 patients were evaluated for this report. Ninety-five patients received BHD, 155 BHD + BCG and 127 patients had DTIC + BCG. The BHD + BCG arm was kept open longer because of possible differences in response and survival in certain subgroups.

The overall remission rate (CR+PR) was 25 percent, with response rate of 31 percent (29/95) in BHD group, 26 percent (41/155) BHD + BCG and 18 percent (23/127) for DTIC + BCG. This difference in response rate was statistically significant (p = 0.05).

There were no differences in duration of response in the three groups with median length in weeks for BHD 27, BHD + BCG 30 and DTIC + BCG 38 weeks (p = 0.79).

The overall median survival was 28 weeks with no evidence of difference between the three therapies (p = 0.66).

Patients between 30 to 60 years of age had response rate of 41 percent (24/58) to BHD treatment as compared to 11 percent (8/71) on DTIC + BCG. This difference was statistically significant (p = 0.02). In patients older than 60 years of age the response rate was higher in the BCG groups, but was not statistically significant.

No difference was found in remission rate among the three groups as related to other characteristics such as performance status, site of metastases, poor or good risk, prior therapy and prior chemotherapy or immunotherapy.

Patients with primary lung metastases had longer remission on BHD + BCG than BHD alone (p = 0.04). Patients treated with DTIC + BCG had better duration of response than the combined chemotherapy with or without BCG (p = 0.02).

Patients with lung metastases (p = 0.03) and primarily nodal involvement (p = 0.05) had longer survival with BHD + BCG than with BHD alone. Also, patients above the age of 60 had significantly (p = 0.01) longer survival on BCG groups than on the chemotherapy alone.

The overall survival of patients older than 30 had better survival than younger patients (p = 0.01), regardless of the types of therapy. Also, significantly better survival was found in patients with good performance status than poor performance status and without major organ involvement (brain, liver, bone or lung) than those with such organ metastases. This last finding may necessitate the stratification according to age, performance status and major organ involvement in Phase III clinical trials in patients with advanced malignant melanoma.

Drug toxicity was comparable in the three groups. Severe nausea and vomiting was reported most frequently. Although the BCG groups reported dermatitis, chills and fever, as evidence of disseminated BCG, disease was noted (Table 2).

Total peripheral lymphocytes were measured and recorded before the start of therapy. There was statistical difference ($p = 0.03$) between the levels of pretherapy peripheral lymphocytes and the overall response rate, regardless of the type of systemic treatment. Patients with total peripheral lymphocytes of less than 1000/mm³ had a response rate of 24 percent, 1000–2000/mm³ had a response rate of 19 percent, while those with lymphocytes of greater than 2000/mm³ had a response of 32 percent. There was no difference in survival of patients as related to the levels of pretreatment total peripheral lymphocytes. No statistical difference in survival was found in patients who had complete or partial of stable disease and different levels of total lymphocytes.

Those patients with increasing disease and lymphocytes less than 1000/mm³ had median survival of 12 weeks, those with 1000–2000/mm³ had median survival of 19 weeks, and patients with total peripheral lymphocytes greater than 2000/mm³ had median survival of 15 weeks ($p = 0.03$).

No difference in the levels of pretherapy total lymphocytes and age, sex, incidence of metastatic sites, number of positive skin to PPD, Varidase, mumps, candida, dermatophyton and PHA were found.

A challenge to a battery of antigens to determine delayed hypersensitivity reaction were performed pretherapy and the results were recorded

Table 2. Type and Degree of Toxicity in the Three Treatment Groups

	BHD					BHD + BCG					DTIC + BCG				
	None	Mild	Mª Mod	S^b Sev	L.^{c} T.	None	Mild	M Mod	S Sev	L. T.	None	Mild	M Mod	S Sev	L. T.
Leukopenia	63	9	17	7	1	120	4	14	17	3	117	2	8	3	0
Thrombocytopenia	83	3	3	8	0	147	0	5	1	4	126	0	1	2	1
Nausea	52	5	35	5	0	82	7	51	16	1	49	8	55	18	0
Vomiting	54	5	33	5	0	85	7	51	14	0	50	8	55	16	1
Dermatitis	96	0	1	0	0	154	0	1	2	0	126	0	1	3	0
Chills/Fever	97	0	0	0	0	147	1	6	3	0	120	1	6	3	0

[a] Mod = moderate.

[b] Sev = severe.

[c] L.T. = life threatening.

(Table 3). Some of the patients who received BCG had repeated PPD testing during their treatment. No statistical significant differences were found between the overall response to therapy and the number of skin tests.

Survival was significantly better in patients with higher number of positive delayed hypersensitivity reaction, regardless of the therapy group (p = 0.05) (Figure 1). Patients with no positive skin tests (69) had a median survival of 26 weeks, those patients with one or two positive tests (138) had median survival of 32 weeks, while patients with three or more sensitive skin tests (74) had median survival of 48 weeks.

No significant difference in survival was found between patients with a negative or positive reaction to PPD (Figure 2), dermatophyton, Varidase or candida albicans. There were statistical differences, however, in the survival of patients with a positive reaction pretherapy to mumps antigen (p = 0.02) or to PHA (p = 0.02) as compared with those with negative tests.

Of those patients that were treated with BCG and chemotherapy arms and had a pretherapy PPD negative (47), 74 percent had changed to positive on a repeat test during treatment. Those 35 patients had a median survival of greater than 63 weeks, while those patients that remained PPD negative during the treatment had a median survival of 31 weeks (p = 0.01) (Figure 3).

No difference in the number of positive skin tests were found as it related to age of patients, sex, incidence of metastatic sites or the total pretherapy peripheral lymphocytes.

Discussion

In the systemic chemotherapy of patients with disseminated malignant melanoma, DTIC is the most extensively studied and consistently active single agent. In collective large studies, it has exhibited 12 percent to 30 percent remission rate.[1-3,13-15]

Table 3. Incidence of Positive Delayed Hypersensitivity Reactions in Disseminated Malignant Melanoma

Type	No. Tested	No. Positive	Percentage
PPD	125	31	25
Dermatophyton	244	66	27
Varidase	240	108	45
Candida	242	128	53
Mumps	195	104	53
PHA	92	41	46

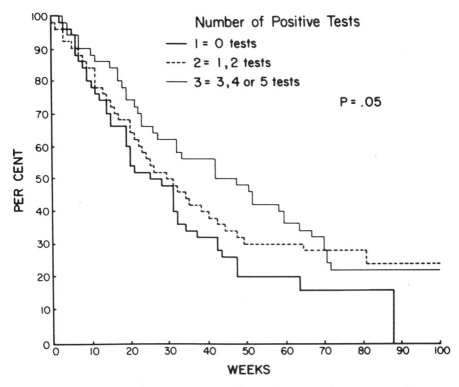

Figure 1. Survival in weeks of patients with malignant melanoma according to number of skin tests positivity.

Combination of DTIC with other agent(s) had been utilized and found to be somewhat more active against advanced melanoma than single agent.[10,11] In 1974 Gutterman et al.[12,16] reported a nonrandomized study using DTIC plus BCG in the treatment of patients with disseminated malignant melanoma. The results were compared with similar historic control at their institution. The remission rate for DTIC + BCG was 27 percent in 89 patients as compared to 15 percent response in a historic control group of 111 patients who received DTIC alone. The response rate of patients with nodal metastases was greater (55 percent) for the chemoimmunotherapy group as compared to 18 percent for the DTIC group. The duration of remissions and survival was significantly longer for patients treated with DTIC and BCG than for those treated with chemotherapy alone in the historic control group.

In a prospective randomized study, Ramseur et al.[17] did not find a difference in the response rate in patients with metastatic malignant melanoma treated with chemotherapy alone or chemoimmunotherapy consisting of methanol extracted residue of Bacillus Calmette-Guérin.

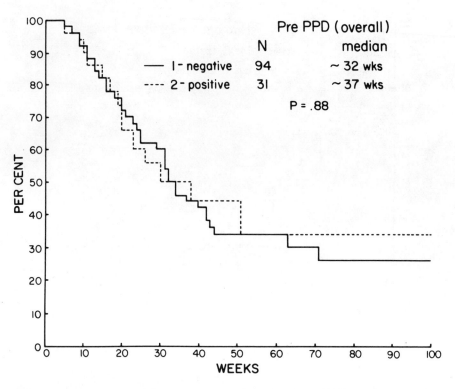

Figure 2. Survival in weeks of patients with pretherapy positive or negative PPD.

In our present prospectively randomized study carried at Southwest Oncology Group Study the response rate to DTIC plus BCG was 18 percent, no different than previously reported remission rate to DTIC alone in malignant melanoma.

At the same time the remission rate to combination of DTIC chemotherapy alone (BHD) or with BCG were superior to that of DTIC and immunotherapy (p = 0.05). Again no advantage of adding BCG to combined chemotherapy was found.

No difference in overall survival in the three groups was observed.

We note the differences in remission rate and survival that we found in certain subgroups. We believe that in future studies there may be a need to stratification according to those characteristics and these subgroup(s) need further study to prove such a difference with one therapy or another.

Adding BCG to the single agent chemotherapy or to combination chemotherapy did not alter drug toxicity, especially those caused by bone marrow suppression.

Many authors[18-22] reported various ranges of delayed hypersensitive responses to challenge of antigens in patients with malignant melanoma at different stages. Incidence of skin reaction to various antigens are found in Table 3.

Patients with higher number of positive tests had statistically longer survival, regardless of the type of therapy they received (Figure 2). Also, of interest, patients who changed from negative PPD pretherapy to positive reaction after chemotherapy had better survival than those patients remaining negative (Figure 3). Pretreatment determination of PPD positively did not influence the overall survival.

We believe that the results of the immune evaluation in patients with disseminated malignant melanoma done at times before systemic therapy are of interest, but did not help in designing future studies and were not consistently predicted prognosis in these patients.

We concluded that the addition of BCG and single agent chemotherapy or to combined chemotherapy is not superior to chemotherapy alone in patients with advanced melanoma.

Figure 3. Survival in weeks of patients treated with BCG and chemotherapy according to during therapy PPD skin test results.

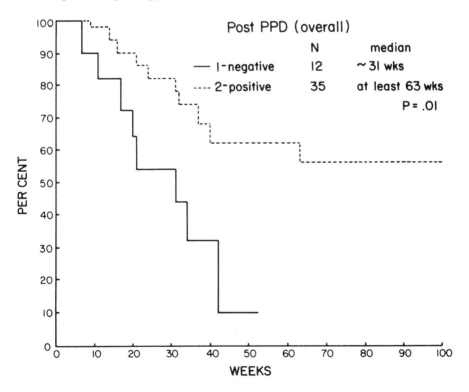

References

1. Nathanson, L, Wolter, J, Horton, J et al.: Characteristics of prognosis and response to an imidazole carboxamide in malignant melanoma. *Clin. Pharmacol. Ther.* 12:955–962, 1971.

2. Luce, JK, Thurman, WG, Isaacs, BL et al.: Clinical trials with the anti-tumor agent 5-(3,3-dimethyl-l-triazeno) imidazole-4-carboxamide (NSC-45388). *Cancer Chemother. Rep.* 54:119–124, 1970.

3. Cowan, DH, Bergsagel, DE: Intermittent treatment of metastatic malignant melanoma with high dose 5-(3,30-dimethyl-l-triazeno) imidazole-4-carboxamide (NSC-45388). *Cancer Chemother. Rep.* 55:175–181, 1971.

4. DeVita, V et al.: Clinical trials with 1,3-Bis-(2-chloroethyl)-nitrosourea (NSC-409962). *Cancer Res.* 25:1876–1881, 1965.

5. Gailani, S, Moon, J: Comparative study of DTIC and combination of BCNU and vincristine in the treatment of metastatic melanoma. *Proc. Am. Soc. Clin. Oncol.* (Abstract) 23, 1971.

6. Moon, J: Combination chemotherapy in malignant melanoma. *Cancer* 26:468–473, 1970.

7. Carter, SK, Newman, JW: Nitrosoureas: 1,3-Bis (2-chloroethyl)-3-1-nitrosourea (NSC-79037, CCNU N)-clinical brochure. *Cancer Chemother. Rep.* Part III, 1:151, 1968.

8. Bloedow, CE: Phase II studies of hydroxyurea in adults: miscellaneous tumor. *Cancer Chemother. Rep.* 40:39, 1964.

9. Thurman, WG et al.: Study of serum B_{12} and folate in patients treated with hydroxyurea. *Cancer Chemother. Rep.* 40:23, 1964.

10. Costanza, ME, Nathanson, L, Lenhard, R et al.: Therapy of malignant melanoma with an imidazole carboximide and dis-chloroethyl nitrosourea. *Cancer* 30:1457–1461, 1972.

11. Cohen, SM, Greenspan, EM, Weiner, MJ, Kabakow, B: Triple combination chemotherapy of disseminated malignant melanoma. *Cancer* 29:1489–1495, 1972.

12. Gutterman, JU, Mavligit, GM: Chemotherapy of disseminated malignant melanoma with DTIC and BCG. *Proc. Am. Assoc. Cancer Research and Am. Soc. Clin. Oncol.*, Abs. #792, p. 182, 1974.

13. Costanza, ME, Nathanson, L: (EOGC). Combination DTIC and methyl CCNU vs single agents in disseminated malignant melanoma: preliminary report. *Proc. Am. Assoc. Cancer Research and Am. Soc. Clinical Research*, Abs. #758, p. 173, 1974.

14. Wagner, DE, Ramiraz, G, Weiss, AJ et al.: Combination phase I–II study of imidazole carboxamide (NSC-45388). *Oncology* 26:310–316, 1972.

15. Luce, JK: Chemotherapy of malignant melanoma. *Cancer* 30:1604–1615, 1972.

16. Gutterman, JU, Mavligit, G, Gottlieb, JA et al.: Chemoimmunotherapy of disseminated malignant melanoma with dimethyl triazone imidazole carboxamide and Bacillus Calmette Guérin. *N. Engl. J. Med.* 291:592–597, 1974.

17. Ramseur, WL, Richards, F,II, Muss, HB et al.: Chemoimmunotherapy for disseminated malignant melanoma: a prospective randomized study. *Cancer Treat. Rep.* 62:1085–1087, 1978.

18. Pritchard, DJ, Ritts, RE Jr, Taylor, WF, Miller, GC: A prospective study of immune responsiveness in human melanoma. I. Assessment of initial pretreatment status with stage of disease. *Cancer* 41:2165–2173, 1978.

19. Catalona, WJ, Chretien, PB: Abnormalities of quantitative dinitrochlorobenzene sensitization in cancer patients: correlation with tumor stage and histology. *Cancer* 31:353–356, 1973.

20. Eilber, FR, Nizze, JA, Morton, DL: Sequential evaluation of general immune competence in cancer patients: correlation with clinical course. *Cancer* 35:660–665, 1975.

21. Morton, DL, Eilber, FR, Malmgren, R, Wood, WC: Immunological factors which influence response to immunotherapy in malignant melanoma. *Surgery* 68:158–163, 1970.

22. Ziegler, JL, Lewis, MG, Luyombya, JMS, Kinyabwire, JWM: Immunologic studies of patients with malignant melanoma in Uganda. *Brit. J. Cancer* 23:729–734, 1969.

Chemoimmunotherapy of Advanced, Recurrent Hodgkin's Disease: For the Cancer and Leukemia Group B

Vincent Vinciguerra, Morton Coleman, Thomas Pajek, Sameer Rafla

Department of Medicine, North Shore University Hospital, Manhasset, New York; Department of Medicine, New York Hospital, New York, New York; Department of Radiation Therapy, Methodist Hospital, Brooklyn, New York

Summary

One hundred and sixty-seven patients have been evaluated for a CALGB randomized treatment study of previously treated advanced Hodgkin's disease. Combination chemotherapy consisted of three arms with or without immunotherapy with MER. CVPP (CCNU, vinblastine, procarbazine, prednisone) was compared with a new combination, BAVS (bleomycin, Adriamycin, vincristine, streptozotocin). The third regimen consisted of alternating cycles of each regimen. At the current analysis, there is no significant difference in complete responses for each regimen, however, the alternating chemotherapy program shows less hematologic and GI toxicity. MER did not improve complete response frequency and actually resulted in significantly poorer survival for patients previously treated with chemotherapy. There was also no benefit with MER for patients with pretreatment positive skin tests. Because of the lack of therapeutic benefit and morbidity due to painful ulcers, MER treatment has been discontinued.

Introduction

The effectiveness of four-drug combination chemotherapy for advanced Hodgkin's disease has been shown repeatedly. Between 60–80 percent of untreated Stage III and Stage IV patients will achieve a complete remission with standard MOPP therapy.[1–3] Complete responses persist in 50–75 percent of these patients at the end of three years.[2] Previous cancer and leukemia Group B (CALGB) experience[4] has confirmed the effectiveness of four-drug programs showing 65 percent complete remission rates in untreated and treated patients. A combination employing CCNU, vinblastine, procarbazine and prednisone has been studied extensively and shown to be highly active when compared with MOPP.[5] Also, a new combination chemotherapy program consisting of bleomycin, vinblastine, doxorubicin (Adriamycin) and streptozotocin (BVDS) has demonstrated effectiveness in MOPP-resistant Hodgkin's disease patients.[6]

Preliminary observations using immunotherapy with the methanol extraction residue (MER) of BCG have suggested therapeutic effect when used with chemotherapy for patients with acute myelocytic leukemia and breast cancer.[7-10]

In 1975 a prospective randomized program was initiated by the CALGB to study combination chemotherapy and MER immunotherapy for previously treated Stage III and Stage IV Hodgkin's disease patients. This report principally discusses the results of the immunotherapy component of the study.

Materials and Methods

Patients with biopsy-proven Hodgkin's disease were studied after appropriate informed consent was obtained. All patients were Stage III or Stage IV and had previous treatment with radiation therapy or chemotherapy or both. Patients were randomized to receive either CVPP, BAVS or alternating form drug combinations with or without MER (Table 1). The doses for the CVPP program were: CCNU 75 mg/m² p.o. Day 1, vinblastine 4 mg/m² IV Days 1 and 8, procarbazine 100 mg/m² p.o. Days 1–14, and prednisone 40 mg/m² p.o. Days 1–14. The doses for BAVS were: bleomycin 5 units/m² IV Days 1 and 8, Adriamycin 50 mg/m² IV Day 1, vincristine 1.4 mg/m² IV Days 1 and 8 and streptozotocin 1500 mg/m² Days 1 and 8. Each two-week treatment period was followed by two weeks of rest and cycles were repeated monthly for 12 cycles.

The immunotherapy was administered monthly on the first day of the cycle with the chemotherapy. Pretreatment recall skin tests were carried out with PPD, dermatophytin and Varidase. A positive skin test was a 3mm or greater area of induration. MER was injected intradermally into nine injection sites preferably using the proximal thighs, upper and lower abdomen and intraclavicular areas. The doses injected ranged from 200 ug of MER to .01 ug. The titration sites were observed for one to three weeks after the initial administration of MER. The smallest dose of MER which produced areas of induration 1 cm in diameter with minimal or no central necrosis was used for subsequent courses of MER. That dose was injected intradermally into each of five sites drained by different

Table 1. CALGB Hodgkin's Disease

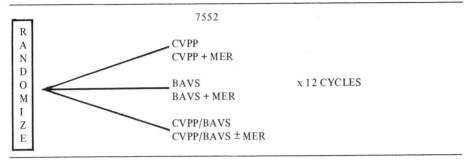

groups of lymph nodes. New injections were at least 1 cm distant from previous injections in the same area.

Complete remissions (CR) required complete regression of measurable lesions and disappearance of all other objective and subjective evidence of active disease. Partial remission (PR) meant an average decrease of measurable lesions to less than 50 percent of the pretreatment values over two successive measurement periods. Patients in PR who were actively continuing on protocol were considered in a special category (PR-cont) since they have the potential of achieving complete response.

Results

One hundred ninety-nine patients have been entered into the study and 167 are currently evaluable (Table 2). Since the program is still active and accruing patients, the results of the chemotherapy arms are coded. For purposes of analysis, the response frequency is separated into patients who received prior chemotherapy and those who did not. The

Table 2. Patient Entries

Coded Chemo.	Immuno	No. Patients Entered	No. Patients Eval.
P	No MER	33	31
	MER	34	27
Q	No MER	34	32
	MER	34	27
R	No MER	33	28
	MER	31	22
	Total	199	167

Table 3. Response by Chemotherapy Program and Prior Treatment

	Patients with no Prior C.T.		
Coded Rx	Total Eval.	CR No. (%)	PR – Cont No. (%)
P	27	16(59)	3(11)
Q	25	19(76)	4(16)
R	15	11(73)	1 (7)

overall complete response frequency for patients not receiving prior chemotherapy was 69 percent while 26 percent of patients previously treated with chemotherapy had complete responses. At the present time, there are no statistical differences comparing the three chemotherapy programs for patients with and without prior chemotherapy (Tables 3 and 4). The complete remissions for patients not receiving prior chemotherapy ranged from 59 percent to 76 percent. For patients who had had any previous chemotherapy, the complete response rates were between 17 percent and 33 percent.

The pretreatment patient characteristics for both immunotherapy groups with no prior chemotherapy are shown in Table 5. There were more patients in the no MER group and a higher percentage of these patients had liver involvement. In the MER group a greater percentage had B symptoms and lung involvement. The pretreatment characteristics for the patients with any prior chemotherapy were similar except for a higher mean age for the patients who did not receive MER (Table 6). The complete response frequency for patients who received no prior chemotherapy was 73 percent in patients not receiving MER and 63 percent for the MER patients. With prior chemotherapy treatment only, 22 percent of patients not receiving MER and 29 percent of MER patients had complete responses (Table 7).

Pretreatment skin testing with PPD, dermatophytin and Varidase was performed in 57 percent of the patients (Table 8). Of the 96 patients

Table 4. Response by Chemotherapy Program and Prior Treatment

	Patients with Any Prior C.T.		
Coded Rx	Total Eval.	CR No. (%)	PR – Cont No. (%)
P	30	5(17)	3(10)
Q	33	11(33)	2 (6)
R	35	9(26)	5(14)

Table 5. Pretreatment Characteristics of Immunotherapy Patient Groups

Characteristics	No Prior C.T.	
	No MER	MER
Total evaluated	40	27
Percent male	53	52
Mean age	34	36
Percent splenectomy	79	69
Percent stage III	32	28
Percent "B" symptoms	45	63
Percent liver involved	22	4
Percent lung involved	26	52
Percent bone marrow involved	17	16

initially skin tested, 24 percent had at least one positive test. The complete response frequency for the patients with at least one positive skin test is 60 percent versus 52 percent for patients with all negative tests ($p = .45$). Also, there is currently no significant difference in complete response frequency whether or not MER is used if the skin tests are not performed, initially positive or initially negative.

The survival for patients who had no prior chemotherapy is not altered by treatment with MER (Figure 1). However, in the prior chemotherapy patient group the patients receiving MER had a significantly poorer survival than those not receiving immunotherapy (Figure 2, $p = .01$).

Skin testing results and time to relapse were also analyzed and are shown in Figures 3 and 4 as time to failure. There are currently no apparent significant differences comparing the no prior chemotherapy

Table 6. Pretreatment Characteristics of Immunotherapy Patient Groups

Characteristics	Any Prior C.T.	
	No MER	MER
Total evaluated	50	48
Percent male	66	58
Mean age	40	33
Percent splenectomy	51	63
Percent stage III	17	11
Percent "B" symptoms	74	66
Percent liver involved	28	34
Percent lung involved	41	40
Percent marrow involved	17	21
Percent prior R.T.	76	75
Percent prior MOPP	52	58

Table 7. Response by Immunotherapy Program and Prior Treatment

Immunotherapy	Total Eval.	CR No. (%)	PR-Cont No. (%)	PR-Off No. (%)
		Patients With No Prior CT		
No MER	40	29 (73)	4 (10)	3 (8)
MER	27	17 (63)	4 (15)	5 (19)
		Patients With Any Prior CT		
No MER	50	11 (22)	9 (18)	15 (30)
MER	48	14 (29)	1 (2)	16 (33)

and prior chemotherapy patient groups and skin testing results with regard to time to failure.

Toxicity for the chemotherapy programs is mainly hematologic for the CVPP regimen and gastrointestinal with nausea and vomiting for BAVS. The toxicity for the alternating combinations has been of intermediate severity compared with the single combinations. MER toxicity has been mainly painful ulcerations (Table 9). The patients with at least one positive skin test experienced greater MER associated morbidity than patients with negative skin tests. The incidence of ulcers was significantly higher for the positive skin tested patients (93 percent) compared with the patients with negative skin tests (42 percent, $p = .02$).

Discussion

One of the most important factors in the evaluation of treatment programs for previously treated Hodgkin's disease patients is whether or not the patients received prior chemotherapy. Those patients not receiving prior chemotherapy had a greater chance of achieving complete remissions

Table 8. Pretreatment Skin Testing Results

Skin Test[a]	No. Not Done	Results		
		No. Eval.	Neg. %	Pos. %
Varidase	75	92	79	21
PPD	73	94	96	4
Dermatophytin	80	87	95	5

[a] Of the 96 patients who received at least one skin test, 24 percent had at least one positive test.

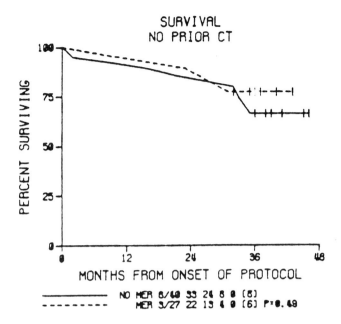

Figure 1.

Figure 2.

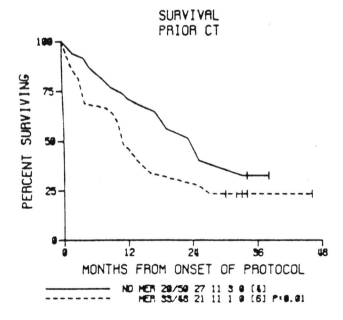

352

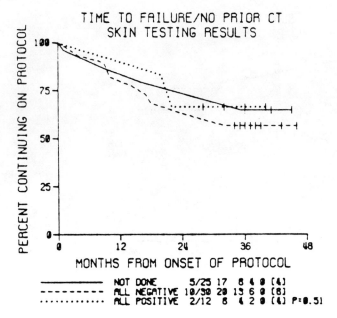

Figure 3.

Figure 4.

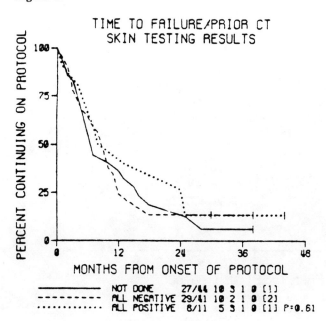

Table 9. Severity of MER Related Toxicities (Percent of Patients)

Complication	Total Eval.	Severity				
		0	1	2	3	4
Fever	60	85	8	7	0	0
Chills	61	95	3	0	2	0
Ulcers	61	34	7	38	21	0
Pain	58	76	10	12	2	0
Other	51	98	0	0	2	0

and the overall complete response frequency for all chemoimmunotherapy regimens was 69 percent. However, the complete responses for patients failing prior chemotherapy were only 26 percent. Our current results show that all three combination chemotherapy regimens are active in patients not previously treated and all are equally poor for patients who received prior chemotherapy. At the present time, no significant difference exists as to overall responses or survival comparing the three chemotherapy programs. The major advantage in the use of the alternating combinations is that there is less toxicity. The severity of the hematologic toxicity of the CVPP and the nausea and vomiting from BAVS is reduced when alternating cycles are used.

The addition of MER to the chemotherapy programs did not increase the complete response frequency. Although there were some differences in the pretreatment characteristics of the patient groups, some of these favored the MER group and others favored the no MER group and would not alter the results. In comparing the no prior chemotherapy group and prior chemotherapy patients no differences in complete responses are seen currently.

Analysis of skin test data suggests that the majority of these patients were immunosuppressed as only 24 percent reacted to one skin test. There was, however, no difference in complete responses whether the patients were skin test positive or negative.

Survival data are currently being evaluated. With followup approaching 48 months, there does not appear to be any improved survival as a result of the addition of MER for patients who had no prior chemotherapy. In the prior chemotherapy patient group, the patients receiving MER had a significantly poorer survival.

The toxicity of the immunotherapy program was severe and led at times to difficulties in patient compliance with the protocol. The major toxic effects of MER were painful ulcers which frequently required months to heal. Using serial dilutions of MER to detect minimal ulcers limited the severity of the toxicity to the immunotherapy. The patients who reacted most severely were those who had at least one positive skin test.

We conclude that the addition of MER failed to demonstrate any significant trend toward improvement in the therapeutic efficacy of the chemotherapy regimens. Because of the significant morbidity associated with this MER schedule, the MER has been discontinued.

References

1. DeVita, VT, Serpick, AA, Carbone, PP: Combination chemotherapy in the treatment of advanced Hodgkin's disease. *Ann. Int. Med.* 73:881–891, 1970.
2. Frei, E et al.: Combination chemotherapy in advanced Hodgkin's disease. *Ann. Int. Med.* 79:376–384, 1973.
3. Goldsmith, MA, Carter, SK: Combination chemotherapy of advanced Hodgkin's disease. *Cancer* 33:1–9, 1974.
4. Nissen, NI et al.: Chemotherapy of Hodgkin's disease in studies by acute leukemia group B. *Arch. Int. Med.* 131:396–407, 1973.
5. Cooper, MR, Spurr, CL, Glidewell, O et al.: The superiority of a nitrosourea (CCNU) containing four-drug combination over MOPP in the treatment of stages III and IV Hodgkin's disease. *Cancer* (in press).
6. Vinciguerra, V, Coleman, M, Jarowski, CI et al.: A new combination chemotherapy for resistant Hodgkin's disease. *JAMA* 237:33–35, 1977.
7. Bekesi, JG, Holland, JF, Cuttner, J et al.: Immunotherapy in acute myelocytic leukemia with neuraminidase treated allogeneic myeloblasts with or without MER. *Proc. Am. Assoc. Cancer Res.* 17:184, 1976.
8. Cuttner, J, Holland, JF, Bekesi, JG: Chemoimmunotherapy of acute myelocytic leukemia. *Proc. Am. Assoc. Cancer Res.* 16:264, 1975.
9. Weiss, DW: MER and other mycobacterial fractions in the immunotherapy of cancer. *Med. Clin. J. Am.* 60:473–497, 1976.
10. Perloff, M, Holland, J, Bekesi, JG: Chemoimmunotherapy of breast cancer. *Proc. Am. Assoc. Cancer Res.* 17:308, 1976.

Immune Responses and Recurrences in Stage II and III Breast Cancer Patients Undergoing Adjuvant Chemoimmunotherapy[a]

Myles P. Cunningham, Joseph A. Caprini, Miguel A. Oviedo, Eli Cohen, Barry Robinson, Edward F. Scanlon

Abraham Lincoln School of Medicine, University of Illinois, Chicago, Illinois; Saint Francis Hospital, Evanston, Illinois; Northwestern University Medical School, Chicago, Illinois; Evanston Hospital, Evanston, Illinois; Northwestern Memorial Hospital, Chicago, Illinois; Vogelback Computing Center, Northwestern Universidy, Evanston, Illinois

Summary

One hundred ninety-four patients who had had mastectomy for breast cancer were given repeated, adjuvant chemoimmunotherapy for one year in one of three treatment groups: L-Pam, cytoxan-fluorouracil-prednisone (CFP), or CFP plus BCG.

Recurrent breast cancer has been identified in 34 percent (13/38) L-Pam patients while for the same interval of enrollment and followup, proportion of recurrences have been 27 percent (13 of 78) for both CFP and CFP-BCG. Curves of recurrence rates for all three groups are now trending toward parallel slopes suggesting that CFP and CFP-BCG are equally effective in delaying appearance of recurrent disease. However, there is presently no statistically significant difference in proportion of recurrence among the three groups. PHA analysis and skin testing for DNCB and recall antigens failed to predict recurrences in all patients as well as in each treatment group.

No difference in proportion of recurrence, survival, morbidit) or peripheral white blood cell and platelet counts have been identified in

[a]This study was supported by the National Institutes of Health Contract (N.C.I.) NO1-CB-53917.

the CFP and CFP-BCG groups, regardless of menopausal status, tumor burden or other stratification factors suggesting no additive benefit of BCG to adjuvant polychemotherapy.

Introduction

Interest in adjuvant chemotherapy for breast cancer goes back many years and was directed initially at free circulating cancer cells, presumably dislodged during surgical manipulations of tumor.[1] Modern concepts of tumor pathogenesis consider that occult micrometastases already are present at first diagnosis in most instances of breast cancer and such occult metastases may be more than usually sensitive to either chemotherapeutic or immunologic manipulation. The early, encouraging reports by Fisher[2] and Bonadonna[3] using single and multiple drug adjuvant chemotherapy for breast cancer plus the developing use of immune manipulations in the care of patients with leukemia, melanoma and lymphoma[4-8] prompted us to attempt an evaluation of various chemotherapy programs with and without BCG in patients with loco-regionally advanced breast cancer.

Materials and Methods

From July 1, 1975, to June 30, 1979, 194 patients who had had either modified or radical mastectomy for Stage II or Stage III breast cancer were assigned to one of three treatment groups and received adjuvant chemotherapy or chemoimmunotherapy for one year. Prior to randomization, patients were stratified according to tumor size, presence of unfavorable local signs, extent of nodal involvement, menopausal status and treating institution (Table 1). To assure balance in the treatment arms with respect to prognostic factors, the minimization procedures described by Taves,[9] Pocock and Simon[10] were used to assign patients to one of three groups. To further assess comparability between treatment groups, a tumor burden index was formulated, derived by multiplying the greatest diameter of the tumor by the number of positive axillary nodes. Tumor burden, so defined, was found to be comparable for all three treatment groups.

The treatment groups consisted of L-phenylalanine mustard (L-Pam, Group I), cytoxan-fluorouracil-prednisone (CFP, Group II) and CFP-BCG (Group III). Patients received chemotherapy for five consecutive days once every six weeks for one year postoperatively. One half the patients receiving multi-drug therapy were inoculated with BCG, Tice strain by multi-puncture (Tine technique) on Days 21 and 28 of cycles I and II and Day 28 of each succeeding cycle (Figure 1).

Table 1. Stratification Factors and Distribution Among Treatment Groups in 194 Patients with Stage II and III Breast Cancer

| | Treatment Groups | | | |
	I	II	III	TOTALS
Factor 1 - Tumor size:				
Less than 3 CM	15	38	35	88
Greater than or equal to 3 CM	23	40	43	106
Factor 2 - Unfavorable local signs:				
Present	9	15	18	42
Absent	29	63	60	152
Factor 3 - Extent of nodal involvement:				
One to three nodes	23	45	45	113
Four or more nodes	15	33	33	81
Factor 4 - Menopausal status:				
Premenopausal	9	28	27	64
Postmenopausal	29	50	51	130
Factor 5 - Hospital:				
Evanston Hospital	13	32	34	79
Saint Francis Hospital	11	18	18	47
Northwestern Memorial Hospital	14	28	26	68

Each patient underwent a complete physical examination prior to enrollment, every six weeks during the first postoperative year and every three months thereafter. All patients received a comprehensive laboratory screening evaluation including chemistry survey, mammogram, chest X-ray and bone scan prior to initiating chemotherapy and at yearly anniversary dates thereafter.

CBC and platelet analyses were performed on Days one and 21 of each cycle and chemotherapeutic dose modifications were performed to achieve a WBC nadir of 1500–3000.

The first 105 patients enrolled underwent skin testing to the neoantigen DNCB and to four skin recall antigens prior to and at the completion of nine cycles of chemotherapy. The recall antigens were mumps, candida, varidase and PPD. Fifty-eight of the early patients also underwent serial phytohemagglutination (PHA) assays throughout the year of chemotherapy.

Enrollment to the L-Pam arm was ended with 38 patients at 112 weeks because of a perceived, high incidence of early recurrence. However, all patients assigned to the L-Pam arm completed nine full cycles of chemotherapy and all patients entering the study thereafter were enrolled in either the CFP or CFP-BCG.

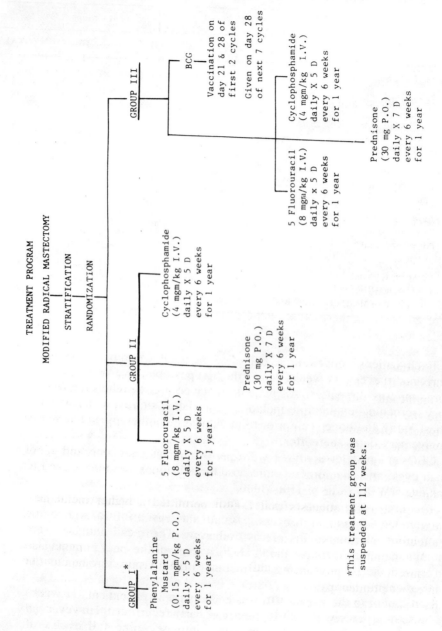

Figure 1. Treatment schema.

Statistical Analysis

The statistical analyses were carried out on a treatment failure time distribution (disease-free interval), proportion of recurrences and recurrence rate. Treatment failure time distributions were calculated by the actuarial method described by Berkson and Gage.[11] The test statistic to evaluate the failure time distributions among the treatment arms was the Gehan modification of the Wilcoxon test for censored data.[12] The proportion of recurrence and recurrence rates were subjected to a chi-square statistic associated with a contingency table and Cox's F statistic, respectively.

Results

Recurrences

All patients have been followed an average duration of 25 months with a range of followup of three to 46 months. Patients enrolled during the first 112 weeks (the L-Pam interval) have been followed an average of 36 months with a range of 24 to 46 months.

To date, recurrent cancer has been identified in 39/194 patients, a ratio of 20 percent; there have been 13 deaths from breast cancer and four deaths unrelated to breast cancer. Recurrent disease has been found in 34 percent (13/38) of L-Pam patients, while for the same interval of enrollment and followup, the incidence of recurrence is 27 percent (10/37) for CFP and 25.6 percent (10/39) for CFP-BCG. These ratios are not significantly different ($\chi^2 = .56$, p = .756). When all patients are followed to the present time, recurrence proportions for Groups II and III are exactly the same at 17 percent (13/78 in each group). When compared with the recurrence proportion for L-Pam treated patients (34 percent), Group II and III recurrence ratios are not quite significantly different (p = .0653). It now appears that ultimate recurrence incidences are quite similar for the three treatment groups. However, attention to recurrence curves strongly suggests that L-Pam permitted a higher incidence of early recurrences and that, conversely, CFP and CFP-BCG were equally effective in extending disease-free intervals (Figure 2).

When analyzed for recurrence proportions with respect to menopausal status, no difference among the three treatment groups can be identified in either premenopausal or postmenopausal patients (Figures 3 and 4). In particular, the recurrence curves in premenopausal patients are almost concordant among the three treatment groups. In postmenopausal patients, there is a trend to early identification of recurrent disease in the L-Pam treatment group, but no statistically significant difference in recurrence proportion is seen at 200 weeks.

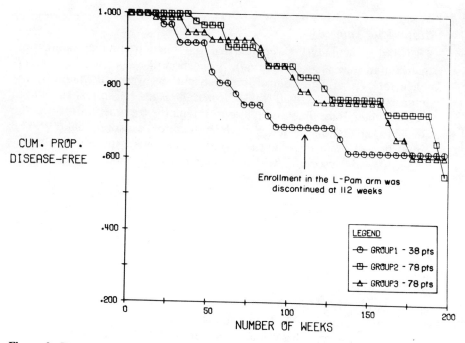

Figure 2. Recurrence curves for entire study population—194 patients.

Figure 3. Recurrence curves in 64 premenopausal patients.

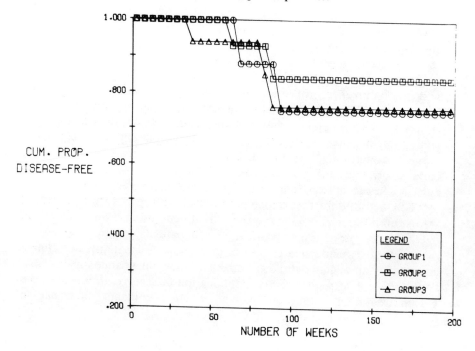

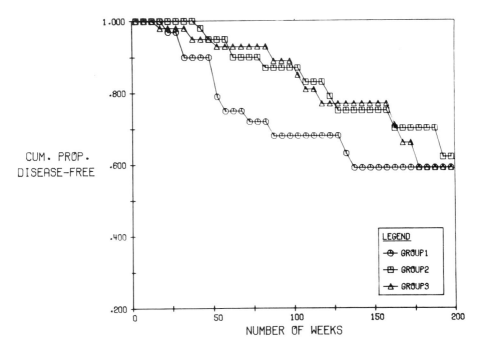

Figure 4. Recurrence curves in 130 postmenopausal patients.

Skin Test Data

One hundred and five patients were evaluable for results of skin testing. Approximately 50 percent of patients had at least one positive response to each antigen (Table 2), while 89 percent had at least one positive response to any antigen (Table 3).

When skin test reactivity was measured against cancer recurrence, no correlation could be identified (Table 2). This lack of correlation between skin test reactivity and recurrent disease was true not only for the entire population, but also for each individual treatment group as well as for

Table 2. Results of Skin Testing and Corresponding Recurrence Proportions

Skin Test	(+)	(%)	Proportion of Recurrence (%)	(−)	(%)	Proportion of Recurrence (%)
DNCB	62	59%	33.87%	43	41%	23.25%
Mumps	64	39%	15.87%	41	61%	51.21%
Candida	43	41%	30.23%	62	59%	29.03%
Varidase	69	66%	33.33%	36	34%	22.22%
PPD	56	53%	28.57%	49	47%	30.61%

(+) Response = 1 positive reaction to antigen at any time.

Table 3. Reactivity to Skin Tests

		Recurrence Proportion
No. patients negative to all antigens	= 12 (11%)	33%
No. patients showing at least one positive reaction to any antigen	= 93 (89%)	29%

p = .6573.

each antigen. In particular, recurrence rates were not statistically different among DNCB positive and negative patients (Table 4). Curiously, the few (13) patients who had at least one positive response to every antigen—i.e., a singularly reactive subgroup—had the highest proportion of recurrent cancer, 62 percent (Table 5). This difference was statistically significant (p = .007), but can probably be explained on the basis of the small number of patients.

PHA Results

Serial measurements of PHA were performed on 58 patients enrolled during the first 18 months of the study. These results could be grouped according to changes in the index measured at various intervals throughout the year of chemotherapy and drawn at the beginning of a cycle prior to administration of chemotherapy. Patients were classified as to increasing, decreasing or unchanging indices (Table 6). About one half of the group showed an increase in PHA assays. No difference in incidence of recurrence could be identified in each of the three groups (Table 7), nor could differences in recurrences be recognized when analyzed in each group according to treatment modality although the latter numbers are quite small (Table 8). A somewhat higher number of patients with larger tumor burdens was found in the group showing increases in PHA assay (Table 9). One might speculate that as both surgery and chemotherapy reduced tumor burdens, PHA ratios tended to rise.

Table 4. Reactivity to DNCB and Corresponding Recurrence Proportions

	(+) Skin Test		(−) Skin Test	
	No.	%	No.	%
No recurrence	41	66%	33	77%
Recurrence	21	34%	10	23%
Totals (105)	62	(59%)	43	(41%)

p = .2410.

Table 5. Proportion of Recurrence in Patients Highly Reactive to Antigens

		Proportion of Recurrence
No. of patients with at least one (+) reaction to all antigens	= 13	62%
No. patients not (+) to all antigens	= 92	25%

p = .0069.

BCG Response

Most, but not all, applications of BCG result in local skin reactions characterized by small pustules, vesicles and erythema. We thought it worthwhile to measure cancer recurrence against the frequency of positive skin reactions to BCG as well as against the frequency of negative reactions. These analyses suggest that the greater number of recurrences tend to occur in patients having the most frequently positive skin responses to BCG (Table 10). Conversely, all 12 recurrences occurred in patients having either no negative skin responses (nine) or only two negative responses (Table 11).

Toxicity

Toxicity was moderate, generally well tolerated and limited to alopecia, nausea, fatigue and mild marrow depression. One patient of the 194 suffered a severe episode of leucopenia-thrombocytopenia associated with sepsis which required hospitalization. She recovered and has remained free of disease. Toxicity was further limited by dose attenuation, where appropriate, but almost all patients completed nine full cycles of chemotherapy. Toxicity was not appreciably different between treatment groups except that fatigue and alopecia were more severe in polychemotherapy patients while thrombocytopenia was more intense in L-Pam

Table 6. Results of PHA Assays

		PHA Groups		
		Increase	Decrease	No Change
Group I	(16)	4	7	5
Group II	(23)	12	8	3
Group III	(19)	14	1	4
Total	(58)	30 (52%)	16 (28%)	12 (20%)

Table 7. Proportion of Recurrence in PHA Groups

	PHA Assays		
	Increase	Decrease	No Change
Recurrences Total = 17	9	5	3
Proportion of recurrence	9/30=33%	5/16=31%	3/12=25%

treated patients (Figure 5). Except for local skin reaction, no difference in toxicity was identified in patients receiving BCG in addition to chemotherapy.

Discussion

The proper role of adjuvant chemotherapy for Stages II and III breast cancer is still uncertain. Although the initial reports of the cooperative chemotherapy trials were promising,[2,3] a longer experience has failed to show any significant benefit except for premenopausal women with limited axillary node metastases.[13,14] The proper role of immunotherapy is even more obscure. Gutterman et al.[15] noted longer remission-induction and survival for patients with advanced breast cancer treated with a combination of fluorouracil-Adriamycin-cytoxan (FAC) plus BCG when compared with a similar group of patients treated with FAC alone.[16] The same group reported an increased two-year survival in patients with Stages II and III breast cancer receiving FAC-BCG as adjuvant treatment when compared with a group of recent historic controls.[17]

In a study similar to our own, Ahmann[18] and colleagues identified L-Pam as distinctly inferior to CFP or CFP plus radiotherapy, but only in premenopausal patients. Disease-free intervals were significantly shorter

Table 8. Recurrence by Treatment in PHA Group

Treatment	Groups	PHA Assay		
		Increase	Decrease	No Change
Group I	(6)	1	3	2
Group II	(7)	5	2	0
Group III	(4)	3	0	1
	(17)	9	5	3

Table 9. Recurrent Cancer in PHA Groups Analyzed for Tumor Burden

| PHA Groups | Range of Tumor Burdens[a] | |
	Recurrences	Nonrecurrences
Increase	1.9 - 234.0	0.6 - 84.0
Decrease	3.0 - 63.0	1.4 - 24.5
No change	8.0 - 60.0	1.8 - 22.0

[a] Tumor burden index defined as number of positive nodes X greatest diameter of primary tumor.

Table 10. Recurrence Classified by Positive Skin Reaction to BCG

No. of Positive Skin Reactions to BCG	No. of Patients	No. of Recurrences
0	1	1
1	2	0
2	4	0
3	2	0
4	5	0
5	1	1
6	3	1
7	3	0
8	5	1
9	15	4
10	10	2
11	13	2

Table 11. Recurrence Classified by Negative Skin Reaction to BCG

No. of Negative Skin Reactions to BCG	No. of Patients	No. of Recurrences
0	43	9
1	11	0
2	4	3
3	2	0
4	1	0
5	0	0
6	2	0
7	1	0

366

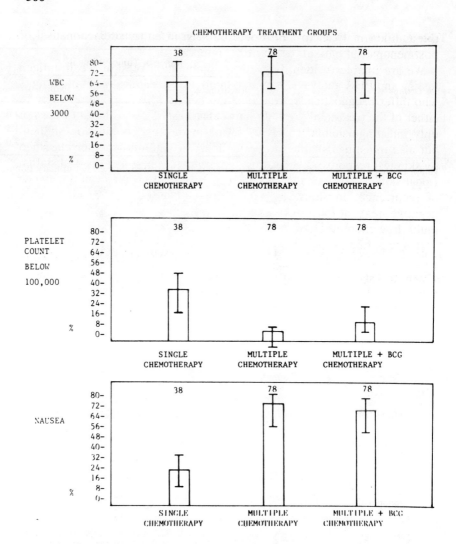

Figure 5. Toxicity in chemotherapy groups.

for premenopausal patients treated with L-Pam versus those treated with CFP with or without radiotherapy and mortality tended to be higher. No such differences prevailed in postmenopausal patients.

In a comparable number of premenopausal patients, we detect no difference among L-Pam, CFP and CFP-BCG treated patients. Differences in recurrence proportions were confined to postmenopausal patients where a higher number of recurrences in the L-Pam group was detected at 26 months but not at 48. The data are also at variance with the clinical trials of both Bonadonna and Fisher.[13,14] No benefit from the addition of BCG to CFP could be seen in either premenopausal or postmenopausal patients at any time interval.

We are unable to identify, with a combination of skin recall antigen testing and PHA analyses, any immunologically unique subset of patients who differ prognostically from one another or who respond uniquely to either of the treatment arms. In particular, results of CFP-BCG were not only indistinguishable from CFP alone in the total population studied, but also indistinguishable in every subset of patients whether classified by skin test response, PHA ratios, treatment group or menopausal status. Local skin reaction or the lack of it to BCG had no effect on incidence of recurrence. In short, we can ascribe no effect, either positive or negative, (except local skin reactions) to the use of BCG when added to multi-drug chemotherapy.

It is tempting to speculate, based on the improved, cumulative disease-free interval in the multi-drug groups, that either more drugs or more effective drugs in combination or more sophisticated immune manipulations would permit longer disease-free intervals. However, until all patients presently enrolled in clinical trials are followed to significant observations on *survival,* the merit of such theses must remain essentially conjectural.

References

1. DeLarue, NC: The free cancer cell. *Can. Med. Assoc. J.* 82:1175–1183, 1960.

2. Fisher, B, Carbone, P, Economou, SG et al.: L-phenylalanine mustard in management of breast cancer. A report of early findings. *N. Eng. J. Med.* 292:117–122, 1975.

3. Bonadonna, G, Brusamolino, E, Valagussa, P: Combination chemotherapy as an adjuvant treatment on operable breast cancer. *N. Eng. J. Med.* 294:405, 1976.

4. Mathé, G, Amiel, JL, Schwarzenberg, L et al.: Active immunotherapy for acute lymphoblastic leukemia. *Lancet* 1:697, 1969.

5. Mathé, G: Active immunotherapy. *Adv. Cancer Res.* 14:1–36, 1971.

6. Morton, DL, Eilber, SR, Holmes, EC et al.: BCG immunotherapy of malignant melanoma: summary of a seven-year experience. *Ann. Surg.* 180:635–643, 1974.

7. Bast, RC, Zbar, B, Borsos, T, Ratp, H: BCG and cancer. *N. Eng. J. Med.* 290:1413–1420 and 1458–1469, 1974.

8. Sokal, JE, Aungst, CW, Snyderman, M: Delay on progression of malignant lymphoma after BCG vaccination. *N. Eng. J. Med.* 291:1226–1230, 1974.

9. Taves, DR: Minimization: a new method of assigning patients to treatment and control groups. *Clin. Pharm. Ther.* 15(5):443–453, 1974.

10. Pocock, SJ, Simon, R: Sequential treatment assignment with balancing for prognostic factors in the controlled clinical trail. *Biometrics* 31:103–115, 1975.

11. Berkson, J, Gage, R: Calculation of survival rates for cancer. *Proc. Mayo Clin.* 25:270, 1950.

12. Gehan, E: A generalized Wilcoxon test for comparing arbitrarily single-censored samples. *Biometrika* 52:203–224, 1965.

13. Bonadonna, G, Rossi, A, Valagussa, P et al.: CMF program for operative breast cancer with positive axillary nodes. *Cancer* 39:2904–2915, 1977.

14. Fisher, B, Glass, A, Redmond, C et al.: L-phenylalanine mustard (L-Pam) in the management of primary breast cancer: an update of earlier findings and a comparison with those utilizing L-Pam plus 5-fluorouracil (5-FU). *Cancer* 39:2883–2903, 1977.

15. Gutterman, JU, Cardenas, JO, Blumenschein, GR et al.: Chemoimmunotherapy of advanced breast cancer. Prolongation of remission and survival with BCG. *Br. Med. J.* 2:1222–1225, 1976.

16. Blumenschein, GR, Cardenas, JO, Freireich, EJ, Gottlieb, JA: FAC chemotherapy for breast cancer. *Proc. Am. Soc. Clin. Oncol.* March, 1974.

17. Bezdar, AU, Gutterman, JU, Blumenschein, GR et al.: Intensive postoperative chemoimmunotherapy for patients with Stage II and Stage III breast cancer. *Cancer* 41:1064–1075, 1978.

18. Ahmann, D, Scanlon, PW, Bisel, HF et al.: Repeated adjuvant chemotherapy with phenylalanine mustard of 5-fluorouracil, cyclophosphamide, and prednisone with or without radiation, after mastectomy for breast cancer. *Lancet,* April 29, pp. 893–896, 1978.

Review of Multiple Nonspecific Immunotherapeutic Agents in Combination with FAC Chemotherapy of Stage IV Breast Cancer

George R. Blumenschein, Gabriel Hortobagyi,
Aman U. Buzdar, Alfred Distefano,
Jordan U. Gutterman, Evan M. Hersh

Medical Breast Section, Department of Medicine, The University of Texas System Cancer Center M.D. Anderson Hospital and Tumor Institute, Houston, Texas; Immunology Section, Department of Developmental Therapeutics, The University of Texas System Cancer Center M.D. Anderson Hospital and Tumor Institute, Houston, Texas

Summary

The sequential investigation of nonspecific immunotherapeutic agents (Bacillus Calmette-Guérin (BCG), methanol extracted residue of BCG (MER), levamisole, levamisole plus BCG combination and *C. parvum*) in combination with 5-fluorouracil, Adriamycin and cyclophosphamide (FAC) have demonstrated a remission duration and an overall survival benefit for patients who respond to chemotherapy as compared with those patients treated with FAC chemotherapy alone. Duration response improvement between responders treated with FAC plus immunotherapy as compared with those treated with FAC alone is five months. The survival duration benefit for FAC and immunotherapy treated responders as opposed to FAC alone treated patients is on the order of eight to 10 months. No remission induction benefit is evident from the use of nonspecific immunotherapy in combination with FAC.

A sequential repetition of the original FAC study without immunotherapy conducted five years following the initial FAC study confirmed the remission duration and survival associated with FAC chemotherapy administered without nonspecific immunotherapy. While nonspecific immunotherapy provides remission duration and survival advantage to chemotherapy treated patients, this advantage is dependent upon the effectiveness of chemotherapy and its ability to induce significant reduction in tumor burden. Benefits to be derived from nonspecific immunotherapy are therefore totally dependent upon other effective tumor reducing therapeutic measures.

Introduction

Over a five-year period, M.D. Anderson investigators have conducted a number of clinical studies of the use of nonspecific immunotherapy in combination with multiple drug chemotherapy for the treatment of metastatic breast cancer. [1-5]

The chemotherapy has consisted of variations of the 5-fluorouracil, Adriamycin, cyclophosphamide, (FAC)[6] treatment program and has included, in addition, methotrexate and vincristine.

Adriamycin in each therapeutic program has been used in a dose of $50mg/m^2$ every 21 days in combination with cyclophosphamide. The nonspecific immunotherapeutic or immunomodulating agents investigated in these trials were Bacillus Calmette-Guérin (BCG) (lyophylized Pasteur or Connaught),[1] levamisole (LMS),[2] *Corynebacterium parvum* (CP),[3] methanole extraction residue of BCG (MER),[4] Pseudomonas vaccine (PV)[3] (a heptavalent lipopolysaccharide preparation from Pseudomonas aeruginosa) and BCG plus LMS in combination.[5]

Details of the separate chemoimmunotherapy programs are shown in Table 1. Additional information about the separate combination chemotherapy programs may be found in respective references.

Table 1. Dose, Route, and Schedule of Immunotherapy (I.T.) Used in Combination with Chemotherapy (C.T.) for the Treatment of Metastatic Breast Cancer

C.T.	I.T.	Dose	Route	Schedule
FAC	BCG	6×10^8 organisms	Scarification	Day 9, 13, and 17 of 21-day cycle
FAC	LMS	$100mg/m^2$	p.o.	Day 9, 10, 13, 14, 17, and 18 of 21-day cycle
FAC	CP	$2mg/m^2$	i.v.	Day 9, and 16 of 21-day cycle initially and every 63 days 14-day intensive course
VAC FUM	MER	$0.5mg/m^2$	Subcutaneous	Day 8 and 15 of each VAC course and Day 9, 16, and 23 of each FUM course
FAC + M	PV	$0.5mg/m^2$	Subcutaneous	Day 7, 12, and 17 of 21-day cycle
FAC	BCG +	6×10^8 organisms	Scarification	Day 9, 13, and 17
	LMS	$100mg/m^2$	p.o.	Day 9, 10, 13, 14, 17, and 18 of 21-day cycle

Evaluation of Response

In these studies a complete remission (CR) was defined as complete disappearance of all objective and subjective evidence of disease including complete recalcification of bone lesions on X-ray; a partial remission (PR) was interpreted as a 50 percent or greater reduction in the product of the greatest diameter of measurable lesions and/or partial recalcification of bone metastasis. Patients with less than 50 percent reduction or less than 25 percent increase in tumor size for a period of at least two months were considered to have stable disease provided no new lesions appeared during that time; progression or relapse was defined as more than a 25 percent increase in existing tumor masses or the appearance of any new lesions.

Remission duration was determined from the date remission was achieved until the date of progression or relapse. Survival was measured from the start of treatment to the date of death or the last followup examination.

Comparative Treatment Group

For the purpose of more rapid accumulation of information about the therapeutic effect and the toxicity of these nonspecific immunomodulating agents, these clinical trials were conducted in sequence and compared with the original FAC study. Because of criticism of this clinical trial strategy and because 14 responding patients were excluded from the initial FAC study (1973), a second FAC (1978) study was conducted five years after the first. The results of this repeat trial of FAC compare exactly with the initial FAC (1973) in response rate (73 percent *vs* 75 percent), median duration of response (nine months) (Figure 1) and median duration of survival, sixteen months. When comparisons in this text are made with the results of FAC chemotherapy without immunotherapy, they refer to FAC (1973) confirmed by this later trial.

The Chi-Square test was used to compare response rates in different trials. The Kaplan and Meier method was used to calculate and plot remission and survival curves[7] and a generalized Wilcoxon test with a two-tailed analysis was used to test differences between remission and survival curves.[8]

Results

There was no significant variation in CR and PR among the chemoimmunotherapy trials, with significant numbers of evaluable patients and acceptable evaluable/entered patient population, e.g., FAC BCG, FAC LMS, VAC-FUM MER, and FAC LMS BCG (Table 2). In these studies, CR ranged from 14 to 22 percent and PR ranged from 44 to 59 percent.

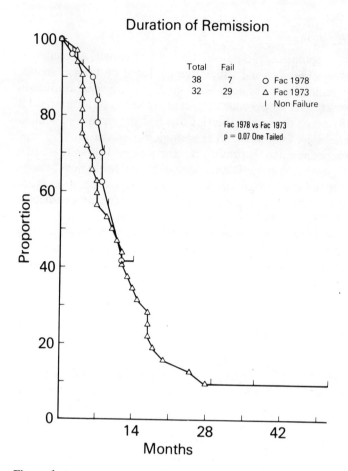

Figure 1.

The median duration of remissions in these chemoimmunotherapy clinical studies compared favorably with FAC alone (Figure 2).

Comparisons between chemoimmunotherapy trials showed no advantage from any single or combined nonspecific immunomodulators for prolonging remissions.

The median remission time was three to five months greater for metastatic breast cancer patients treated with chemoimmunotherapy (12.5 to 14 months) than was the remission time for FAC alone treated patients (nine months) (Table 3). While there was never a significant difference in median length of complete remission between FAC patients and chemoimmunotherapy patients, approximately one in five CRs are enjoying continued complete remissions beyond two years. Unfortunately, patients in this category who received FAC alone in the original

Table 2. Metastatic Breast Cancer Rate of Response

	FAC No. Pts. (%)	FAC BCG No. Pts. (%)	FAC LMS No. Pts. (%)	FAC CP No. Pts. (%)	VAC-FUM MER No. Pts. (%)	FAC + M PV No. Pts. (%)	FAC BCG + LMS No. Pts. (%)
Number of evaluable patients	44	105	114	14	96	16	117
Complete remission	6(14)	20(19)	15(13)	1(7)	21(22)	3(19)	19(16)
Partial remission	26(59)	60(57)	57(59)	6(43)	42(44)	11(69)	66(56)
Stable	12(27)	19(18)	26(23)	6	23(24)	2(12)	27(23)
Progressive	—	6(6)	6(5)	—	10(10)	—	5(4)
CR + PR	32(73)	80(76)	82(72)	7(50)	63(66)	14(88)	85(72)

FAC = 5-fluorouracil, Adriamycin, cyclophosphamide; BCG = Bacillus Calmette-Guérin; LMS = levamisole; CP = *Corynebacterium parvum*; MER = methanol extraction residue of BCG; PV = Pseudomonas vaccine.

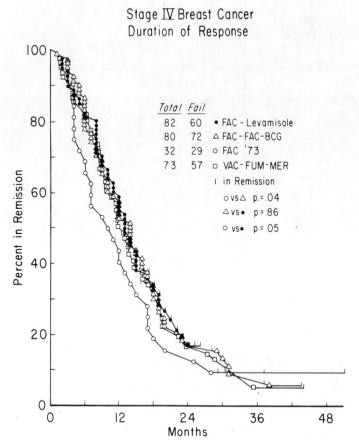

Figure 2.

study are too few to make a valid comparison, and the more recent FAC alone trial has not sufficiently matured to make observations about the possible influence of nonspecific immunotherapy on the prolongation of complete remission for a subset of patients.

Survival would be assumed to be a less reliable parameter for comparison among these trials begun over a four-year period (1973-1977) and conducted over six years. During this time, modest yet productive gains have been made in second line chemotherapy and it could be assumed that this has given some survival advantage to patients in more recent studies. The similar fifteen to sixteen month median survival of the original FAC (1973) and the more recent FAC (1978) argue against this assumption. Median duration of survival for responders treated with chemoimmunotherapy (23.8 to 28.6 months) exceeded by more than seven months the median duration of survival of the FAC alone treated group of patients (Table 3).

Patients who did not achieve CR or PR in any of these studies had shortened survivals which were not benefited by the addition of nonspecific immunotherapy.

Toxicity

It was in the area of toxicity that the greatest distinctions could be drawn between the nonspecific immunotherapy programs. Toxicity secondary to FAC chemotherapy has been thoroughly described. [1,5]

Each immunotherapeutic agent had its unique side effects. Those associated with BCG were mild and consisted mainly of local soreness, pruritus, low-grade fever and ill-defined flu-like syndrome for 12 to 24 hours following each scarification. All of these symptoms were self-limited. After prolonged administration of BCG, local and systemic reaction became stronger, especially in responding patients. In 30 percent of these patients the dose of immunotherapeutic agent was reduced to prevent excessive reaction. A generalized rash with a histologic picture of hypersensitivity vasculitis occurred in three patients. No disseminated BCG disease was observed.[1]

Levamisole was extremely well tolerated and the incidence of side effects associated with this drug was small. Nausea and vomiting were the most commonly observed symptoms while a variety of other subjective and objective disturbances were reported by a small number of patients. A dose reduction of levamisole had to be carried out in seven percent of the patients to decrease or eliminate excessive gastrointestinal or neurologic side effects. Only five percent of patients had to discontinue levamisole for reasons related to toxicity.[2] Immunotherapeutic side

Table 3. Median Duration Remission and Survival FAC and FAC Plus Nonspecific Immunotherapy

	Median Duration Remission (Mo.)	Median Survival of Responders (Mo.)
FAC '73	9	16
FAC '78	9	15+
FAC BCG	14	23.8
FAC LMS	13	28.6
VAC-FUM MER	12.5	24
FAC BCG + LMS	14	28+

effects associated with the BCG and levamisole combination program could be separated into the respective immunotherapeutic agents.[5]

The administration of MER was complicated by severe local and occasionally severe systemic toxicity. More than 70 percent of patients developed ulceration at the site of the subcutaneous injection of MER. For this reason, 16 patients received only one dose. The draining ulcers persisted for many months with a median duration of approximately three months. Their presence required frequent alteration of schedule and reduction of dose. Two patients developed superinfection of the extensive ulcerative lesions related to MER. One patient had incapacitating pain related to the ulceration for a two-week period.[4]

C. parvum had associated temperature elevations which required analgesics and occasional hypothermic measures to maintain body temperature at or below the 103° F level. Because the FAC C. parvum trial was limited because of early exhaustion of the supply of Corynebacterium parvum, sufficient and comprehensive data are not available about its toxicity.[3]

The pseudomonas vaccine study was complicated by extreme hematologic toxicity associated with the use of L-Asparaginase and methotrexate. An unacceptably high incidence of sepsis associated with granulocytopenia resulted in a significant number of patients being withdrawn from this protocol early in its course. For example, only 15 of 20 patients who received the pseudomonas vaccine took a second course of chemotherapy at the initially prescribed dose. By the fourth course, more than half of the patients had been removed completely from the study. Toxicity that was related to pseudomonas vaccine was also significant. It consisted of pain and tenderness at the site of injection, and fever and chills. Because of this, the dose and schedule of the pseudomonas vaccine was altered significantly. At the end of six months only 12 percent of the patients initially begun on FAC methotrexate pseudomonas vaccine remained on the study.[3]

Discussion

In the trials reviewed, the addition of nonspecific immunotherapy to effective chemotherapy for metastatic breast cancer has resulted in modest, but definite therapeutic benefit. Patients treated with FAC plus nonspecific immunotherapy, who achieve at least a 50 percent reduction in measured metastatic breast cancer volume, have significantly longer remissions and survivals than do patients receiving FAC chemotherapy alone.

Unfortunately, these kinds of results have not been observed consistently in numerous other trials of combination chemotherapy and nonspecific immunotherapy for metastatic breast cancer.[9-17] As a result, a healthy skepticism prevails about the general clinical application of nonspecific immunotherapy for breast cancer.[18]

The reason or reasons for the widely conflicting results reported from trials of BCG, *C. parvum*, MER and levamisole in combination with chemotherapy are unclear. Obvious difficulty arises because the data have not been reported uniformly in a manner which allows comparison of dose, dose rate and total dose of both chemotherapeutic and immunotherapeutic agents. Because of its significant relationship to response[19] the distribution of tumor burden in populations of breast cancer patients undergoing clinical study needs careful definition. Identification of this parameter is another critical factor missing in reports of many of these trials.

After careful consideration of the large number of patients reported in this review, it is clear that uniform therapy of metastatic breast cancer with effective drugs, in therapeutic doses, administered at optimum dose rate, over a significant period of time results in a very predictable PR and CR in a population of patients. While the addition of nonspecific immunotherapy to this program does not result in altered remission rate, it does prolong the duration of the remissions. For these same patients longer survival appears to be an accompanying benefit. When tumor is not influenced significantly by chemotherapy, nonspecific immunotherapy gives no apparent therapeutic advantage.

References

1. Hortobagyi, G et al.: Combination chemoimmunotherapy of metastatic breast cancer with 5-fluorouracil, Adriamycin, cyclophosphamide, and BCG. *Cancer* 43(4): 1225-1233, 1979.

2. Hortobagyi, G et al.: Combined chemoimmunotherapy for advanced breast cancer: a comparison of BCG and levamisole. *Cancer* 43(3):1112-1122, 1979.

3. Hortobagyi, G et al.: Chemoimmunotherapy of metastatic breast cancer with 5-FU, doxorubicin, cyclophosphamide, methotrexate, *Corynebacterium parvum* and pseudomonas vaccine. *Cancer Treatment Report* (in press), 1979.

4. Hortobagyi, G et al.: Alternating noncross-resistant combination chemotherapy and active nonspecific immunotherapy with BCG or MER-BCG for advanced breast cancer. *Cancer* (in press), 1979.

5. Hortobagyi, G et al.: Response of disseminated breast cancer to combined modality treatment with chemotherapy and levamisole with or without Bacillus Calmette-Guérin. *Cancer Treatment Reports* 62(11):1685-1692, 1978.

6. Blumenschein, GR et al.: FAC chemotherapy for breast cancer, *Proc. Am. Assoc. Clin. Oncol.* 15:193, 1974.

7. Kaplan, EL, Meier, P: Nonparametric estimation from incomplete observations. *J. Am. Stat. Assoc.* 53:457-481, 1958.

8. Gehan, EA: A generalized Wilcoxon test for comparing arbitrarily singly-censored samples. *Biometrica* 52:203–223, 1965.

9. Haskell, C et al.: Cyclosphamide, methotrexate and 5-fluorouracil with and without

Corynebacterium Parvum in the treatment of metastatic breast cancer. In: Crispen, RG, ed. *Neoplasm Immunity: Solid Tumor Therapy,* Franklin Institute Press, Philadelphia, 1977.

10. Israel, L: A randomized study of chemotherapy versus chemotherapy and immune therapy with *Corynebacterium parvum* in advanced breast cancer. In: Milano, A, ed. *Conferences, Symposium, Workshops of the XI International Cancer Congress,* Vol. I, 1974.

11. Klefstrom, P: Levamisole in addition to chemotherapy in advanced breast cancer. In: Rainer, H, ed. *Immunotherapy of Malignant Diseases,* Springer-Verlag, New York, 1978.

12. Mayr, AC et al.: Randomized trial in advanced breast cancer using combination chemotherapy with or without *C. parvum:* preliminary results. In: Rainer, H, ed. *Immunotherapy of Malignant Diseases,* Springer-Verlag, New York, 1978.

13. Mercurio, T et al.: A comparison of 5-fluorouracil, Adriamycin, cytoxan (FAC) chemotherapy with chemoimmunotherapy using *C. parvum* ± BCG in advanced breast cancer. *Proc. Am. Assoc. Clin. Oncol.* 19:349, 1978.

14. Muss, HB et al.: Chemo- versus chemoimmunotherapy in advanced breast cancer. *Proc. Am. Assoc. Clin. Oncol.* 19:337, 1978.

15. Muss, HB et al.: Chemo- versus chemoimmunotherapy in advanced breast cancer. *Proc. Am. Assoc. Clin. Oncol.* 20:356, 1979.

16. Pinsky, CM et al.: *Corynebacterium parvum* as adjuvant to combination chemotherapy in patients with advanced breast cancer: preliminary results of a prospective randomized trial. In: WD, Terry, Windhorst, D, eds. *Immunotherapy of Cancer: Present Status of Trials in Man,* Vol. 6, Raven Press, New York, 1978.

17. Yanagihara, R et al.: *Corynebacterium parvum* plus combination chemotherapy for patients with advanced breast cancer. *Proc. Am. Assoc. Clin. Oncol.* 20:336, 1979.

18. Terry, WD: Concluding remarks. In: WD, Terry, Windhorst, D, eds. *Immunotherapy of Cancer: Present Status of Trials in Man,* Vol. 6, Raven Press, New York, 1978.

19. Swenerton, KD et al.: Prognostic factors in metastatic breast cancer treated with combination chemotherapy. *Cancer Research* 39:1552-1562, 1979.

Panel Discussion

JOSEPH SOKAL: Dr. Hollinshead, when you go from stage I disease to disseminated disease you have the problem of patients with disease at multiple metastatic sites. Some of these patients may have one tumor that might respond to specific immunotherapy because it has the right antigen and another tumor may evade the immunologic effect because it has changed its surface antigens. What do you think about this and how much of a problem is it going to be? What can we do about it?

ARIEL HOLLINSHEAD: In answer to your question, Dr. Sokal, we have to understand that the immunoevasive properties on the cell surface are so numerous that to use whole cells is no longer tenable. 97% of the cell surface components are normal. What happens on the surface of the tumor cell is unbelievable in terms of the number of immunoevasive properties. Therefore, as the tumor advances and as the properties increase, we gain more of the suppressor substances. These suppressor substances are now known and we chemically characterized them as DNA nuclear proteins. They increase very rapidly. They are so enormous in number in oat-cell carcinoma that the patient is overwhelmed before he starts. Now, the constant modulation and redistribution of these cell surface components; the loss in alteration, aggregation and agglutination, the fluctuation in the microvilli, and so on make it so mandatory to separate only the one to two percent of the total cell surface that is tumor associated in the correct manner for use in specific active immunotherapy. It is no longer tenable to use whole cells and the human committees will no longer permit it.

CARL PINSKY: Dr.Wallack, you use an oncolysate. Do you separate the tumor-specific antigen from the mix?

MARC WALLACK: We extract tumor cell membrane that is affected with the tumor cell surface. What we're doing in the laboratory, now, is using either sodium chloride or potassium chloride extractions in order to modify the tumor cell.

PINSKY: I understand that; but assuming what Dr. Hollinshead said is correct that 97% of the cell surface which you use is not appropriate, I wonder how you and Dr. McCune deal with this issue of highly purified TAA that Dr. Hollinshead is now using in clinical trials.

HOLLINSHEAD: Dr. Wallack is in my laboratory and we've talked about this very seriously.

PINSKY: Dr. McCune, do you have any comments?

CRAIG MCCUNE: I think using the antigens in their natural state on the cell surface versus trying to take subcellular fractions is an important controversy. There is no factual evidence to resolve it. I think the reason there is a great deal of interest in whole cells as a natural presentation of the antigens is because that model has been tested successfully in animals, as well as the fact that there are three documented human studies with regression of advanced diseases. Although it may be an argument in concept, the presence of regressions shown by Laucius and the people at UCLA and our own studies strongly support using whole cells as a simpler, lower risk way of presenting the antigens. The problems, certainly, with using subcellular fractions are the ability to pick the right portion and the added complexity of the procedures introduces considerable risk. When more studies are done with subcellular fractions to determine whether they can produce regressions in advance disease then we can make a better comparison.

PINSKY: What it basically comes down to is a practical versus a highly theoretical approach. I do think we should end this discussion of purifying the antigen, especially, if one can find it, versus using whole cell on the assumption that there has to be an antigen there. If we could have the next question?

DAVID SALKIN: Dr. Hollinshead, I think, mentioned that there was a sense of well-being that accompanied some of her favorable cases. Is that right, Dr. Hollinshead? I would caution everyone to be very careful about that sense of well-being. I not only had it in my favorable cases but in my unfavorable cases that were hopeful. I see it continually among the Laetrile cases where the disease is progressive, in urine injection therapy where the disease is progressive and also in psychosurgery that is done in the Phillipines. I even believe, mind you unscientifically, that I think I have seen a couple of cases where the progression was slowed down a little following that sense of well-being. I would be very cautious in using these so-called emotional or psychological factors as an index.

PINSKY: Even before the report from Dr. Hollinshead and others, most of us were aware of the sense of well-being that just treating a patient can induce even when the disease is progressing. Therefore, it is very good that we also saw objective evidence, X-rays and so forth in these presentations.

HOLLINSHEAD: Yes, we use this only as one of the many clinical comments in context.

MELVIN DODSON: Dr. Hollinshead, in most of your early work the tumor-associated antigen extract that you used was allogeneic. In the cases you presented today, was the TAA allogeneic? When you did surgery, were you making extract from these particular tumors that were being surgically removed or was this your tumor-associated allogeneic extract?

HOLLINSHEAD: These are two randomized trials. One in melanoma and one in lung. One lot of material is used for each of them for a large number of patients. It is allogeneic. I just presented the melanoma antigen work at the Tumor Markers Meeting in London; but, unfortunately there was not enough time today. But, we've gone full cycle in proving tumor relatedness. I would be very glad to discuss this with you.

DODSON: Well, I think this brings back the subject of the tumor-associated antigens. What are they? How do we know that they are tumor-associated?

HOLLINSHEAD: I have a series of slides showing the rim around the tumor. We have monoclonal antibody and we have exchanged our work with five different melanoma groups, etc. We have gone full cycle. The other comment about augmented antigens; we don't really know which of those other antigens are associated with different forms of disease.

PINSKY: I would like to enable other speakers to comment on this question. There are some who used autologous tumor cells and presented good data and of course there are those who used allogeneic tumor cells. Again, it comes down to the theoretical versus the practical. In certain trials, such as the one Dr. Hollinshead described, it would be impossible to insist upon autologous tumor cells.

DODSON: I understand that. I wish to point out, for example, that Order published some work on a tumor-specific antigen in Hodgkin's disease and this turned out to be transferrin. There have been reports of tumor-associated antigens in ovarian tumors and they turned out to be an increased concentration, by a factor of ten, of normal ovarian tumor antigens. I am constantly concerned about this fact.

HOLLINSHEAD: That is why we enter these workshops and cross compare.

WALLACK: One of the things we've done, fortunately, is to use both autologous and allogeneic tumor cell vaccines. I cannot treat a patient with recurrent disease for a long period of time until progression of disease or whatever with the patient's own tumor cells. It is impossible. What we did, with Kaprowski at the Wistar Institute, was to take the lines that we used to make our allogeneic vaccines and reacted them with his monoclonal antibodies in a radioimmune assay. We're showing tremendous cross-reactivity among the various lines we used for our allogeneic vaccines with his monoclonal antibody. We've done the same experiment with the oncolysates. We see absorption of the monoclonal antibody to the oncolysates.

JOSEPH SOKAL: Dr. Vinciguerra, I think I can answer in part the question of whether you were giving MER at the optimal time. You were probably not; but obviously you were getting an immunologic affect or you wouldn't have the toxicity you had. The fact that you had reactions to the agents proves your getting an immunologic event. We ran two single institution studies pooling Hodgkin's and other lymphomas in Stage III and IV disease. The population was comparable to yours except we had different diagnoses. We found in our first study, which was done between 1965 and 1967, no difference in survival between patients who received BCG and patients who did not receive BCG. Most patients received only one or two BCG vaccinations. Later in the 1970's we decided to do the study again with a more intense regimen, similar to your regime, using larger doses of BCG and more frequent administrations. Again, we found no difference in survival between controls and patients given BCG. However, in a similar group of patients with Stage I and II disease, who were also part of the study, we did find a definite BCG effect, $P = .01$, for delayed progression of disease. So, I think, the combined experience of a number of centers, suggests that immunotherapy is more likely to be effective in patients with limited disease. This appears to be true for BCG, MER and I suspect it will also turn out to be true for other agents. We had a limited experience with *C. parvum* which also showed no affect in advanced disease.

SAMUEL MCILVANIE: We've been working on this problem, too. We found that if we wait 72 hours after chemotherapy before giving BCG we get better percentage conversion and better T-cell response.

VINCENT VINCIGUERRA: The main objection that we found to MER is its toxicity.

KENNETH RAMMING: Dr. McCune, did you inject any of your patients directly with *C. parvum?*

CRAIG MCCUNE: Directly into cutaneous nodules?

RAMMING: Yes.

MCCUNE: No.

RAMMING: The reason I ask is because we have not had much success with tumor cell vaccines. We haven't used *C. parvum*. We are having a fair experience, now, with patients who have been injected pre-operatively in the lung and elsewhere with BCG. It is always surprising to me that those patients, and they now number over one hundred, have not shown any evidence of other metastatic disease regression. You have a model with a large number of patients with a lot of disease on board and you are adding more disease and you get a regression.

MCCUNE: I think there are some interesting animal models that compare injecting the tumor nodules on the skin of the animals versus giving them a suspension of their tumor cells with the adjuvant. I cannot name the specific paper, at the moment, but I remember it indicating the advantage of giving the cell suspension with the adjuvant evenly distributed throughout the material rather than injecting the lesions, where it would be irregularly distributed.

GEORGE BLUMENSCHEIN: Dr. Cunningham, I don't mean to be repetitious; but, I think when you are dealing with chemotherapy in metastatic breast cancer you have to use drugs that are effective in the management of metastatic breast cancer. L-Pam is a drug that has about a 19% response rate in metastatic disease and one would expect it not to be an active drug. In the use of Adriamycin, which is the most effective single agent in the management of metastatic breast cancer, certain features have to be remembered. It's dose-response-related and it's also schedule-related. If it is used in an inappropriate schedule and in an inappropriate dose, you will not get a good response. In order to reduce microscopic tumor burden to an effective level where you will see some response from nonspecific immunotherapy, you will have to use appropriate chemotherapy. So, I don't think your remarks about adjuvant chemotherapy not being effective in the management of breast cancer are appropriate. You cannot lump all chemotherapy together. You should say that adjuvant chemotherapy with the drugs you used is not effective.

MILES CUNNINGHAM: I think, perhaps, my remarks are misrepresented or were not clear. I was not attempting to say that chemotherapy was not useful. I was trying to say that one has to be very cautious in analyzing the present results on the basis of recurrence rather than survival. Even though the Bonadonna study has shown an effect on survival in pre-menopausal patients with limited nodes, we do not have an untreated control line here and we're comparing single drug versus multi-drug at four years. We don't see a difference and adding BCG to the multi-drug arm doesn't show a difference. This is not to say that it has no effect at all. More important, we may not have identified the proper subset of patients in whom an effect on recurrence may yet develop. I think it is a little premature to assess the effects of these agents when we only have recurrence data on which to base the analysis.

BLUMENSCHEIN: Again, there are several studies which do show absolute improvement in survival that is statistically significant both in premenopausal and post-menopausal women when the appropriate systemic treatment is utilized. I would urge those people who are going into adjuvant studies to ask some of these important questions, to consider the chemotherapeutic aspects of the management of breast cancer as well as the immunotherapeutic aspects. In terms of the no treatment control arm, I think you are fairly comfortable with Bonadonna's retrospective historical control study in which there is no difference between the two. In fact, they match our historical controls in every aspect each time we conducted historical controls. I think we are past that issue of whether or not historical controls in similarly matched patients in Stage II disease is something to worry about. What we need to be concerned with is whether the therapies we are testing are, in fact, effective in prolonging disease-free survival as well as over all survival.

Index

388